Imaging in Internal Medicine

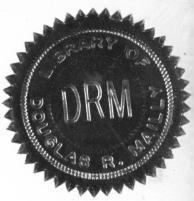

Imaging in Internal Medicine

Edited by
Robert L. Siegle, M.D.

Professor and Chief, Division of Diagnostic Radiology,
Department of Radiology, University of Texas Health
Science Center; Chief of Radiology, Medical Center
Hospital, San Antonio

Little, Brown and Company
Boston/Toronto

To the three generations of my family for
the inspiration they have provided through
their pursuit of excellence.

Contents

Contributing Authors   vi

Preface   vii

1   Gastrointestinal Disease   1
James G. Bova

2   Cardiovascular Disease   45
Ina L. D. Tonkin

3   Respiratory Tract Disease   67
Robert L. Siegle

4   Genitourinary Disease   115
Jack G. Rabinowitz

5   Oncology   139
Janet L. Potter

6   Bone and Joint Disease   151
Robert O. Cone III

7   Endocrine and Reproductive   209
Disease
Janet L. Potter

8   Neurologic Disorders   217
Donald W. Chakeres

9   Medical Complications   249
of Pregnancy
Janet L. Potter

Index   253

Contributing Authors

James G. Bova, D.O.

Associate Professor of Radiology, University of Texas Health Science Center; Chief of Abdominal Imaging Section, Department of Radiology, Medical Center Hospital, San Antonio

Donald W. Chakeres, M.D.

Associate Professor of Radiology, Ohio State University College of Medicine; Chief of Neuroradiology, Ohio State University Hospital, Columbus

Robert O. Cone III, M.D.

Clinical Assistant Professor of Radiology, University of Texas Health Science Center; Attending Radiologist, Southwest Texas Methodist Hospital, San Antonio

Janet L. Potter, Ph.D., M.D.

Assistant Professor of Radiology, University of Texas Health Science Center; Chief, Radiology Service, Audie L. Murphy Memorial Veterans Hospital, San Antonio

Jack G. Rabinowitz, M.D.

Professor and Chairman, Department of Radiology, Mount Sinai School of Medicine; Director, Department of Radiology, The Mount Sinai Hospital, New York

Robert L. Siegle, M.D.

Professor and Chief, Division of Diagnostic Radiology, Department of Radiology, University of Texas Health Science Center; Chief of Radiology, Medical Center Hospital, San Antonio

Ina L. D. Tonkin, M.D.

Professor of Radiology and Pediatrics, The University of Tennessee, Memphis; Attending Cardiovascular Radiologist, LeBonheur Children's Medical Center, Memphis

Preface

Radiology is the "star wars" of medicine. Imaging information, derived from both ionizing and non-ionizing radiation, can provide a virtually limitless array of pictures. Radiologists are challenged to match the expansion of the field. Medical students and specialists in other fields have even greater difficulty selecting and interpreting the relevant from the extraneous information obtainable from radiologic procedures.

In this textbook we have attempted to provide more radiographic information relevant to problems in internal medicine than is available in textbooks of internal medicine, but we have also tried to discriminate and not overwhelm readers with valueless detail. We have used Stein's INTERNAL MEDICINE as the basis for this radiology text, but it will also complement other internal medicine textbooks.

IMAGING IN INTERNAL MEDICINE was written for medical students, house staff, and practitioners of internal medicine. As such, this text has certain features that distinguish it from conventional radiology textbooks. First, we have avoided radiologic jargon and used terms that all physicians should understand. Second, we have oriented the text toward disease processes rather than radiographic features. Using this approach, we hope to improve the integration of the radiologic material with the rest of medical knowledge, rather than overemphasize the radiologic material as an end unto itself. Finally, we have attempted to curtail our natural tendencies to create grand, expensive texts that usually cost more than the medical or surgical books that they were designed to complement; at the same time, we have worked to maintain the high quality of the radiographic reproductions. They are, after all, the essence of the book.

R.L.S.

1. Gastrointestinal Disease

James G. Bova

This chapter includes evaluation of the alimentary canal, liver, gallbladder, bile ducts, and pancreas. There are a great number of disease entities that could be encountered and described radiologically; however, only those relevant to students and house staff physicians are shown in this text.

Because of the many imaging modalities available and the complexity of diagnostic algorithms, it is important that attending physicians be knowledgeable and consult with radiologists so that there is an efficient and appropriate plan for the diagnosis and treatment of the clinical problems discussed in this chapter.

The Abdominal Plain Film

One of the most commonly ordered tests for the work-up of patients with abdominal pain is the conventional radiograph of the abdomen (also called the KUB or flat plate). Clinicians should be specific in the terminology they use for ordering the x-ray studies they need. In most institutions, an acute abdomen series includes supine and erect views of the abdomen and an upright view of the chest. Because subdiaphragmatic air from a perforated viscus is a sign frequently looked for, the upright view of the chest must include the diaphragm and be obtained after the patient has been erect for 5 minutes so that small amounts of air have time to rise to the upper abdomen. The chest x-ray is also used for identifying a pneumonia in a lung base as a possible cause of abdominal pain. If erect views cannot be done, recumbent (usually supine) chest and left lateral decubitus (the patient lies left side down for 5 minutes) abdominal views are substituted.

An organized approach to the interpretation of abdominal radiographs is recommended so that all essential findings are seen. Develop your own plan, but be sure it includes organ and bony structures, gas patterns, fluid, and calcifications. Knowledge of the normal anatomy is essential and is assumed here, so that abnormal findings can be highlighted.

GAS PATTERNS. In the ambulatory patient there is normally a small amount of intestinal gas. The actual amount varies from person to person as well as by time since the last meal and time of day. The bowel should not be distended and the cecum should be less than 9 cm in diameter. Patients who are bedridden, especially if they are not eating a normal diet, tend to have more gaseous distention of the bowel.

Ileus. Ileus (paralytic ileus or adynamic bowel) may be either a focal or diffuse process whereby the patient swallows air but there is no effective peristalsis. Usually the viscus dilates symmetrically. The amount of distended bowel found depends on both the time interval from onset and the extent of paralysis. Focal adynamic segments are seen adjacent to inflammatory diseases such as pancreatitis or appendicitis. A diffuse adynamic pattern is most

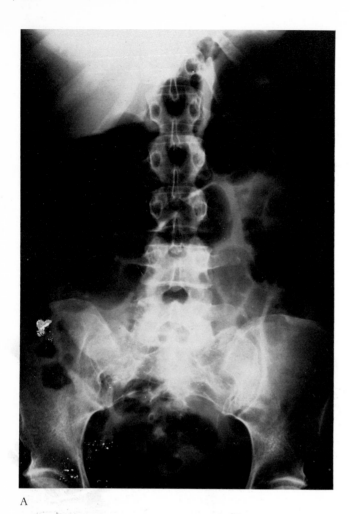

A

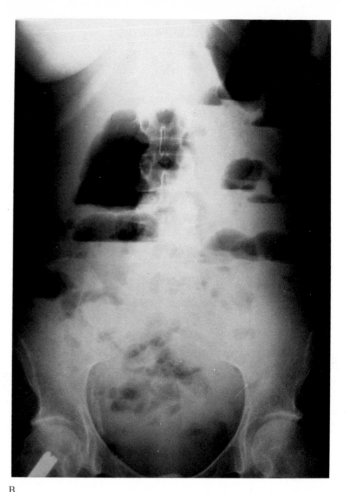

B

Fig. 1-1. Postoperative ileus. A. Supine abdomen: symmetric, moderate gaseous distention of small and large bowel. B. Erect abdomen: several scattered air/fluid levels within small and large intestinal loops. Films obtained 12 hours later showed no change.

commonly seen postoperatively (Fig. 1-1). Small to moderate amounts of fluid may collect within the paralyzed loops of bowel and cause air-fluid levels. Serial abdominal films show a pattern that does not change very much until the gut resumes its normal activity.

Bowel Obstruction. The radiographic findings of bowel obstruction depend on the length of time from the onset of obstruction, the level of obstruction, and whether the obstruction is partial or complete. Early in a high-grade partial or complete small bowel obstruction moderate distention of the obstructed loops, along with some fluids, is seen. Gas is still present in the colon, but is less than that seen in the small intestine. Within hours there is a progression of findings. The obstructed loops dilate more and fluid accumulates further (Fig. 1-2). The air-fluid interfaces appear at different levels on the erect film due to the increased peristalsis early in obstruction, as the gut tries to force its contents pass the obstructed site (the hyperactive phase). The bowel beyond the obstruction eventually empties itself of gas and stool. Late in this process there is massive dilation and accumulation of fluid; the bowel fatigues (the paresis phase) and differential air-fluid levels are not seen. In contrast to an ileus, progressive changes appear on sequential films. Findings in a colonic obstruction (Fig. 1-3) are very similar, except that the changes are initially and more prominently seen in the large bowel. The extent of small bowel distention depends on the competency of the ileocecal valve.

Except in the case of cecal (Fig. 1-4) or sigmoid volvulus (Fig. 1-5), the cause of intestinal obstruction is not usually seen. The most common cause of small intestinal obstruction is an adhesion. For the colon the most common causes are carcinoma or sigmoid volvulus.

Toxic Megacolon. Toxic megacolon is an uncommon dilatation of the large bowel caused by severe transmural inflammation. It is most commonly seen with ulcerative colitis but has also been associated with granulomatous colitis, amebic colitis, ischemic colitis, and pseudomembranous colitis. Because patients with toxic megacolon are very ill and usually lie supine, the most dilated portion of the bowel is the transverse colon (Fig. 1-6). It measures 6 cm or greater at the level of maximum distention because of its anterior location within the abdominal cavity. Besides the dilatation, the haustrations are thickened due to edema, and occasionally pseudopolyps caused by the ulcerated mucosa can be seen within the lumen. This condition can progress to necrosis and perforation.

Pneumoperitoneum. Pneumoperitoneum (extraluminal air) is most easily identified as crescent-shaped collections of air under the diaphragm (Fig. 1-7). As little as 2 cc of air can be identified if the proper technique is used. Other manifestations of pneumoperitoneum include air outlining the edge of the liver, falciform ligament, or wall of a loop of bowel that has gas in its lumen (known as the dou-

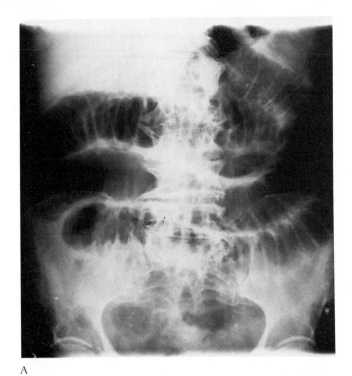

A

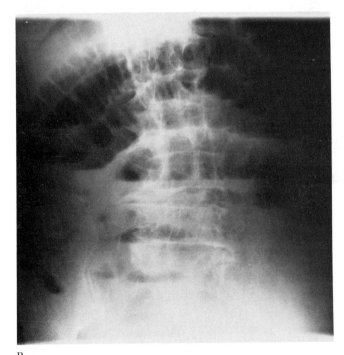

B

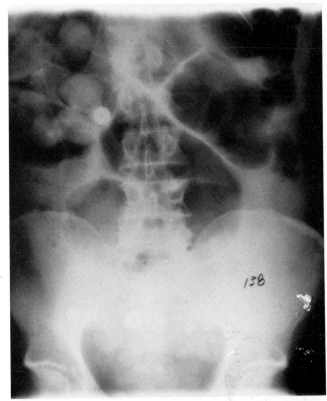

A

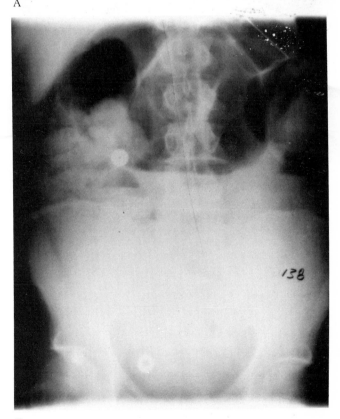

B

Fig. 1-2. Small bowel obstruction caused by adhesions. A. Supine abdomen: markedly dilated proximal small bowel loops in a "step-ladder" configuration. Note that the colon is collapsed and poorly visualized. B. Erect abdomen: significant air/fluid levels seen only within the distended jejunum. Films from 12 hours earlier showed only an ileus pattern.

Fig. 1-3. Colonic obstruction caused by carcinoma. A. Supine abdomen: marked gaseous distention of colon; very little is seen in the small bowel. B. Erect abdomen: air/fluid levels identified in the large bowel.

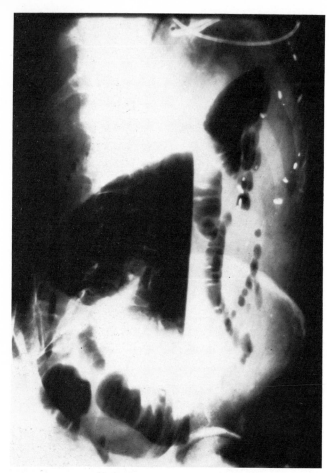

Fig. 1-4. A left lateral decubitus view shows the typical pattern of cecal volvulus. The cecum is severely dilated, with dilatation and air/fluid levels seen within the small bowel proximal to the ileo-cecal valve. The axis of the cecum is generally directed toward the left upper quadrant.

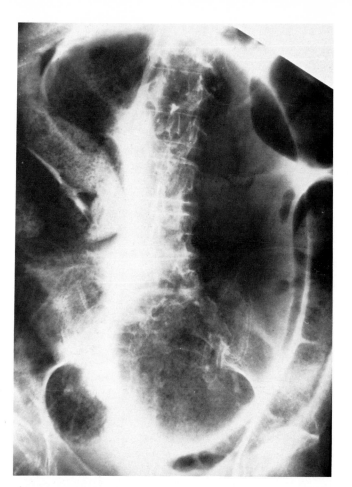

A

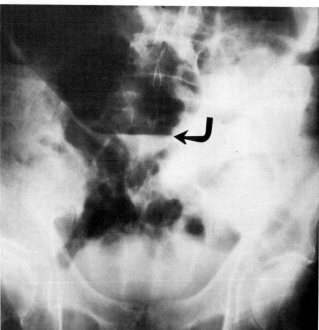

B

Fig. 1-5. Characteristic features of sigmoid volvulus are shown on these supine (*A*) and erect (*B*) films. A dilated loop of sigmoid is seen rising out of the pelvis. The axis of this loop tends to be toward the epigastrum or right upper quadrant. An air/fluid level is located at the point of volvulus (arrow). The colon, proximal to the volvulus, is very distended.

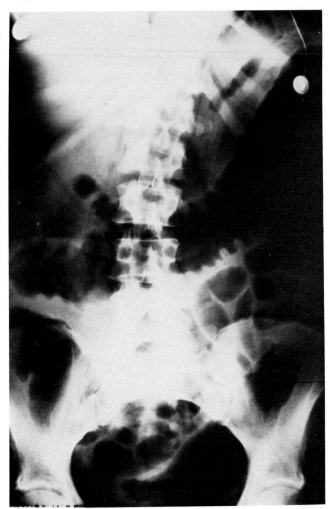

Fig. 1-6. Toxic megacolon. A supine radiograph in this patient with ulcerative colitis shows the typical dilated transverse colon with blunting and thickening of the haustrations.

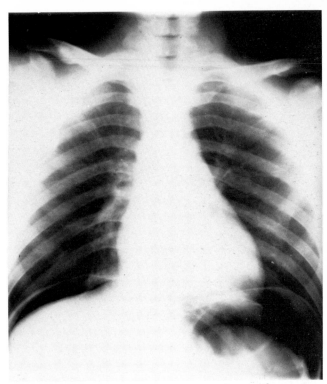

Fig. 1-7. Pneumoperitoneum. This upright PA chest was obtained after an exploratory laparotomy. Air under the thin hemidiaphragms is easily identified.

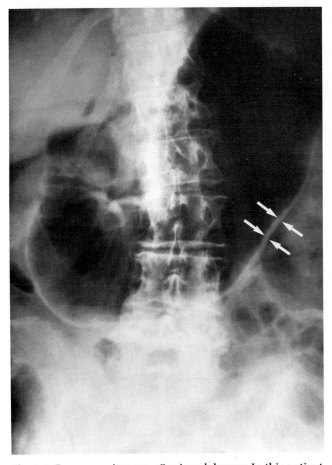

Fig. 1-8. Pneumoperitoneum. Supine abdomen: In this patient with a perforated ulcer, air is seen inside and outside the gastric lumen allowing sharp visualization of both sides of the bowel wall (*arrows*). This is called the *double wall sign*.

ble wall sign) (Fig. 1-8). The most common cause of pneumoperitoneum is recent abdominal surgery, whereby air is trapped within the abdomen when the incision is closed. This gas may be seen postoperatively for up to two weeks. Other causes include viscus perforation due to ulcer, neoplasm, or trauma. The origins for retroperitoneal air are essentially the same, except for rectal perforations and diverticulitis. The gas dissects along tissue planes, especially the psoas muscle margins, and is recognized on radiographs as sharply defined linear lucent streaks (Fig. 1-9).

Abscesses. Confined infections caused by gas-forming organisms (most commonly *Escherichia coli*) or fistulous communication with the gut can be identified radiographically (Fig. 1-10). These infections usually present as ill-defined, mottled collections of air, sometimes with an ovoid mass effect. Another common pattern is a round, slightly irregular lucency with an air-fluid level. The most frequently seen abscesses on plain film are those associated with appendicitis, diverticulitis, pancreatitis, and postoperative infections.

Intramural Air. Occasionally gas may be found in the bowel wall. It occurs in two forms, cystic and linear. The

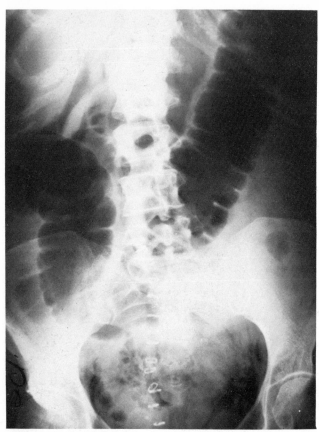

Fig. 1-9. Extraperitoneal air. Linear, lucent streaks of gas are shown outlining tissue plains in the pelvis of this patient with traumatic perforation of the rectum.

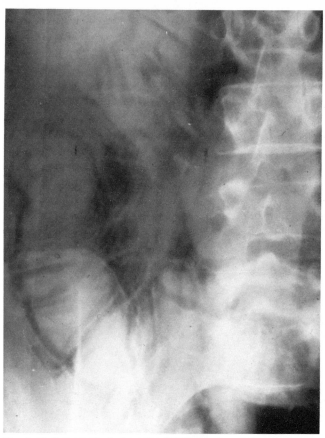

Fig. 1-11. Pneumatosis intestinalis (linear form). Lupus vasculitis with ischemia caused these intramural linear streaks of gas that conform to the outline of the colon.

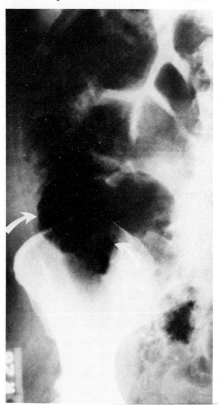

Fig. 1-10. Intraabdominal abscess. A round, irregular collection of gas caused by appendicitis with a periappendiceal abscess can be seen in the right lower quadrant (*arrows*).

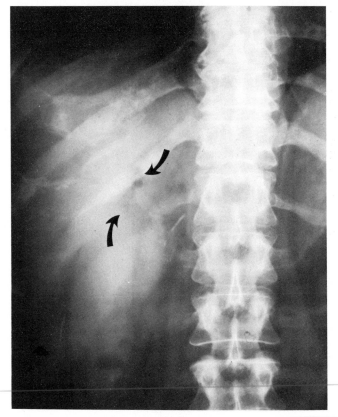

Fig. 1-12. Hepatobiliary air. The central tubular branching lucencies (*arrows*) seen here were caused by a duodenal ulcer eroding into the common bile duct.

cystic type is seen in a benign condition known as *pneumatosis cystoides intestinalis*. This condition is associated with obstructive airway disease but its exact cause is not known. The colon is the most common site of involvement. These air sacs can rupture, causing a rare benign case of pneumoperitoneum. Linear intramural air is more serious than cystic and indicates a loss of mucosal integrity (Fig. 1-11). This loss of integrity in the mucosa is due to severe inflammation or ischemia. Mesenteric vascular insufficiency has many causes that include atherosclerosis, shock, congestive heart failure, emboli, and vasculitis such as those found in the collagen vascular diseases. Infection with a gas-forming organism may also cause this.

Hepatobiliary Air. Tubular, branching lucencies may be seen in the liver (Fig. 1-12). If they are persistent and centrally placed near the porta hepatis they most likely represent air in the bile ducts. The most common cause for this finding is a previous operative biliary-enteric anastamosis (e.g., choledochoduodenostomy). These lucencies also appear if a duodenal ulcer has perforated into the biliary system or a gallstone has eroded into the duodenum or colon. Fleeting, peripherally placed tubular air is more ominous because it represents gas in the portal venous system (Fig. 1-13). The pathogenic mechanism is necrosis of the bowel wall with escape of luminal air into the portal veins. This finding is associated with a high mortality rate.

CALCIFICATIONS. A majority of patients over the age of 40 have some type of calcification in the abdomen or pelvis but outside of the osseous structures. The most frequently encountered abdominal calcification is the phlebolith, a concretion within a vein that has no pathologic significance. Arterial calcifications are commonly seen in the elderly and in diabetics. Abdominal aortic aneurysms are sometimes identified on plain films of the abdomen (Fig. 1-14), especially if a cross-table lateral view is added. On the frontal projection a curvilinear calcification appears lateral to the lumbar spine. On the lateral view the anterior and posterior walls can be seen and measurements obtained. If the diameter between the two walls of calcification is greater than 3 cm, it is considered aneurysmally dilated.

Gallstones and appendicoliths are identified on radiographs in fewer than 15 percent of patients who have them. Gallstones may be solitary or multiple; when multiple they are usually faceted. They are seen in the right upper quadrant (Fig. 1-15). An appendicolith appears as a solitary, ovoid radiopacity in the right lower quadrant or anywhere in the true pelvis (Fig. 1-16).

Miscellaneous types of calcifications that may be seen include those of chronic pancreatitis (Fig. 1-17), granulomas of the liver and spleen, and occasional renal, ureteral, or bladder calculi. Although these last three structures are not part of the gastrointestinal tract, abnormalities in them may cause abdominal pain.

FLUID. The most common free-fluid collections encountered in the abdomen are ascites and blood. Ascites is most frequently seen in patients with cirrhosis of the liver, while the accumulation of blood is usually due to blunt trauma causing damage to the liver and/or spleen. Obliteration of the normally sharp edge of the right lobe of the liver and fluid in the paracolic gutters that medially displaces the ascending or descending portions of the colon are found in small to moderate amounts of free fluid. A massive quantity of fluid is manifested by a hazy "ground

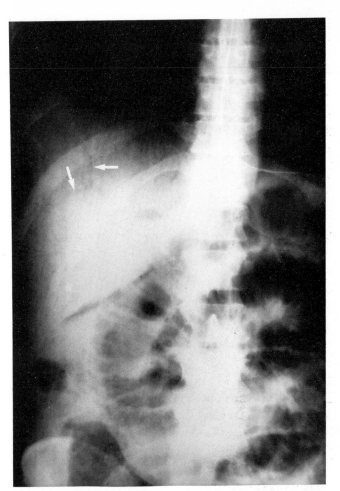

Fig. 1-13. Portal venous gas. Small, tubular lucencies in the periphery of the liver (*arrows*) were found in this patient who subsequently died of a bowel infarction.

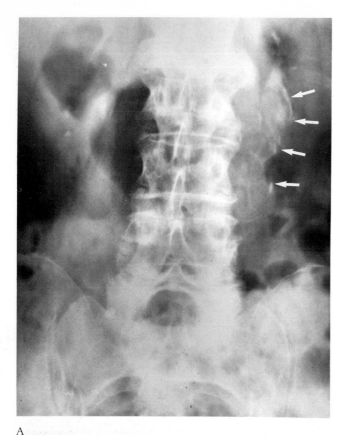

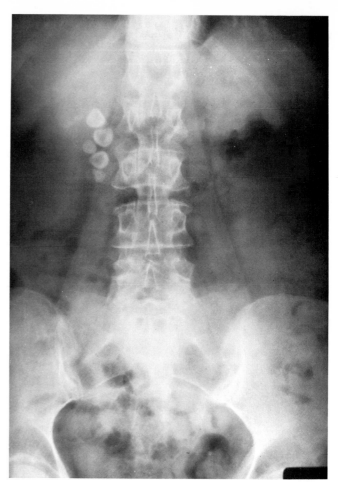

Fig. 1-15. Gallstones. Multiple, faceted calculi are easily identified in the right upper quadrant.

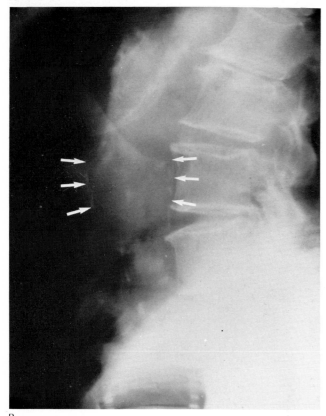

A

B

Fig. 1-14. Calcified abdominal aortic aneurysm. A curvilinear calcification is seen lateral to the lumbar spine on the frontal supine view of the abdomen (*arrows*) (*A*) and anterior to the spine (*arrows*) on the lateral view (*B*). The anterior-posterior dimension of the aneurysm can be measured when both walls are calcified.

glass" appearance of the abdomen and the central location of air-filled loops of bowel that float to the superior aspect of the abdominal cavity when the patient is in the supine position (Fig. 1-18).

Diseases of the Esophagus

The normal esophagus (Fig. 1-19) is a smooth, tubular structure that extends from the hypopharynx to the gastroesophageal junction. The anatomy and function of the esophagus are best evaluated by barium swallow. Peristalsis is observed with fluoroscopy and can be recorded on videotape for repeated viewing. Significant gastroesophageal reflux is identified as a large amount of barium going from the stomach to the mid- or proximal esophagus. Vigorous maneuvers to elicit reflux are not advocated because of too many false positives. An accuracy rate of only 30–40 percent should be expected. Dysphagia and heartburn are the most common indications for studying the esophagus.

INFLAMMATION. Peptic Esophagitis. Repetitive reflux of acidic gastric contents may initiate mild to severe inflammation of the mucosa, and ulcerations with scarring and

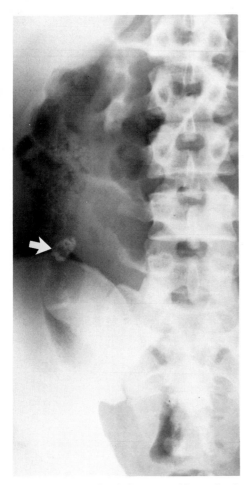

Fig. 1-16. Appendicolith. An ovoid opacity (*arrow*) was observed in the right lower quadrant in this patient with appendicitis. It can usually be differentiated from a phlebolith by its larger size and ovoid configuration.

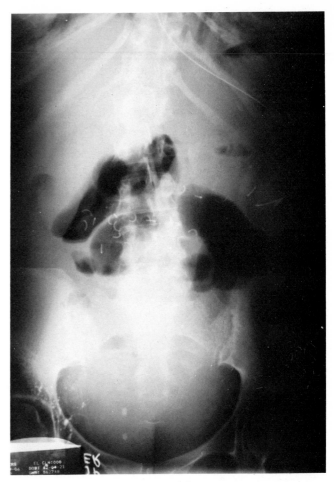

Fig. 1-18. Massive ascites. Ascites from any cause may become massive. Edges of organs become obscured, there is a hazy "ground glass" appearance, and air filled bowel loops float into the center of the abdomen.

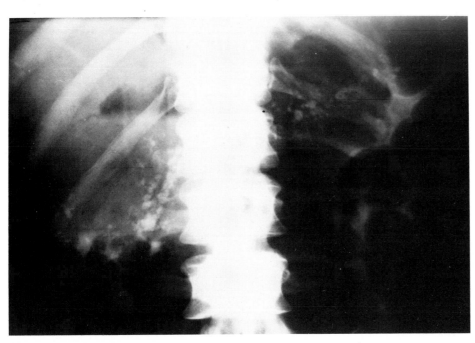

Fig. 1-17. Chronic pancreatitis. Irregular calcifications of varying shape scattered in the distribution typical of chronic alcoholic pancreatitis.

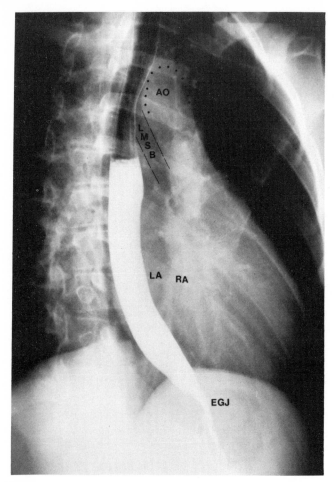

Fig. 1-19. Normal esophagus. An upright, full length view demonstrates the difference between single (distal) and double (proximal) contrast techniques as well as the relationship of the esophagus to adjacent structures. Note the smooth mucosal surface of the proximal portion with the double contrast technique. AO = aorta, LMSB = left mainstem bronchus, LA = left atrium, RA = right atrium, EGJ = esophagogastric junction.

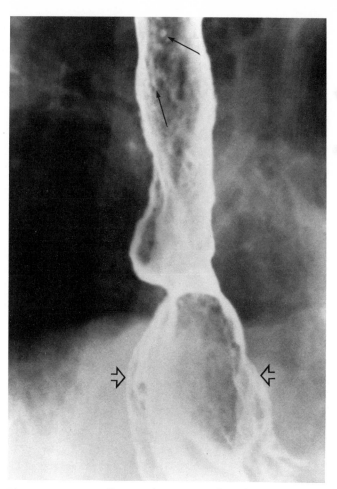

Fig. 1-20. Severe reflux esophagitis. Besides a hiatal hernia (*open arrows*), there are irregular narrowing and small ulcerations (*arrows*) of the distal esophagus.

stricture may result (Fig. 1-20). Ulcers are round or linear and tend to be located along the longitudinal axis of the esophagus near the gastroesophageal junction; however, these ulcers can occasionally occur more proximally. A hiatal hernia may be present but is not a prerequisite for reflux. A common complication of inflammation is the transformation of the esophageal squamous epithelium into a gastric-like columnar mucosal lining (Barrett's esophagus). This is a histologic diagnosis that is only suggested radiologically by seeing a large, round esophageal ulcer or a very proximal stricture (Fig. 1-21).

Radiation Esophagitis. Small ulcerations and smooth, tapered narrowing within a radiation therapy port are typical for this kind of inflammation. A permanent stricture may result.

Medication-induced Esophagitis. This uncommon entity presents with odynophagia. A focal ulceration is caused by a tablet or capsule that is "stuck" on the mucosa, usually in the proximal esophagus above the aortic arch. The offenders are most often potassium supplements, antiarrythmics, or antibiotics that are taken at bedtime but are not followed by a sufficient amount of fluid to wash them

into the stomach. Radiographically there is a discrete small ulcer that may be associated with mild narrowing.

Corrosive Esophagitis. Accidental or intentional ingestion of corrosive materials (e.g., lye) can cause extensive damage to the esophagus and stomach. The mucosa is severely ulcerated and inflammation can progress through the entire thickness of the wall and perforate into the mediastinum. Strictures are the consequence; they are usually long and sometimes multiple.

INFECTION. The esophagus can be infected by fungi, viruses, tuberculosis, and bacteria. The most commonly seen infections are *Monilia* and *Herpesvirus* organisms, and these usually occur in patients whose immune systems are compromised. Example situations include organ transplants, acquired immune deficiency syndrome (AIDS), and cancer therapy. Occasionally patients who have been receiving a prolonged course of antibiotics may get a secondary infection. This diagnosis can be suggested on barium swallow but requires culture and sometimes biopsy for confirmation.

Monilial Esophagitis. Radiographically, monilial esophagitis presents as small, raised plaques on the mucosa (Fig. 1-22). These may be solitary, or multiple and diffuse. There

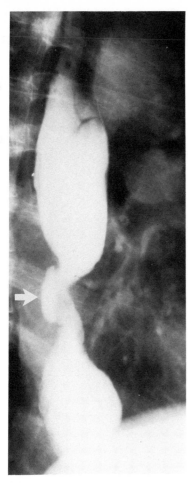
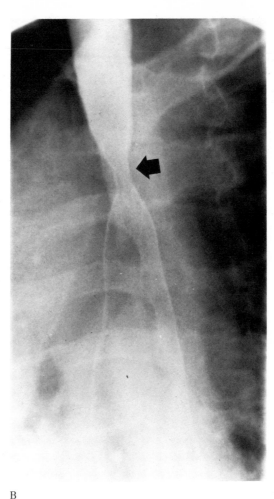

A   B

Fig. 1-21. Two characteristic appearances for Barrett's esophagus. A. Large, round ulcer (*arrow*) and narrowing in the distal esophagus. B. Smooth, short segmental stricture (*arrow*) in the proximal third of the esophagus.

is a tendency for involvement of the proximal esophagus. Edematous longitudinal folds and spasm may be seen in conjunction with small filling defects. Ulcers are not a typical finding in this disease.

Herpes Esophagitis. The dominant abnormalities found on barium swallow are small, solitary or multiple, well-defined mucosal ulcerations (Fig. 1-23) that may occur anywhere along the esophagus.

MOTOR DISORDERS. Normal peristalsis consists of a longitudinal and circumferential muscular contraction wave that completely empties the esophagus and is initiated by the act of swallowing. Thus, the contraction begins in the cervical portion of the esophagus just below the pharynx and proceeds caudad in a smooth, uniform manner. Occasionally, shallow nonperistaltic contractions (tertiary waves) can be seen in normal patients but should not be a dominant pattern that impairs emptying.

Diffuse Esophageal Spasm. Diffuse esophageal spasm (DES) may cause chest pain similar to that of myocardial origin. However, DES is uncommon, and the diagnosis difficult to make. DES should be diagnosed when deep, nonperistaltic waves that tend to be persistent are seen. Asking patients

if they are having any symptoms when these prominent contractions are seen is very useful. When this pattern is very marked, multiple outpouchings simulate diverticulosis.

Achalasia. The characteristic findings of achalasia are esophageal dilatation, absent peristalsis, poor emptying in the upright position, and a smooth, tapered ("beak-like") appearance at the gastroesophageal junction (Fig. 1-24). Barium may mix with undigested food, creating an irregular pattern. A dilated air-filled esophagus with an air-fluid level is seen on chest x-ray. These findings are actually late manifestations of achalasia, because it is rarely discovered early. The differential diagnosis includes Chagas' disease, reflux stricture, and infiltrating tumor.

Scleroderma. Inconsistent normal peristalsis with incomplete emptying of the esophagus is the earliest abnormality in scleroderma, which is a collagen vascular disease. With time the esophagus develops into a mildly to moderately dilated tube with absent peristalsis. The gastroesophageal junction becomes patulous and allows spontaneous gastroesophageal reflux. The sequelae of reflux esophagitis described earlier may then occur.

NEOPLASMS. Benign. These masses are an infrequent and usually incidental finding. Leiomyoma, seen as a round, smooth mass that has a sloping, obtuse interface with the esophageal wall, is the most common benign tumor seen.

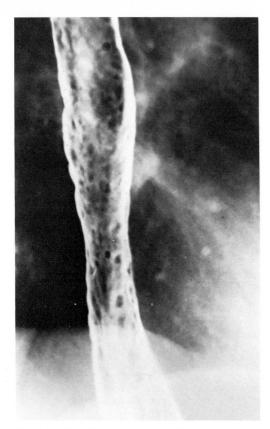

Fig. 1-22. Monilial esophagitis. Characteristic multiple, scattered round or ovoid plaques in a patient with AIDS.

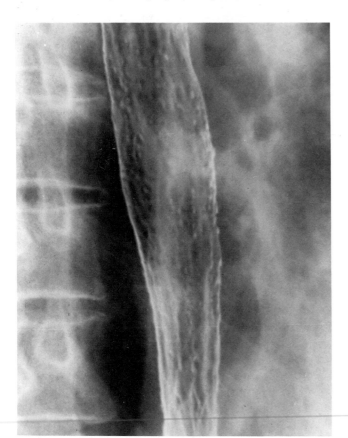

Fig. 1-23. Herpes esophagitis. Multiple, small, discrete mucosal ulcers can be easily identified. This patient was undergoing chemotherapy for leukemia.

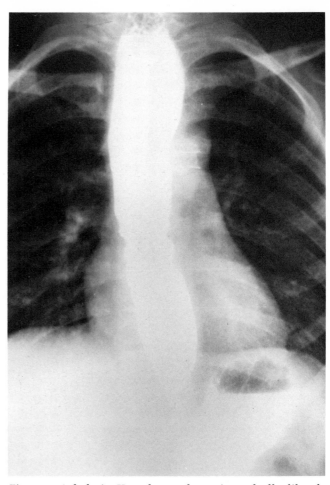

Fig. 1-24. Achalasia. Here the esophagus is markedly dilated with a "beak-like" configuration of the gastroesophageal junction. There is absence of normal peristalsis and delayed emptying. Shallow, nonperistaltic contractions (tertiary waves) are seen.

Other rare benign tumors include fibromas, neuromas, lipomas, and neurofibromas.

Malignant. Squamous cell carcinoma is the most frequent histology and tends to occur in the mid- to distal esophagus (Fig. 1-25). Gastric adenocarcinomas can cross the gastroesophageal junction and invade the esophagus or arise de novo in the columnar epithelium of a Barrett's esophagus.

The radiographic features of malignant lesions vary from small polypoid or plaque-like mucosal masses to large, irregular, ulcerating circumferential tumors. Unfortunately, most patients present at an advanced stage and are found to have the latter.

MISCELLANEOUS DISORDERS. Hiatal Hernia. There are two types of herniation of the stomach associated with the esophageal hiatus formed by the crura of the diaphragm; these are sliding and paraesophageal hernias.

The more common type is the sliding hiatal hernia, which is the cephalad movement of the gastroesophageal junction to a position in the mediastinum superior to the diaphragm. This movement is caused by laxity of the phrenicoesophageal ligamentous attachments to the crura. It is identified on barium studies as obvious gastric folds

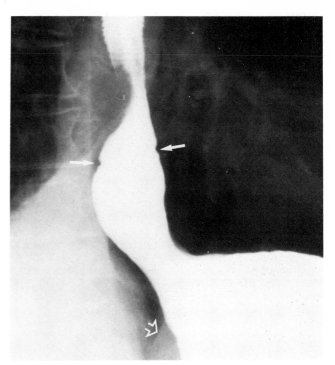

Fig. 1-26. Sliding hiatal hernia. A mucosal ring (*arrows*) identifies the esophagogastric junction, which is seen above the diaphragm (*open arrow*) during the Valsalva maneuver. Reflux is also present.

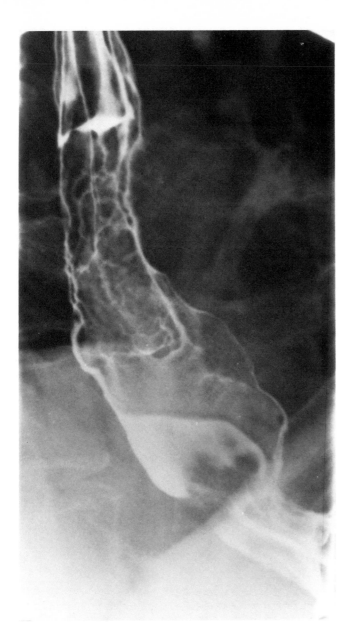

Fig. 1-25. Squamous cell carcinoma of esophagus. An irregular fungating mass in the distal third of the esophagus. There is also loss of the normal smooth mucosa, and the lumen is narrowed.

in the lower mediastinum, sometimes with the presence of a thin, horizontal, lucent line representing a rim of redundant mucosa that creates a ring-like narrowing (Fig. 1-26). This is called a B-ring or Schatski ring, which radiographically locates the squamocolumnar (esophagogastric) junction. Although their exact cause is not known, these rings are probably acquired. They are considered stenotic when less than 2 cm in diameter. At fluoroscopy the hernia can be accentuated with the Valsalva maneuver and reduced with normal quiet breathing. Reflux is frequently associated with but not caused by a sliding hiatal hernia, which can become quite large and fixed in position. Reflux and esophagitis can occur just as often without a hernia, however.

The paraesophageal hernia is seen as all or some of the stomach herniating up next to the esophagus in the hiatus or through a defect in the crus of the diaphragm. The gastroesophageal junction remains in its normal position (Fig. 1-27). In contrast to the sliding type, these hernias are infrequently associated with reflux. However, they are prone

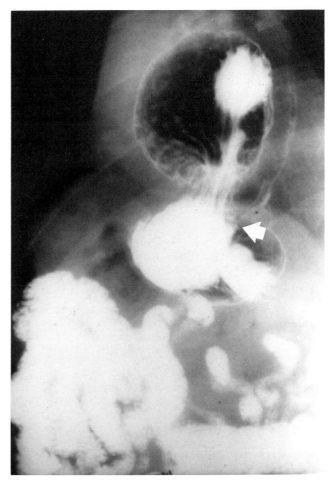

Fig. 1-27. Paraesophageal hernia. The stomach is herniated up into the chest, but note the normal location of the esophagogastric junction below the diaphragm (*arrow*).

to volvulus with obstruction and may create a life-threatening clinical situation.

Webs. These thin rims of mucosal redundancy are similar to the B-ring described above but occur most commonly in the cervical portion of the esophagus. They may cause dysphagia. The etiology is considered congenital; however, webs can arise in areas of chronic mucosal inflammation. Although webs are thought to be a part of the Plummer-Vinson syndrome, they are most likely incidental findings.

Diverticula. These outpouchings of the esophagus are most commonly acquired and are either pulsion or traction in origin. The midesophagus is the usual location for traction diverticula caused by adhesions from mediastinal inflammation. The pulsion phenomenon of increased intraluminal pressure also contributes to their formation. True pulsion diverticula occur above strictures and in the posterior hypopharynx (Zenker's diverticulum). True congenital lesions arise from the posterior aspect of the epiphrenic portion of the distal esophagus. Diverticula are significant only when they become large enough to trap food or are perforated during endoscopy.

Mallory-Weiss Tear and Esophageal Rupture. A longitudinal tear of the mucosa at or near the gastroesophageal junction (Mallory-Weiss tear) can occur during violent vomiting or retching. Radiographic diagnosis is rare, but a tear would be seen as a small linear collection of barium. Esophageal rupture represents an extension of this process so that it involves the entire thickness of the wall, allowing swallowed material to spill into the mediastinum. Widening, air within the mediastinum, and a left pleural effusion are seen on chest x-ray. If a contrast study is indicated to confirm the diagnosis, water soluble contrast should be used instead of barium in order to avoid additional inflammation and granulomatous mediastinitis. The contrast extravasates along irregular mediastinal planes.

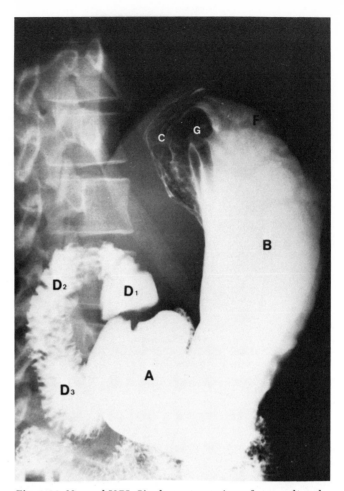

Fig. 1-28. Normal UGI. Single contrast view of stomach and duodenum. A = antrum, B = body, C = cardia, D1, D2, D3 = duodenum (D1 = bulb), F = fundus, G = gastroesophageal junction.

Diseases of the Stomach and Duodenum

The most commonly utilized radiologic method for evaluating the stomach and duodenum is the biphasic upper gastrointestinal series (Biphasic UGI) (Fig. 1-28). The essential elements for this study are gaseous distention, coating with high-density barium for double contrast mucosal detail followed by low-density barium, and manual palpation for single contrast examination of luminal contours.

The stomach is anatomically divided into the cardia, fundus, body, antrum, and pylorus. Functionally, the fundus and body act as a reservoir while the antrum empties the stomach by peristalsis. The duodenum is divided into four parts, extending from the pylorus to the ligament of Treitz. The first portion is called the duodenal bulb. The second through fourth portions are located in the retroperitoneum.

INFLAMMATION. An inflammatory reaction may be initiated by endogenous (i.e., peptic) or exogenous (i.e., food, medication, or corrosive ingestion) chemical stimuli. The severity of the inflammation is dosage-related and determines the radiologic findings. If there is only mild super-

ficial inflammation, no abnormality is seen. The next stage is a grossly edematous mucosa (as with gastritis or duodenitis) with thickened folds, which can proceed to erosions and ulcerations and may progress through the full thickness of the bowel wall to perforate it. An erosion is a small excavation of the mucosa, in which a small amount of barium may collect; thus it can be identified as a tiny collection of barium surrounded by a small lucent halo of edema. It is usually less than 3 mm in diameter. Erosions are usually multiple and are best seen on the double contrast portion of the examination (Fig. 1-29).

An ulcer is an erosion that has penetrated beyond the muscularis mucosae. Ulcers are seen as larger, better defined, round to oval craters that are lined with barium on the double contrast technique (Fig. 1-30), or are filled with barium on the single contrast part of the study. Ulcers are more easily identified when they are filled with barium.

Approximately 95 percent of gastric ulcers are benign, and most occur along the lesser curve of the body and antrum. The typical benign ulcer is less than 3 cm in diameter, is smooth, projects outside the expected gastric wall, and may have uniform mucosal folds radiating to the ulcer base. When viewed in profile, a radiolucent line or band may be seen across the neck of the ulcer. This is called *Hampton's line* when thin or an *ulcer collar* when thick, and is the most reliable sign for a benign ulcer. Malignant ulcers are actually cancerous masses with ulceration within them (Fig. 1-31), although benign ulcers may be as-

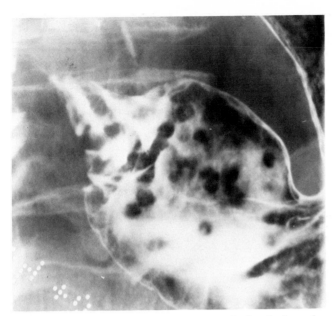

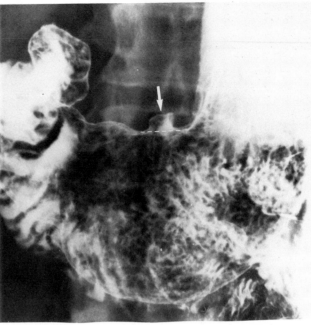

Fig. 1-29. Erosive gastritis. This view reveals the single and double contrast appearance of erosions. These round nodules with small central collections of barium are typical. (Photograph provided by Harvey M. Goldstein, M.D.)

Fig. 1-30. Benign gastric ulcer. A smoothly marginated crater (*arrow*) without a mass, is shown protruding beyond the projected gastric wall (*broken line*).

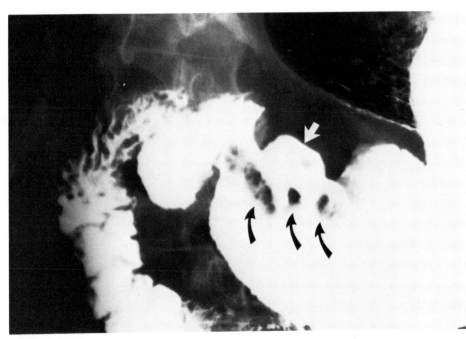

Fig. 1-31. Malignant gastric ulcer. Single contrast view demonstrates a large ulcer crater (*white arrow*) with nodular, mass-like filling defects (*black arrows*) near the ulcer margin.

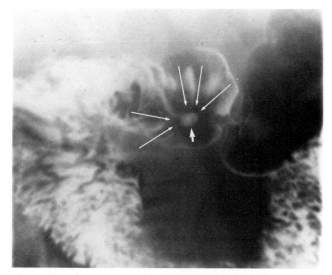

Fig. 1-32. Duodenal ulcer. A smooth, round collection of barium (*short arrow*) is seen in the ulcer crater, surrounded by radiating, edematous folds (*long arrows*).

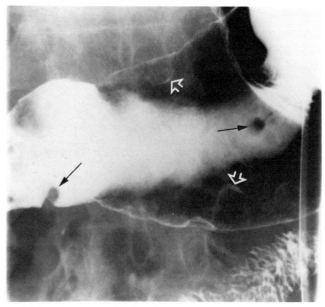

Fig. 1-34. Hyperplastic gastric polyps. Although these lesions are larger than usual, the number and distribution are typical. The polyps are seen as curvilinear white lines (*open arrows*) and as filling defects in the barium pool (*solid black arrows*).

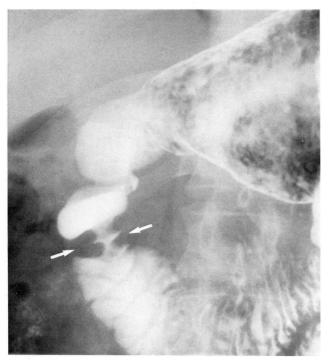

Fig. 1-33. Post-bulbar ulcer. Narrowing of the second portion of the duodenum (*arrows*) is the predominant finding. An ulcer crater is suggested in the middle of the narrowing.

sociated with adjacent cancers. Malignant ulcers are irregular and nodular. Any gastric ulcer that does not meet benign criteria should be considered a carcinoma until proved otherwise. Lesions that do not heal with appropriate therapy are also suspicious. Complete healing can be radiographically confirmed as the absence of any mucosal abnormality or the isolated presence of a surface scar.

The vast majority of duodenal ulcers occur in the duodenal bulb (Fig. 1-32), and all are benign. They are typically round but may also be linear. They are commonly associated with edema and spasm. Postbulbar ulcers are more often identified by narrowing (Fig. 1-33) than by discrete barium collection.

It is more common for inflammatory lesions to heal completely without residual deformity. Narrowing with an irregular outline may be seen when scarring with fibrosis is marked. This scarring may be manifested in the duodenal bulb as a "clover leaf" configuration.

NEOPLASMS. Benign Polyps. The term *polyp* is used to describe any protrusion into the lumen of a growth from the mucosa or submucosa. Polyps anywhere in the gastrointestinal tract appear as curvilinear white lines over the masses on double contrast technique or as rounded radiolucent filling defects on single contrast barium studies. Most are sessile but they can become pedunculated. Gastric polyps are of either hyperplastic or adenomatous origin. Hyperplastic polyps are most common and are usually multiple and scattered in the body or antrum (Fig. 1-34). They are small, rarely greater than 10 mm in size and are not felt to be associated with an increased risk of carcinoma. Hyperplastic polyps represent a regenerative mucosa that is responding to chronic inflammation. In contrast, adenomatous polyps are usually solitary, are found in the antrum, are frequently greater than 10 mm in size, and are considered by some to be premalignant lesions. Such tumors are seen in a small portion of patients with familial polyposis coli and Gardner's syndrome. Hamar-

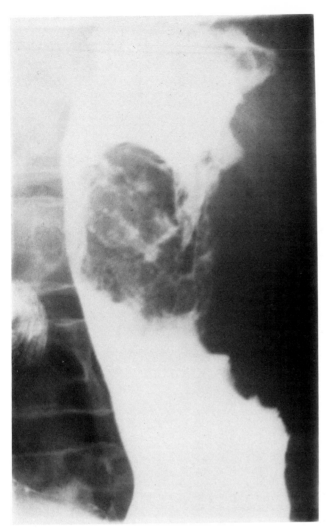

Fig. 1-35. Fungating gastric carcinoma. A large, irregular mass with shallow central ulceration arising from the body of the stomach.

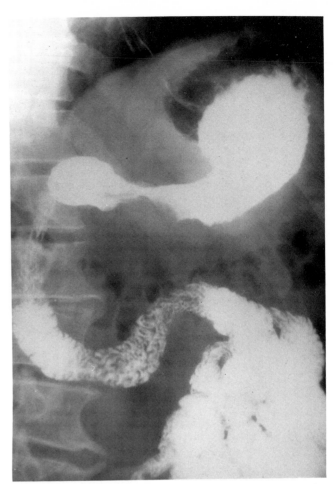

Fig. 1-36. Infiltrating gastric carcinoma (linitis plastica). Diffuse narrowing of the distal stomach characterizes the infiltrative and fibrotic behavior of this tumor. Note the symmetric thickened wall that was seen at the time of surgery.

tomatous gastric polyps are found in Peutz-Jeghers syndrome. Their histology cannot be determined radiographically.

Duodenal polyps occur less commonly than gastric polyps; they are most often adenomatous but the risk of carcinoma is unknown. Other etiologies include Brunner's gland hyperplasia, ectopic pancreas, and nodular lymphoid hyperplasia.

Carcinoma. The radiologic manifestations of gastric adenocarcinoma depend on its type of growth pattern. It may be a slow growing, well-defined polypoid mass or an irregular, fungating mass (Fig. 1-35), or it may infiltrate into the submucosa, extend along the muscle planes, and be associated with a fibrosis (linitis plastica) (Fig. 1-36). Because many of these lesions have a combination of these patterns, barium studies generally underestimate the extent of the tumor. Carcinomas arising from the cardia may invade the distal esophagus and simulate a primary esophageal carcinoma. Although uncommon, blood-borne metastasis (especially from breast or lung cancer) or direct extension from a pancreatic or colonic neoplasm may simulate a primary gastric tumor.

Lymphoma. This type of cancer, which is usually non-Hodgkin's lymphoma, may arise as a primary gastric lesion or may be part of a diffuse process. These lymphomas arise in the lymphoid tissue normally found in the submucosa and infiltrate the gastric wall. The folds become very thickened and nodular and the stomach loses its distensibility (Fig. 1-37). Ulcerations may be seen. This tumor can involve any part of the stomach but does not commonly invade or arise primarily in the duodenum. It is difficult to differentiate gastric lymphomas from gastric adenocarcinomas.

Leiomyoma. Leiomyoma is a common, benign tumor seen frequently at autopsy. It can arise within either the gastric or duodenal wall, but the gastric wall is the more common site. Leiomyomas become significant clinically if the overlying mucosa ulcerates and bleeds or if they become very large and degenerate into sarcomas. On barium studies leiomyomas are seen as round, smooth masses protruding into the lumen. They are usually solitary and the remainder of the stomach is normal.

MISCELLANEOUS DISORDERS. Chronic Atrophic Gastritis. Diagnosis of chronic atrophic gastritis is difficult to make radiologically. It can be suggested when there is a smooth mucosa and absence of the normal rugal pattern, especially in the fundus. These patients should have periodic endoscopy because of the increased risk of carcinoma.

Fig. 1-37. Gastric lymphoma. Histiocytic lymphoma was the cause of the marked, irregular, nodular folds of the entire stomach in this patient.

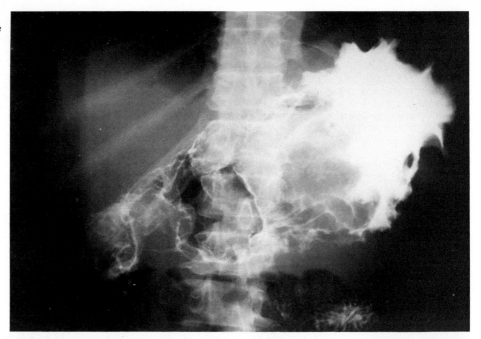

Fig. 1-38. Hypertrophic gastritis. Frontal view of the stomach showing diffuse thickening of the mucosal folds. No ulcerations are seen.

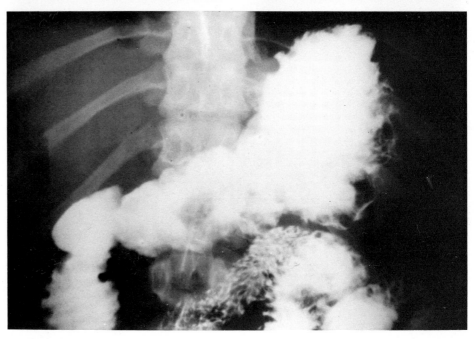

Hypertrophic Gastritis. The hallmark of hypertrophic gastritis is thickening of the mucosal folds in all or part of the stomach (Fig. 1-38). This condition is composed of two entities, hypersecretory gastropathy and Ménétrier's disease. The former is characterized by elevated acid production, whereas the latter has low or normal acid levels but may have protein loss from the mucosal surface. Thickened gastric folds are nonspecific and can be seen in lymphoma, carcinoma, and rare conditions such as sarcoidosis and eosinophilic gastritis.

Corrosive Gastritis. The amount and concentration of ingested material determines the degree of damage in corrosive gastritis and thus the extent of radiographic findings. Narrowing of the antrum, with shallow erosions and ulcerations is typical. Scarring with severe stricture formation may follow.

Bezoar. Nondigestible material may coalesce and form a mobile mass within the stomach. This is seen as a rounded, irregular, mobile tumefaction. Bezoars are of two general types: trichobezoars, composed of hair, and phytobezoars, composed of plant products. Bezoars rarely occur in normal stomachs; they form most commonly in patients who have had previous gastric resection and vagotomy or who have gastric paresis, which has many causes.

Volvulus. It is not uncommon to see the stomach rotated into a transverse position so that it is slightly folded on itself. However, it is rare to develop a frank volvulus with the stomach so twisted on itself that obstruction occurs. There are two types of volvulus: organoaxial, in which the twisting is along the axis between the esophagus and pylorus, and mesenteroaxial, in which the twist occurs along an axis that extends from the lesser to the greater curve. Mesenteroaxial volvulus occurs most often in patients with large paraesophageal hernias.

Zollinger-Ellison Syndrome. In this entity, an islet cell tumor (or gastrinoma) of the pancreas produces markedly elevated levels of gastrin, which stimulate the parietal cells to secrete hydrochloric acid. The most common manifestation is a singular duodenal ulcer. Other findings include thickened gastric folds (due to an increase in the parietal cell mass and inflammation) and single or multiple ulcers in the small bowel beyond the first and second portions of duodenum. Marked intraluminal secretions may be seen.

Diseases of the Small Bowel

In the general practice of medicine, problems with the small bowel portion of the gastrointestinal tract are not common. Moreover, the signs and symptoms tend to be nonspecific. A high index of suspicion and some knowledge about the predilection of disease for certain parts of the small bowel are key to the accuracy of diagnosis.

The small intestine beyond the duodenum is divided into the jejunum and the ileum. Currently, there are two major radiographic methods for examination of these areas: small bowel follow through (SBFT) or enteroclysis (small bowel enema).

The SBFT is usually obtained after an upper gastrointestinal (UGI) series, although it can be done as a separate study if only the small bowel needs to be examined. The patient is given a large amount of barium to drink so that the entire length of intestine can be visualized (Fig. 1-39). Films are obtained at 15 minute intervals and fluoroscopy is done during the study as needed and after barium has reached the cecum and ascending colon. Following the course of only the small amount of barium used for the UGI series is not sufficient to adequately evaluate the jejunum and ileum.

Enteroclysis requires the placement of a tube through the nose or mouth down into the jejunum so that the tip of the tube is beyond the ligament of Treitz. Otherwise, barium refluxes into the stomach, causing vomiting and preventing distention of the bowel. As the intestine is filled and distended, radiographs are taken with fluoroscopic guidance (Fig. 1-40). This procedure requires more time and irradiation than the SBFT, and therefore should only be done for certain indications. They include (1) documented chronic gastrointestinal bleeding but normal evaluation of the esophagus, stomach, duodenum, and colon, (2) Meckel's diverticulum, if the radionuclide study (Meckel's scan) is negative or equivocal, and (3) clinically suspected partial small bowel obstruction but normal or equivocal SBFT.

The normal small bowel folds are thin and delicate. They are more numerous and closely spaced in the jejunum; also, the jejunal caliber is greater than that of the ileum. Although the histology is similar, there is more lymphoid tissue in the terminal ileum than anywhere else in the small bowel.

INFECTION. The following are some commonly discussed organisms that infect the small bowel: *Giardia lamblia*, *Yersinia enterocolitica*, *Strongyloides stercoralis*, cryptosporidiosis, and *Mycobacterium tuberculosis*. Except for the tuberculosis, which causes strictures and fistulas,

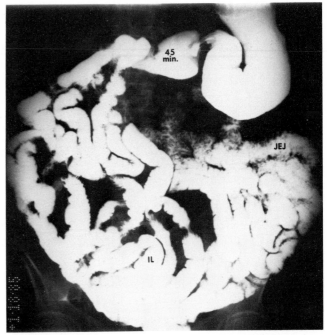

Fig. 1-39. Normal small bowel follow through (SBFT). The folds in the jejunum (JEJ) and ileum (IL) are thin and delicate. No masses are seen and the loops are normal in distribution.

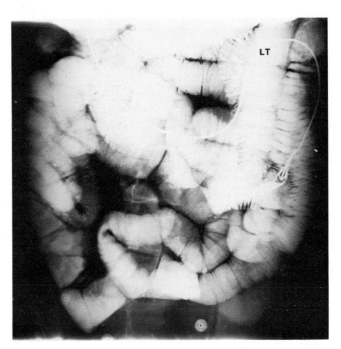

Fig. 1-40. Normal enteroclysis. The intestinal loops are more distended, with better fold definition than on the SBFT (see Fig. 1-39). The tip of the nasogastric tube is well beyond the ligament of Treitz (LT).

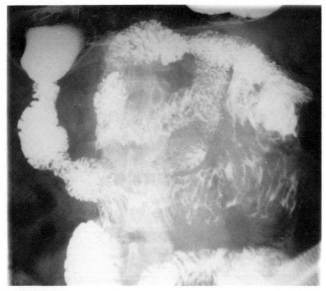

A

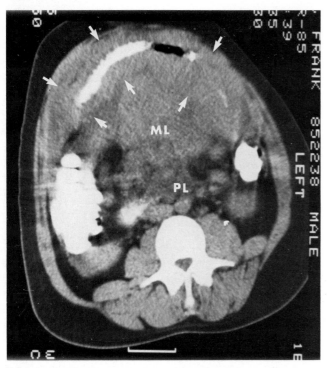

B

Fig. 1-41. A. Non-Hodgkin's lymphoma with marked fold thickening and distortion of the jejunum. A soft tissue mass effect is also suggested. B. CT scan through the same area reveals the bowel wall infiltration (*arrows*) and massive mesenteric (ML) and paraaortic (PL) lymphadenopathy.

these infections are usually acute and result in edema and cellular infiltration of the mucosa and submucosa. Radiographically, these are seen as thickened folds. Cryptosporidium, giardia, and strongyloides predominantly involve the duodenum and jejunum. The other diseases usually involve the distal ileum. In addition to thick folds, those diseases that involve the terminal ileum frequently cause nodular lymphoid hyperplasia as well. *Yersinia enteritis* may simulate Crohn's disease of the terminal ileum.

While in most parts of the United States these infections are uncommon, with the advent of acquired immune de-

ficiency syndrome (AIDS) incidence is increasing, especially of diseases caused by cryptosporidium.

NEOPLASMS. Malignant Neoplasms. In order of frequency, adenocarcinoma, lymphoma, and carcinoid are the most common primary malignancies of the small bowel. The exact order of frequency depends on the series reviewed and the geographic location involved. Adenocarcinomas occur most commonly in the proximal small bowel, with the second and third portions of the duodenum being frequent sites. In contrast, lymphoma and carcinoid tend to occur in the distal ileum. The lymphomas that occur as primary tumors are usually of a nonHodgkin's histology and most are of the diffuse hystiocytic type. Predisposing conditions for lymphoma include celiac sprue and immune deficiency states (e.g., AIDS). Nodular masses, with or without the central ulcerations, are seen in small bowel involvement of Kaposi's sarcoma, a reported complication of AIDS. Diseases associated with adenocarcinomas include regional enteritis (Crohn's disease) and the inherited polyposis syndromes (familial polyposis, Gardner's syndrome, and Peutz-Jeghers syndrome).

Adenocarcinomas appear as lobulated, fungating masses that may have an "apple core" appearance similar to that seen in the colon. The findings in lymphoma vary from nodules and thickened folds (Fig. 1-41) to large ulcerating masses with fistulas. Carcinoids usually present as sessile polypoid masses (Fig. 1-42) that can ulcerate and distort the surrounding bowel because of the associated desmoplastic response.

Benign Neoplasms. Benign adenomas and leiomyomas are the most common benign tumors of the small intestine. These polyps are round, smooth, and sometimes become pedunculated because of the antegrade flow of intestinal contents. Rarely they become a lead point for intussusception. Adenomatous polyps can be associated with familial polyposis and Gardner's syndrome. Hamartomatous polyps of the small bowel are characteristic of the Peutz-Jegher syndrome (Fig. 1-43).

MISCELLANEOUS DISORDERS. Diverticulosis. It is common to see barium collect in smooth outpouchings, which occur especially in the duodenum and proximal jejunum, although they can occur anywhere in the small bowel. The periampullary region in the second and third portion of the duodenum is a frequent site. These outpouchings are only significant in that they may be confused with ulcers, and if they become very large or numerous they can become sites for stasis with bacterial overgrowth and thus cause malabsorption. The cause of these diverticula is unknown but probably is a pulsion phenomenon, with outpouching of the mucosa through areas of weakness in the muscular wall.

Meckel's Diverticulum. Meckel's diverticulum is an entity separate from the diverticula mentioned previously. Its origin is incomplete closure of the omphalomesenteric duct (which connects the hind and foregut with the yolk sac) during embryologic development. It may contain tissue from other parts of the gastrointestinal tract. If this tissue is ectopic gastric mucosa, ulceration may occur and result in bleeding or perforation. Symptoms mimicking appendicitis or bowel obstruction may result.

If Meckel's diverticulum is suspected, a Meckel's scan should be obtained first. This is a nuclear medicine examination in which the radionuclide ^{99m}Tc is injected and

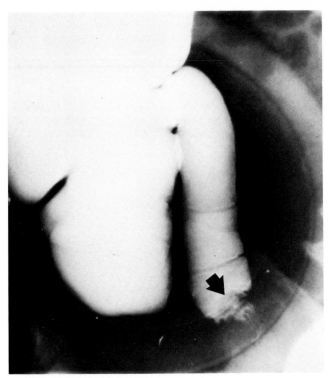

Fig. 1-42. A common location for carcinoid is the terminal ileum, as in this patient with a small, sessile mass (*arrow*).

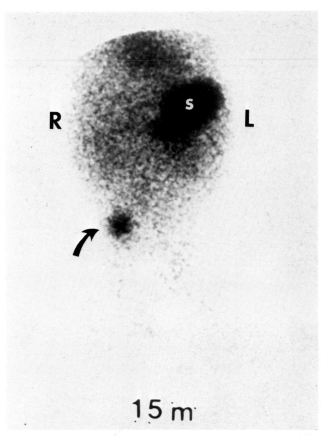

Fig. 1-44. Meckel's diverticulum (radionuclide study). Easily identifiable radionuclide uptake in the normal stomach (S) and in the ectopic gastric mucosa of a Meckel's diverticulum (*arrow*) in the right lower quadrant on this 15-minute frontal scan of the abdomen.

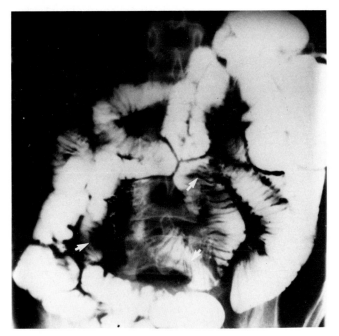

Fig. 1-43. Peutz-Jegher syndrome. Besides buccal pigmentation, multiple hamartomatous polyps of varying size (*arrows*) were found on this examination of the small bowel.

taken up in normal and ectopic gastric mucosa (Fig. 1-44). If this test is negative or equivocal because of insufficient uptake in the diverticulum, then a barium examination with enteroclysis should be done. The diverticulum is typically seen as a 2-inch long, widemouthed outpouching within 2 feet of the ileocecal valve (Fig. 1-45).

Malabsorption. There are many causes of malabsorption. Those diseases in the differential diagnosis for malabsorption that may have radiographic findings include celiac sprue, Crohn's ileitis, lymphoma, short bowel syndrome, extensive diverticulosis, and lymphangiectasia. The most common disorder of malabsorption that has an abnormal small bowel pattern is celiac sprue. This entity usually demonstrates dilatation and dilution of the barium due to excess fluid (Fig. 1-46). However, findings range from normal to extensive thickened folds caused by hypoproteinemia. There is also an increased incidence of lymphoma, which is seen as nodular masses.

Ischemia. Irradiation, collagen vascular disease, arteriosclerosis, embolus, diabetes, and mesenteric infiltration by tumor are some of the more frequent causes of vascular compromise. Edema and hemorrhage cause irregular narrowing of short or long segments of lumen (Fig. 1-47). Infarction and necrosis may result, appearing as air within the bowel wall. Partial or complete obstruction can be a sequela.

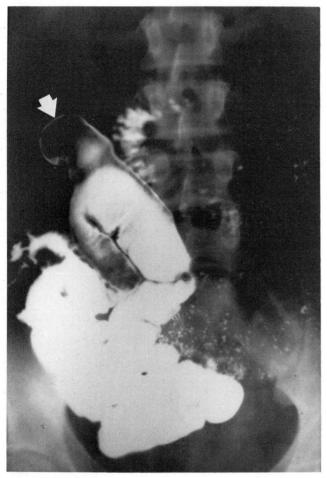

Fig. 1-45. Meckel's diverticulum (barium study). A blind ending, widemouth outpouching (*arrow*) was found on this SBFT.

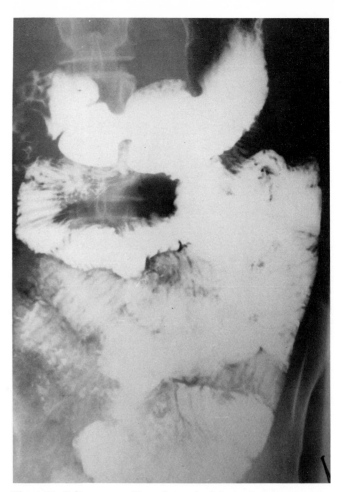

Fig. 1-46. Celiac sprue. Note the typical features (seen as gray, washed-out barium) of dilatation of the lumen and dilution of the barium caused by increased secretions.

Diseases of the Colon

Anatomically, the colon is divided into the cecum, ileocecal valve, ascending colon, hepatic flexure, transverse colon, splenic flexure, descending colon, sigmoid colon, and rectum. For practical purposes, the appendix is also considered part of the colon. The large bowel is generally tortuous in its course and may become redundant. Widely spaced haustrations are characteristic and are normally 2–3 mm thick.

Examination of the large bowel is performed through a tube placed in the rectum. Single or double contrast technique can be used, depending on the indication (Fig. 1-48). The double contrast barium enema (DCBE) is superior for entities where mucosal detail is essential (i.e., polyps or inflamed mucosa as occurs in ulcerative colitis). The single contrast barium enema (SCBE) is accurate for all other problems (i.e., diverticulosis, diverticulitis, appendicitis, extrinsic abdominal masses). When looking specifically for a primary carcinoma, both studies are equally sensitive. When looking for fistulas from the colon, the SCBE should be used. Barium can be used in the patient with suspected large bowel obstruction as long as only a small amount of barium is allowed beyond the obstructed site. The use of water soluble contrast (such as Gastrografin) is reserved for suspected cases of acute perforation.

INFECTION. There are many organisms that may infect the colon. The most common are *Shigella* (in the United States, *S. flexneri* and *S. sonnei*), *Salmonella typhi*, *Entamoeba histolytica*, *Campylobacter fetus*, *Clostridium difficile*, and *Mycobacterium tuberculosis*.

Salmonellosis and Shigellosis. These diseases are usually acquired by fecal-oral or fecal-food-oral contamination. The primary site of enteric involvement is the colon. Radiographic features include lymphoid hyperplasia, ulcerations, edema, and spasm (Fig. 1-49). With treatment the colon returns to normal. Strictures are very rare.

Amebiasis. The right colon, including the cecum, is the most frequent location of ulceration and edema. However, a pancolitis indistinguishable from idiopathic ulcerative colitis may be seen. Strictures and small sessile inflammatory polyps (amebomas) are common.

Campylobacter. A radiographically nonspecific colitis without sequelae is found when campylobacter is present.

Pseudomembranous Colitis. This is an infection usually seen in patients who have been on antibiotic therapy for other conditions. *C. difficile* causes the formation of pseudomembranes and severe inflammation that are identified as mucosal edema and elevated plaque-like lesions (Fig. 1-50). Perforation and stricture formation may occur, but usually the colon returns to normal.

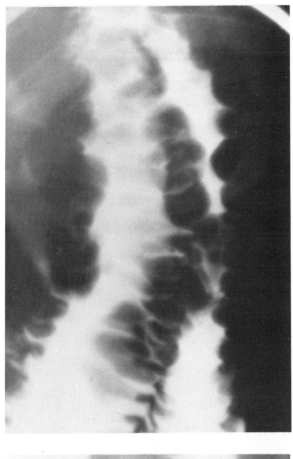

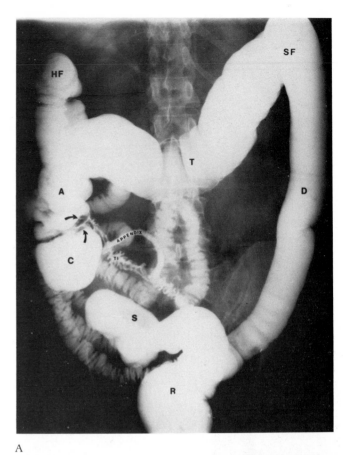

A

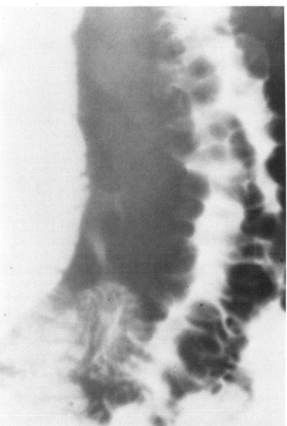

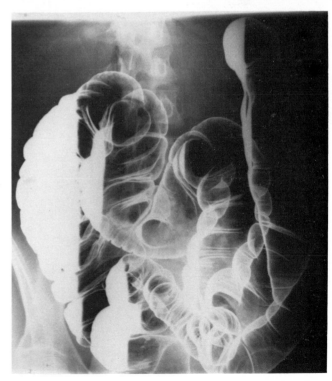

B

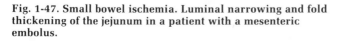

Fig. 1-47. Small bowel ischemia. Luminal narrowing and fold thickening of the jejunum in a patient with a mesenteric embolus.

Fig. 1-48. Normal barium enema. A. Single contrast study. The colon and appendix are filled with barium and there is reflux into the terminal ileum (*arrows*). R = rectum, S = sigmoid colon, D = descending colon, SF = splenic flexure, T = transverse colon, HF = hepatic flexure, A = ascending colon, C = cecum, TI = terminal ileum. B. Double contrast study. Note the smooth mucosal surface.

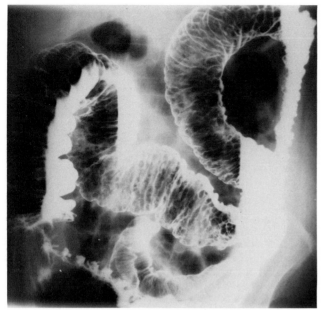

Fig. 1-49. Infectious colitis. Diffuse spasm, haustral edema, and nodular lymphoid hyperplasia with small ulcers were the major findings in this patient with a salmonella infection.

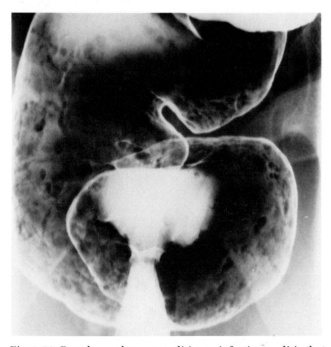

Fig. 1-50. Psuedomembranous colitis, an infectious colitis that is manifested by mucosal plaques (pseudomembranes), not ulcerations. (Photograph provided by Harvey M. Goldstein, M.D.)

Tuberculosis. The radiographic findings are typically those of an indolent process. This results in areas of focal narrowing, especially in the cecum. Nodular masses and fistulas may occur. Tuberculosis is notorious for simulating Crohn's disease and sometimes primary colon carcinoma. Uncommonly, an acute pancolitis is encountered.

OBSTRUCTION. The two most common causes of large bowel obstruction are volvulus and primary carcinoma.

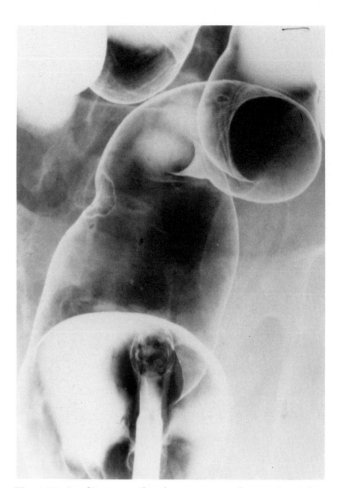

Fig. 1-51. A solitary sessile adenomatous polyp on the right lateral wall of the rectum.

The sigmoid colon is the most frequent site for both of these entities. Other causes include metastatic disease, diverticulitis, stricture caused by ischemia or inflammatory bowel disease, ventral or inguinal hernia, and intussusception. The last of these is very rare in adults and when seen is due to a benign or malignant neoplasm.

The diagnosis of colonic obstruction is usually made on a clinical basis with the use of plain films of the abdomen for confirmation (see section on abdominal plain films). Volvulus of the cecum and sigmoid have characteristic findings and rarely require contrast studies. If a barium enema is performed, a pointed "beak" is seen at the point of the bowel twisting on itself. However, other than the general signs of colonic obstruction, other etiologies have to be sought with a barium enema.

Neoplasms. *Benign Neoplasms.* As in the stomach, polyps in the colon are most commonly either hyperplastic or adenomatous. According to autopsy studies the incidence of adenomas in the general population is approximately 12 to 15 percent. Double contrast barium enema and colonoscopy have a sensitivity of 90 to 95 percent. If both are done in the same patient, this figure rises to 95 to 98 percent. The DCBE is especially helpful in detecting lesions located at the flexures; these lesions are either sessile or pedunculated (Fig. 1-51). Stalk formation is a reliable sign of benignincy. If one polyp is found, there is a 25 to 40 percent chance of finding one or more additional lesions. In familial polyposis and Gardner's syndrome the colon is usually carpeted with polyps (Fig. 1-52) and the physician must search carefully for the presence of cancer.

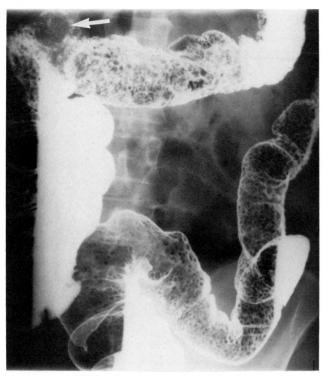

Fig. 1-52. Familial polyposis. Hundreds of polyps are seen carpeting the colon. These tend to be of uniform size but note the large polyp in the hepatic flexure (*arrow*) in which invasive carcinoma was found.

Villous adenomas are a specific histologic type of adenoma and have a high incidence (25–50%) of malignant transformation. These are most commonly seen in the right colon and rectum. About one-fourth have a characteristic frond-like or soapsuds appearance (Fig. 1-53).

Lipomas of the colon are common, but less so than adenomatous or hyperplastic polyps. They are seen as round, smooth masses and are found most frequently in the right colon, especially around the ileocecal valve. On computed tomography they can be seen as tumors with very low attenuation values (negative CT numbers). Other less common benign tumors of the colon are juvenile hamartomatous polyps and leiomyomas.

Malignant Neoplasms. Adenocarcinoma is by far the most common lesion. It is usually seen as an irregular circumferential narrowing ("apple core") (Fig. 1-54). In addition to the carcinoma, one or more polyps are found in 25 to 40 percent of patients affected and synchronous cancers occur in 2 to 3 percent. Next in frequency is lymphoma, which usually occurs in the cecum because of the abundance of lymphoid tissue in that area. After the appendix and ileum, the rectum is a common location for carcinoid tumors. These are identified as smooth, submucosal masses.

Miscellaneous Disorders. *Diverticulosis and diverticulitis.* Mucosal outpouchings between hypertrophied smooth muscle related to aging, disordered motility, and diet are very common in western man. At least 50 percent of those over 50 have this problem. In most patients the symptoms

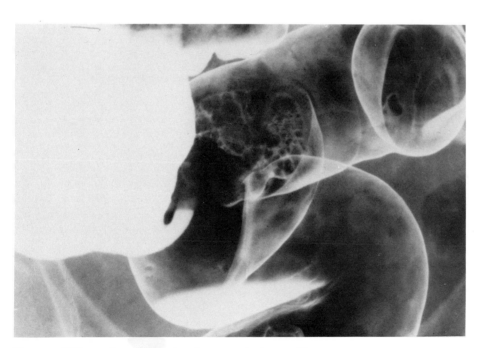

Fig. 1-53. Villous adenoma. Barium between the large villous fronds in this lesion of the sigmoid creates the characteristic soapsuds appearance seen in 25 percent of these tumors. (Case provided courtesy of Harvey M. Goldstein, M.D.)

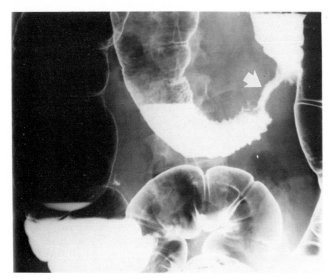

Fig. 1-54. Carcinoma of the colon. The circumferential narrowing caused by this neoplasm simulates an apple core (*arrow*).

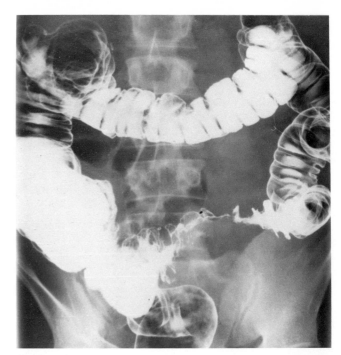

A

are minor. Diverticula can occur anywhere in the colon or appendix, but they do predominate in the left colon and can become quite marked in the sigmoid. One to three isolated right colon diverticula are usually congenital in origin.

When a diverticulum becomes inflamed the process may proceed transmurally and perforate. This is called *diverticulitis*. The perforation is almost always locally confined. An extrinsic and intramural inflammatory mass, with or without an abscess cavity, is the hallmark for the radiologic diagnosis (Fig. 1-55). Diverticulitis can occur anywhere in the colon, and when occurring on the right side may simulate appendicitis. Complications include stricture, obstruction, fistulas, and bleeding. The diagnosis is made clinically in a majority of patients, with subsequent evaluation with a barium enema 2 to 3 weeks after the acute episode.

Ischemia. Mesenteric vascular disease can be divided into two major forms, occlusive and nonocclusive. The nonocclusive disease is most common and is seen in such low-flow and vasoconstrictive states as congestive heart failure, aortic stenosis, shock, cardiac arrhythmias, and the use of vasoconstrictive drugs.

Mesenteric vascular occlusion can result from an embolus (e.g., left atrial myxoma, mitral valvular disease, arterial embolus from elsewhere) or thrombus (e.g., atherosclerosis, birth control pills). Because of the extensive collateral pathways available, the damage is limited. However, when blood flow is decreased enough, edema and hemorrhage into the bowel wall occur. This is the pathologic mechanism for "thumbprinting", which causes rounded indentations of the colon that are seen either on plain films or barium studies (Fig. 1-56). Thumbprinting can occur anywhere in the colon, although it very rarely occurs in the rectum because of its extensive collateral network. The transverse colon and sigmoid are frequent sites for ischemic changes. Bleeding and strictures are frequent complications.

Pneumatosis coli. (See p. 5, Intramural Air).

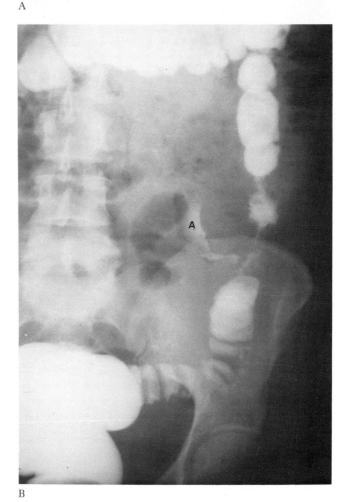

B

Fig. 1-55. Diverticulitis. A. Marked narrowing of the sigmoid colon by an extrinsic and intramural mass is a common feature. B. Sometimes barium is seen entering an abscess cavity (*A*).

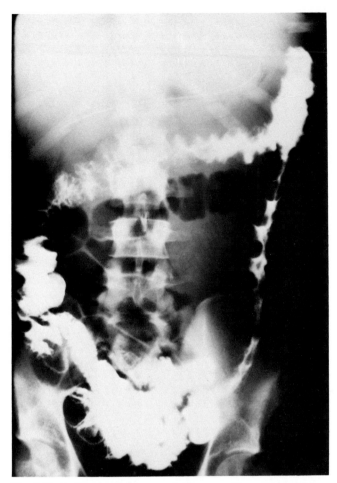

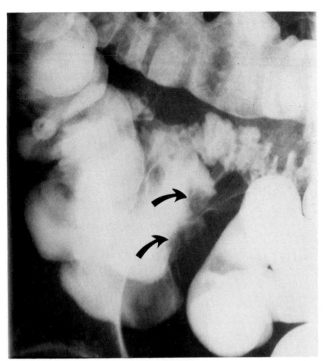

Fig. 1-57. Appendicitis. The appendix is not visualized and an intramural mass is seen at the tip of the cecum (*arrows*).

Fig. 1-56. Ischemia. Submucosal edema and hemorrhage in the transverse and descending colons create the submucosal indentations that are referred to as thumbprinting because they are usually about the size of the tip of the thumb. (Photograph provided by Harvey M. Goldstein, M.D.)

Disorders of Appendix. *Inflammation.* Appendicitis is a very common disorder that does not require many diagnostic studies. A barium enema is used only when there is doubt about the diagnosis, and sometimes this does not answer the question.

A SCBE is performed when needed. If the appendix is well visualized and normal in appearance, appendicitis is excluded. If the appendix is not seen and there is an intramural or extrinsic mass on the cecum, the diagnosis is confirmed (Fig. 1-57). If the appendix is not seen and no mass effect is identified, appendicitis can neither be ruled out nor confirmed. In these equivocal cases computed tomography is sometimes helpful in identifying inflammation. Rarely, appendicitis can cause small or large bowel obstruction. In some individuals the appendix is located cephalad and posterior to the cecum and ascending colon (this is known as retrocecal appendix). Inflammation in this location may simulate acute cholecystitis or pyelonephritis.

If the appendix becomes obstructed (usually from inflammation), mucus production may create a mass called a *mucocele.* This infrequent entity is seen as an indentation on the cecum.

Neoplasm. Mucinous adenocarcinoma and carcinoid are the only significant tumors of the appendix. These appear

as masses like those seen elsewhere in the gastrointestinal tract or nonvisualization of the appendix, and may distort the cecum, causing bowel obstruction.

Idiopathic Inflammatory Bowel Disease

The two entities included in this section are granulomatous ileitis and colitis (e.g., Crohn's disease, regional enteritis) and ulcerative colitis. Two important aspects of these disorders should be emphasized. First, in spite of typical or characteristic features of each, their radiographic findings in the colon may overlap and a definitive radiologic diagnosis cannot be made in some patients. Second, extraintestinal manifestations (e.g., arthritis, sclerosing cholangitis) may occur in both. It is beyond the scope of this chapter to describe each of these and their significance; only the pertinent bowel manifestations are considered.

CROHN'S DISEASE. The small bowel is the part of the intestinal tract most commonly involved by this granulomatous process. The most subtle abnormality seen is the aphthous ulcer. This is a small, superficial ulcer surrounded by a halo of edema (Fig. 1-58). Eventually, the inflammation involves the full thickness of the gut and is associated with fibrosis. This combination leads to the major radiologic finding, which is narrowing of the lumen (Fig. 1-58). Other common features include deep, irregular ulcers and fistulas. When the ulcers elongate and spread they also tend to criss-cross each other, creating a cobblestone appearance. Pseudopolyps, which are areas of spared mucosa surrounded by ulceration (Fig. 1-59), or postinflammatory polyps caused by hyperplasia of the

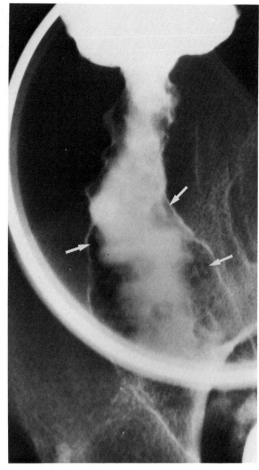

A

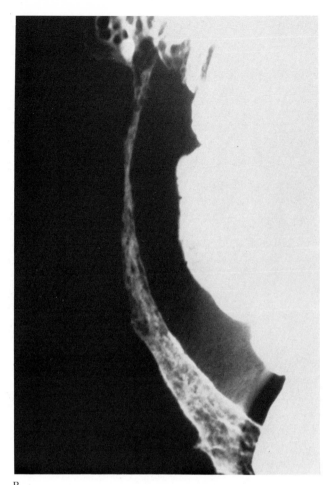

B

Fig. 1-58. Crohn's ileitis. A. Multiple aphthous ulcers (*arrows*) in the ileum. B. Subsequent progression of inflammation and fibrosis resulting in narrowing. (Photographs provided by Theodore Hopens, M.D.)

mucosa as it attempts to repair itself, may be seen. Focal areas of mucosal inflammation called inflammatory polyps are also encountered. All of these are also seen in ulcerative colitis.

Although the most common site of involvement is the terminal ileum, any part of the intestinal tract may be involved, including the esophagus. The antrum of the stomach and duodenum have been reported to be involved in up to 25 percent of patients with bowel involvement elsewhere, but this figure is much higher than my own experience and that of others have proved.

Pathologically, inflammation and fibrosis are not uniform or circumferential in most patients. The radiologic changes reflect this characteristic as "skip areas" and abnormalities on one side of the lumen and not the other. Short or long segments of disease may be seen. Fistulas can occur anywhere and represent an extension of the granulomatous process. These may connect to other loops of bowel or to other organ systems, the genitourinary tract being a frequent site. Fistulas may also lead to abscess cavities.

Complications that can be demonstrated radiographically include small, or, less commonly, large bowel obstruction, abscesses, toxic megacolon, obstructive uropathy, carcinoma, and rarely, bleeding.

The usual radiologic evaluation includes a UGI series with careful small bowel follow-through and DCBE. If fistulas from the colon are being sought, then a single contrast barium enema should be done. Occasionally, computed tomography is helpful to stage the extent of an inflammatory mass and to search for abscess cavities.

Radiographic findings tend to be progressive, and improvement is rarely seen.

ULCERATIVE COLITIS. In contrast to Crohn's disease, ulcerative colitis (UC) involves the mucosa of the colon and is not a transmural process. The exception to this is found in patients who develop toxic megacolon. In these patients the inflammation becomes severe and includes the full thickness of the wall. Also distinct from Crohn's disease is the pattern of involvement in UC; ulcerative colitis begins in the rectum and proceeds in a uniform manner to affect the remainder of the colon circumferentially. Although there is usually a pancolitis, only the rectum or sigmoid colon may be diseased.

Ulcerations are the radiographic hallmark and are frequently seen with the collar button configuration (Fig. 1-60). Barium collects in an ulcer crater that forms just below the undermined mucosal surface. Ulcers can get larger, deeper, and more irregular. When this happens, distinguishing these ulcerations from the ulcers seen in Crohn's colitis may be difficult. A granular mucosal pattern without ulcers is frequently identified and is characteristic of UC (Fig. 1-61). The symmetry, lack of skip areas, and fistulas help to differentiate UC from Crohn's. When pancolitis is present, dilatation of the terminal ileum caused by reflux of inflammatory contents across a patulous ileoce-

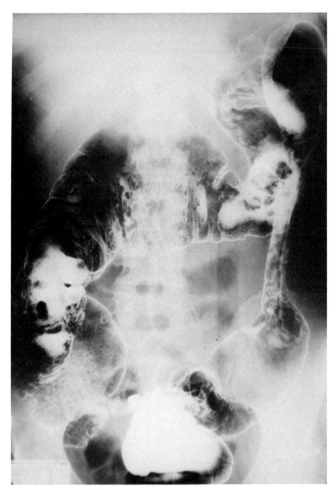

Fig. 1-59. Granulomatous colitis. Besides asymmetry and interval segments of normal ("Skip") areas, multiple pseudopolyps are present in the cecum and the ascending and transverse portions of the colon.

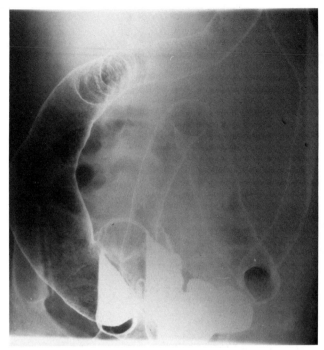

Fig. 1-61. Chronic ulcerative colitis. The colon has become tubular with loss of haustrations. The mucosal surface is granular, and small postinflammatory polyps are seen. The ileocecal valve is patulous and the terminal ileum is dilated ("backwash ileitis").

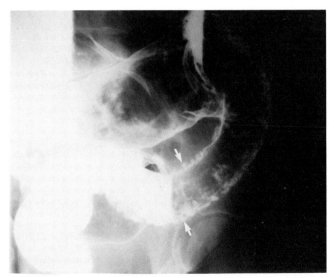

Fig. 1-60. Acute ulcerative colitis. Barium collected beneath the undermined mucosa creates ulcerations with a "collar button" configuration (*arrows*).

cal valve (backwash ileitis) may occur (Fig. 1-61). This is found more commonly in chronic rather than acute UC.

The three types of polypoid lesions mentioned under Crohn's disease actually occur more commonly in UC. Filiform postinflammatory polyps are characteristic of UC and may come and go over the course of the disease.

Complications of ulcerative colitis include bleeding, strictures, toxic megacolon, and carcinoma. Clinicians should be careful in identifying a smooth stricture as benign, because UC carcinomas may be of the scirrhous type and simulate benign disease.

The DCBE, which is more sensitive than the single contrast method, is the diagnostic procedure used most frequently for UC. However, in approximately 10 percent of cases a colon may be shown as normal radiographically but be abnormal histologically.

Diseases of the Liver

The majority of hepatic diseases encountered in the practice of medicine are inflammatory or metabolic and therefore do not commonly require imaging procedures. Primary and secondary neoplasms and abscess are the most common entities in which some form of radiologic evaluation is necessary. There are many techniques available: sonography, computed tomography, radionuclide scanning, magnetic resonance imaging, and angiography. This chapter identifies common problems in which these techniques are useful, and in what sequence they should be performed.

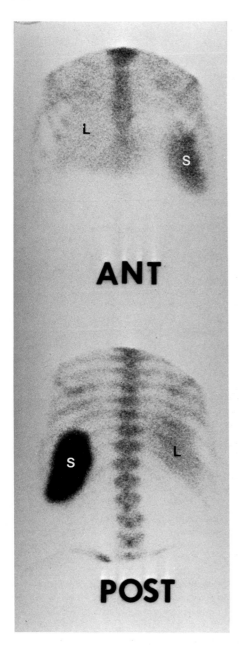

Fig. 1-62. Cirrhosis with portal hypertension. A liver-spleen scan (⁹⁹ᵐTc-sulfur colloid) demonstrates the characteristic picture of poor uptake in the liver (L), increased uptake in the enlarged spleen (S) and "shunting" of the radionuclide to the bone marrow of the spine and ribs. (Photograph provided by Ralph Blumhardt, M.D.)

CIRRHOSIS AND PORTAL HYPERTENSION. Alcohol abuse is the most frequent cause of cirrhosis and the associated complications of portal hypertension and liver failure. The diagnosis is made on a clinical and histologic basis, although it can be strongly suggested on a radionuclide liver-spleen scan with ⁹⁹ᵐTc sulfur colloid (Fig. 1-62). Otherwise, physicians become radiologically involved for evaluating three related problems: bleeding esophageal varices, ascites, and hepatocellular adenocarcinoma (hepatoma).

Either endoscopy or barium swallow can be done to identify the presence of varices. The former is more sensitive but the latter is significantly less expensive. Varices are identified on barium studies as wavy, longitudinal, thickened folds in the distal esophagus (Fig. 1-63) that may extend into the cardia of the stomach. Varices are best seen on collapsed mucosal views, because with distention the blood is pressed out of the dilated veins.

Ascites is the accumulation of fluid within the peritoneal cavity. This fluid can be easily and accurately identified with sonography (Fig. 1-64). Small amounts of fluid collect in the hepatoduodenal space (Morrison's pouch) and the pelvis, but large amounts can be seen throughout the abdomen.

Cirrhosis is the most common predisposing condition for the formation of a hepatoma. Cirrhosis can be clinically suspected by the worsening of liver function, increasing ascites, and abdominal pain. An elevated serum alpha-fetoprotein is a marker for the presence of this primary liver tumor. While it is frequently detected on liver-spleen scans, computed tomography is the most sensitive imaging method; magnetic resonance imaging may be the procedure of choice in the future. A CT guided biopsy is useful for confirming the diagnosis. Angiography is used preoperatively when resection is contemplated.

ABSCESS. The etiologies of liver abscesses fall into two major categories; amebic and pyogenic. The former are more common and are caused by *Entamoeba histolytica*. The latter are associated with biliary tract obstruction or bacterial seeding from extrahepatic intestinal infections and are usually caused by coliform or streptococcal bacteria. Pyogenic infections are most frequently found in the right lobe of the liver, probably because of the greater volume and streaming of blood to that side. Multiple abscesses tend to be of pyogenic origin.

I recommend the use of sonography as the primary imaging test when a liver abscess is suspected. The abscess is seen as a cystic mass that may have internal echoes (Fig. 1-65). Abscesses are usually solitary, but may be multiple or septated. Their size varies, with 1–2 cm being the lower limit of accuracy. Sonography can also be used to monitor the results of therapy and as a guide for needle aspiration. Clinicians should use CT when unsure of the presence, size, or exact location of an abscess. The abscess is seen as a lucent mass that does not enhance with intravenous contrast (Fig. 1-66). Occasionally, air is identified within pyogenic abscesses.

MASSES. Cysts. These fluid collections may be either congenital or acquired. As with most abnormalities in the liver, cysts are detected more frequently in the right lobe. They can be seen on any of the imaging modalities that show space-occupying lesions. Simple solitary cysts are commonly found now because of the widespread use of ultrasound and CT; they are incidental and rarely of clinical significance.

Single or multiple liver cysts are commonly identified in patients with adult polycystic kidney disease (APKD), as are cysts within the pancreas and spleen. Cysts in APKD patients are not clinically important unless they become very large, bleed, or become infected.

Echinococcal (hydatid) cysts are acquired due to infestation with *Echinococcus granulosus* or *Echinococcus multilocularis*. These tend to have a typical appearance by sonography or CT. Many daughter cysts are seen within a larger cystic mass. Because of the possibility of anaphylactic shock caused by spilled contents, percutaneous needle biopsy should be avoided. However, a 22-gauge thin needle aspiration could probably be performed safely.

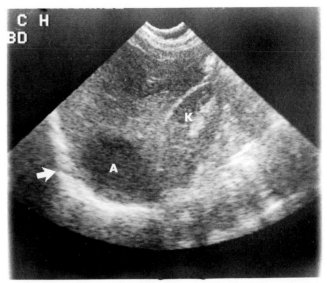

Fig. 1-65. Sonogram of amebic abscess shows a large hypoechoic mass (A) in the right lobe of the liver near the diaphragm (*arrow*). K = right kidney.

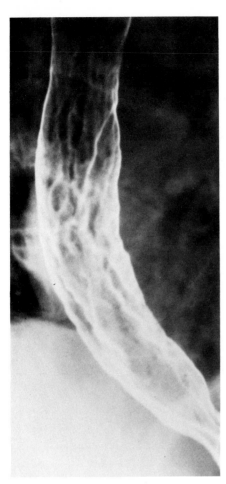

Fig. 1-63. Esophageal varices. Serpiginous folds in this double contrast view of the distal esophagus represent submucosal dilated veins.

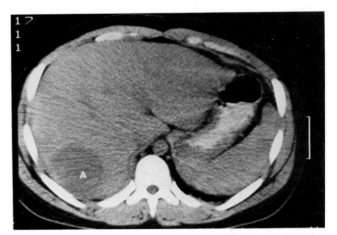

Fig. 1-66. CT scan of amebic abscess (same patient as in Fig. 1-65) reveals a low density mass (A) that did not enhance with intravenous contrast.

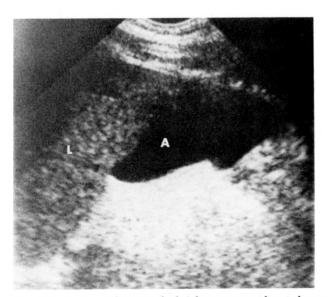

Fig. 1-64. Ascites. Ultrasound of right upper quadrant shows ascites (A) under the right lobe of the liver (L).

Benign Neoplasms. This category includes cavernous hemangioma, adenoma, and focal nodular hyperplasia. Cavernous hemangioma is by far the most common benign neoplasm of the liver. It is found commonly in the periphery of the right lobe of the liver and is of variable size. Calcification may occur. Cavernous hemangioma is seen as an echogenic mass at sonography. On CT it is found as an irregular, low-density mass that has a specific enhancement pattern when intravenous contrast is given (Fig. 1-67). Soon after injection the periphery enhances with subsequent filling-in of the mass, so that it becomes isodense with the rest of the liver. When this pattern is seen, no further evaluation is needed. A ^{99m}TC-tagged RBC scan can identify these tumors as an area of increased activity on delayed images. Also, cavernous hemangiomas will show as tumors with bright signal intensity with magnetic resonance imaging. If necessary, thin needle aspiration or arteriography can be done for confirmation.

Liver cell adenomas are rare, are encountered in women of childbearing age, and are associated with the use of oral contraceptives. The major dangers are hemorrhage or rupture. Malignant transformation is doubtful. This benign lesion can be identified on any of the usual imaging modal-

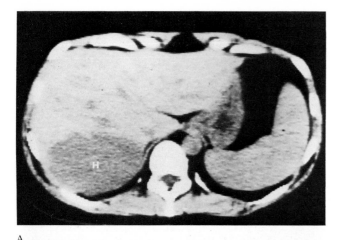

A

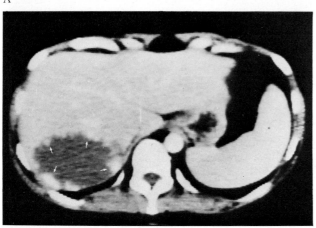

B

Fig. 1-67. Cavernous hemangioma. A. A large low density mass (H) in the right lobe of the liver is seen on the unenhanced CT scan. B. Scan obtained shortly after IV bolus injection demonstrates characteristic peripheral enhancement (*arrows*). Subsequent, delayed scan shows "filling in" of contrast, so that the lesion is almost isodense with the remainder of the liver. (Photographs provided by Harvey M. Goldstein, M.D.)

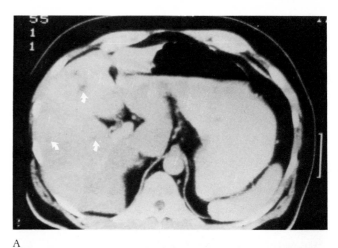

A

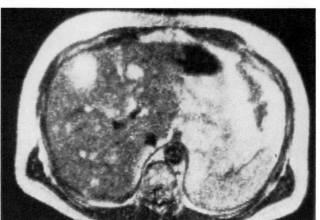

B

Fig. 1-68. Liver metastases. A. Initial CT scan after intravenous contrast reveals multiple subtle lesions in both lobes (*arrows*). B. Magnetic resonance imaging (MRI) of the same patient shows many, more clearly defined masses with high signal intensity. Source: Heiken, J. P., et al. Hepatic metastases studied with MR and CT. *Radiology* 156:423–427, 1985.

ities for the liver. Because there are no Kupffer cells, a liver cell adenoma is seen as a "cold" defect on the sulphur colloid liver/spleen scan. Because of the hemorrhage that may occur, cystic masses are commonly identified on ultrasound or CT. Arteriography is reserved for preoperative evaluation, at which time a hypervascular mass is most commonly seen.

Focal nodular hyperplasia is also associated with the use of oral contraceptives. In contrast to liver cell adenomas, Kupffer cells are present in this disease. Therefore, the mass may have a variable uptake so that the area of focal nodular hyperplasia may be seen as slightly decreased or increased radionuclide uptake on the liver/spleen scan. Because these lesions rarely bleed, cystic spaces on ultrasound or CT are not seen. However, these lesions may have a characteristic central focal scar. Because the vascularity of these lesions is variable, they range from hypovascular to hypervascular at the time of arteriography.

Malignant Neoplasms. The most common malignant mass found in the liver is the metastatic lesion. There are many primary cancers that can metastasize to the liver, especially gastrointestinal tract tumors. Because most primary

tumors are staged with computed tomography, and this modality is the most sensitive technique that is readily available, its use is recommended for this problem. The scan should be obtained both with and without intravenous contrast. Lesions that are even partially vascular may become isodense with the liver and be missed if intravenous contrast is not used. Metastatic lesions can also be identified on ultrasound and on the standard radionuclide liver/spleen scan. The various sensitivities for detecting metastatic lesions are 85 percent for liver/spleen scan, 85 to 90 percent for ultrasound, and 90 to 95 percent for CT. In the future, magnetic resonance imaging may be the procedure of choice for detecting liver metastases (Fig. 1-68). Angiography rarely plays a role in this clinical problem; it is usually reserved for preoperative staging or catheter placement for chemotherapy.

The appearance of metastatic lesions varies according to the imaging modalities utilized. On radionuclide liver/spleen scan lesions are seen as photopenic defects (Fig. 1-69). On ultrasound (Fig. 1-70) and CT they are usually solid, but may become necrotic and have cystic centers.

The most common primary malignancy of the liver is hepatoma (Fig. 1-71). Most hepatomas are found in patients with alcoholic cirrhosis and can be detected by the imaging modalities mentioned above. However, in addi-

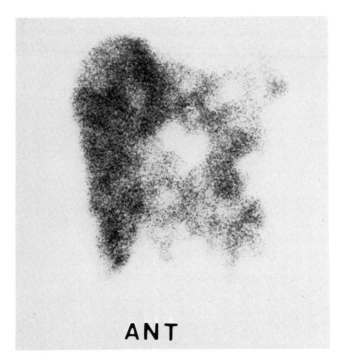

Fig. 1-69. Radionuclide study of liver metastases (colon carcinoma). Anterior view of ^{99m}Tc-sulfur colloid liver-spleen scan demonstrates many photopenic defects in both lobes of the liver.

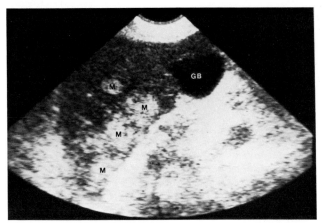

Fig. 1-70. Multiple echogenic masses (M) are easily identified in this sonogram of liver metastases. GB = gallbladder.

tion to focal solitary or multiple masses, hepatomas may present as diffuse infiltration. This last form is usually the most difficult to detect and confirm.

A useful technique in evaluating liver masses is percutaneous needle aspiration biopsy, which can be done under CT or ultrasound guidance. Small caliber needles are used (20- to 23-gauge) with excellent results and a very low complication rate. This procedure facilitates both diagnosis and patient care.

MISCELLANEOUS DISORDERS. Hemochromatosis. In hemochromatosis, there is abnormal deposition of iron within the liver. Hemochromatosis can be a primary metabolic disorder or can be secondary to systemic iron overload. Eventually, damage is caused, and cirrhosis may result. The liver has increased density on CT scan (Fig. 1-72). Because of the paramagnetic properties of iron and its effect on the parameters measured in the magnetic resonance im-

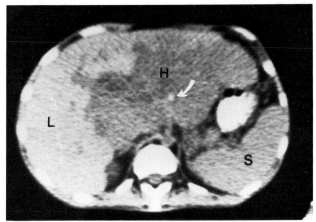

Fig. 1-71. Hepatoma. CT scan of a tumor mass (H) in the left lobe of the liver (L). A small calcification (*arrow*) is a common finding in this tumor. S = spleen.

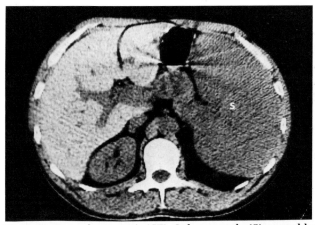

Fig. 1-72. Hemochromatosis (CT). Splenomegaly (S) caused by portal hypertension, in addition to the marked increased density of the liver. The density of the liver and spleen are normally very similar to each other.

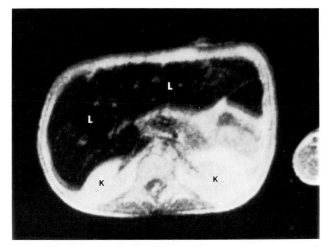

Fig. 1-73. Hemochromatosis (MRI). Because of iron's paramagnetic and binding properties, the liver (L) will lack signal and therefore appear black on a magnetic resonance scan. K = kidney. (Photograph provided by Dennis Balfe, M.D.)

aging, the liver is seen as an organ without signal intensity (i.e., it is black in appearance) (Fig. 1-73). Both CT and MRI can be used to follow the therapy of this disorder.

Fatty Infiltration. There are a number of causes for abnormal deposition of fat within the liver, including alcoholic liver disease, diabetes mellitus, steroid administration, Cushing's disease, hyperalimentation, and pancreatitis. Sonographic findings include enlargement of the liver with increased echogenicity. On CT there is a decrease in the density of the liver (see Fig. 1-67). Magnetic resonance imaging shows an increase in signal intensity in the areas of fatty deposition. While in moderate to severe cases this diagnosis is not difficult, physicians are cautioned in one variation of this process. Fatty infiltration may be focal and simulate neoplastic disease, and at times this requires percutaneous needle aspiration biopsy to confirm the presence of fat.

Budd-Chiari Syndrome. This venoocclusive disorder is elusive. Its diagnosis is difficult and mainly one of exclusion of other etiologies for the clinical presentation. The liver/ spleen scan may show evidence of diffuse hepatocellular disease and portal hypertension with preserved or increased radionuclide uptake in the caudate lobe owing to variation in drainage of the liver. Venography is sometimes used to establish the patency or thrombosis of hepatic veins. Rarely, occlusion of hepatic veins may be identified on sonographic evaluation.

Diseases of the Gallbladder and Bile Ducts

Of all the modalities available to evaluate the biliary system, the most commonly used is sonography. Depending on the clinical picture and sonographic findings, CT, hepatobiliary radionuclide scans, endoscopic retrograde cholangiography (ERCP), and percutaneous transhepatic cholangiography (PTC) may be performed. Angiography is rarely utilized. The role of magnetic resonance imaging is indeterminate at this time.

JAUNDICE. There are many causes for this clinical sign, including the major categories of hepatitis, biliary obstruction, metabolic diseases, and peripheral red cell destruction. The category that involves the radiologist most often is that of biliary obstruction. Commonly encountered etiologies include choledocholithiasis, chronic pancreatitis (with or without pseudocysts), metastatic disease to the porta hepatis, pancreatic carcinoma, and cholangiocarcinoma.

Sonography for biliary obstruction is very accurate. The presence of obstruction and its intrahepatic or extrahepatic location can be readily identified (Fig. 1-74). Computed tomography is also accurate (Fig. 1-75), but is more expensive and less accessible to many individuals. Its major advantages are anatomic detail, ability to further assess etiology and staging (including the presence of metastatic disease), and the fact that percutaneous biopsy can be performed at the same time. The most common approach to obstructive jaundice has been sonography followed by direct visualization of the bile ducts, by either the percutaneous transhepatic (PTC) or endoscopic (ERCP) route. De-

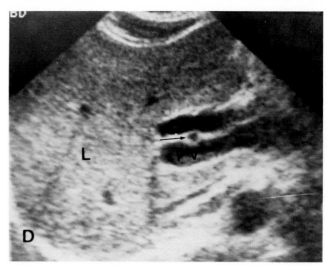

Fig. 1-74. Common bile duct obstruction. This real-time sonogram of the right upper quadrant shows typical dilatation of an obstructed common bile duct (CBD). It lies anterior to the portal vein (PV) and right hepatic artery (*arrow*). L = liver. D = diaphragm.

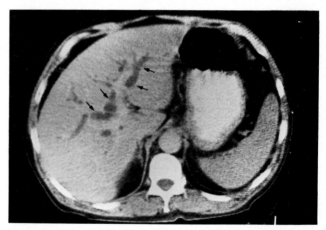

Fig. 1-75. Dilated bile ducts. The arrows indicate dilated intrahepatic bile ducts on this enhanced CT scan through the right lobe of the liver. The portal veins are filled with contrast and are almost isodense with the liver.

pending upon what is found at that time, a CT scan is commonly obtained. Computed tomography is not recommended when calculi are found as the cause of obstruction.

INFLAMMATORY AND CALCULOUS DISEASE. Cholecystitis. Cholecystitis can be divided into acute and chronic forms. Cholelithiasis is present in 95 percent of cases, and acalculous acute cholecystitis occurs in the remaining 5 percent. Sonography is the first and many times only test required for diagnosis (Fig. 1-76). Its accuracy for detection of gallstones is 97 percent, equalling and frequently superseding the diagnostic ability of the standard oral cholecystogram. In addition to the detection of the presence of gallstones, complications such as bile duct obstruction or perforation and abscess formation can be evaluated. Because cystic duct obstruction is seen in the acute setting, a radionuclide hepatobiliary scan (^{99m}Tc HIDA, DISIDA, etc.) can be used. With this examination, if the gallbladder is not visualized, cystic duct obstruction is confirmed (Fig.

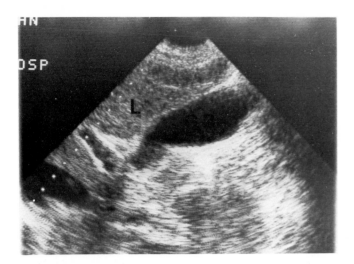

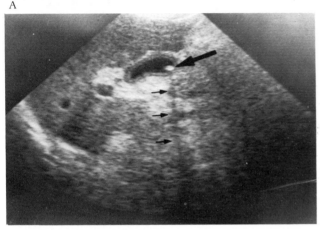

Fig. 1-76. Sonography shows the normal gallbladder (GB) as an ovoid fluid-filled structure free of echoes, adjacent to the right lobe of the liver (L). B. Acute cholecystitis with cholelithiasis (sonogram). An echogenic mass (*large arrow*) with posterior acoustic shadowing (*small arrows*) is a gallstone within an edematous gallbladder, represented by a thickened wall with a "halo" appearance.

1-77). However, this finding is not specific in that it may be caused by chronic disease as well as by prolonged fasting, hyperalimentation, or any other situation involving gallbladder stasis.

Bile duct stones are best identified with intraoperative or postoperative T-tube or endoscopic retrograde cholangiography. Sometimes the presence of bile duct stones can be seen on ultrasound or computed tomography.

Sclerosing Cholangitis. This disease of progressive inflammation and stricture of intra- and extrahepatic bile ducts is most commonly associated with inflammatory bowel disease, usually ulcerative colitis. The cholangiographic findings are multiple areas of stricture between areas of normal to slightly dilated caliber in both the intrahepatic and extrahepatic bile ducts. Over time, these strictures progress and may become confluent. Differentiating this process from primary cholangiocarcinoma is very difficult. In fact, the incidence of cholangiocarcinoma is increased in patients suffering from cholangitis. Initial and follow-up evaluation is by endoscopic retrograde cholangiography. Biliary sonography is normal in this disease.

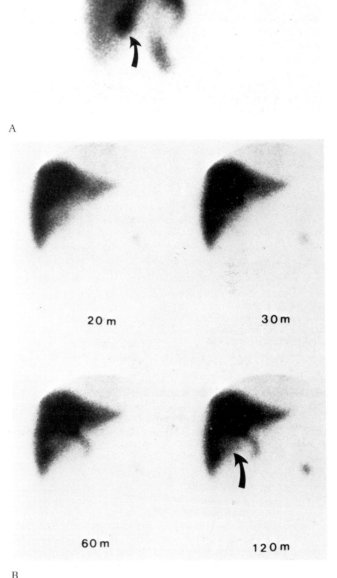

Fig. 1-77. Radionuclide Hepatobiliary Scan. A. A 30-minute scan performed with 99mTc-DISIDA reveals normal hepatic uptake and excretion into the bile ducts, duodenum, and gallbladder (arrow). B. Acute cholecystitis. Scans carried out to 120 minutes fail to show uptake in the gallbladder. Instead, they reveal a defect (*arrow*) caused by cystic duct obstruction by acute inflammation. (Photographs provided by Ralph Blumhardt, M.D.)

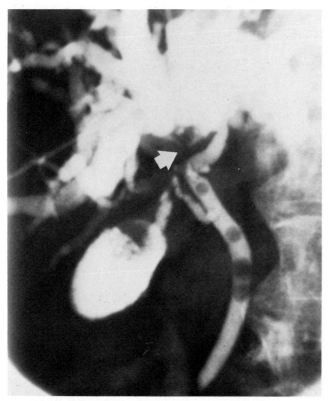

Fig. 1-78. Cholangiocarcinoma at bifurcation (Klatskin's tumor). In addition to calculi seen in the gallbladder and common bile duct, there is marked dilatation of the intrahepatic bile ducts caused by a primary tumor at the bifurcation (*arrow*).

Ascending Cholangitis. This is usually a clinical diagnosis. However, these patients occasionally require sonography, CT, or cholangiography. On CT or ultrasound multiple, small abscesses associated with the biliary tree may be seen. Abscess cavities as well as areas of narrowing of the intrahepatic bile ducts can be identified by cholangiography.

Gallstone Ileus. This is a complication of chronic cholecystitis with cholelithiasis whereby a large gallstone erodes into the duodenum, passes into the distal small bowel, and causes a small bowel obstruction, usually near the ileocecal valve. The classic triad of findings on plain abdominal radiographs are (1) biliary air, (2) small bowel obstruction, and (3) calcified gallstone. However, the most common presentation is small bowel obstruction in an elderly patient. The other abnormalities are not commonly seen.

NEOPLASM. Cholangiocarcinoma. Cholangiocarcinoma is a primary adenocarcinoma of the bile ducts. This tumor usually arises within the larger bile ducts, either at the bifurcation (Klatskin's tumor) (Fig. 1-78) or in the extrahepatic bile ducts. This diagnosis may be difficult to make by sonography or at CT because the tumor tends to be locally infiltrating and may not give a discrete mass. Obstructed bile ducts are found. The principal cholangiographic finding is narrowing, but sometimes irregularity and a mass effect are also present.

Carcinoma of the Gallbladder. Fortunately, this is an uncommon tumor. It is seen most often in association with gallstones. Carcinoma of the gallbladder presents in two major fashions. The first is as an incidental finding at the time of cholecystectomy, and the prognosis is good in these patients. The other is usually at an advanced stage where there is significant tumor mass and obstruction of the biliary system, and in this latter stage the findings are essentially the same as those for primary cholangiocarcinoma.

MISCELLANEOUS DISORDERS. Hyperplastic Cholecystoses. Hyperplastic cholecystoses includes two entities, adenomyomatosis and cholesterolosis.

Adenomyomatosis. This is an abnormal thickness of the muscular layers and enlargement of the mucosal glands. The enlarged mucosal glands and the tubular connection with the lumen are called Rokitansky-Aschoff sinuses. This disorder may cause colic-like symptoms. However, inflammation of the wall of the gallbladder is not seen in this disease. The finding of inflammation and gallstones is purely coincidental. Radiographically, adenomyomatosis is seen as a focal mass in the fundus of the gallbladder or as an area of narrowing of the gallbladder associated with the Rokitansky-Aschoff sinuses.

Cholesterolosis. Here, macrophages within the mucosa of the gallbladder accumulate cholesterol esters and small amounts of precholesterol and fatty acids. Functionally, the gallbladder is normal. However, these small cholesterol polyps, which may be seen as small filling defects on oral cholectestography or at the time of sonography, may become the nidus for gallstone formation. The gross pathologic appearance of the inside of the gallbladder with these yellow deposits simulates that of the surface of a strawberry. Therefore, this disease has sometimes been referred to as "strawberry gallbladder".

Choledochal Cysts. There are many types of focal areas of dilatation of the extra- or intrahepatic bile ducts that create cyst-like spaces. The most common type is a fusiform to sacular dilatation of the common bile duct. The bile duct becomes an area of stasis. Calculi may occur and there is an increased incidence of cholangiocarcinoma in unoperated patients. Presentation is usually at a young age, with jaundice and occasionally right upper quadrant pain. A cystic mass with or without adjacent bile duct dilatation is identified at sonography. The gallbladder can easily be found separate from this abnormality. The same findings are seen on CT. The cholangiographic findings are as expected where a large cystic dilatation of the common bile duct is found. Occasionally, ^{99m}Tc hepatobiliary scintigraphy is helpful in the differential diagnosis of a cystic mass in the right upper quadrant. On delayed images the radionuclide accumulates within the cyst.

Diseases of the Pancreas

Prior to the development of ultrasound and CT (Fig. 1-79), the pancreas was very difficult to evaluate radiologically. These technologic advances have had a major impact on the diagnosis, treatment, and knowledge of the natural history of the various diseases of the pancreas, and this is especially true of pancreatitis and its complications. Angiography and radionuclide examinations are not widely used. Barium studies are now indicated only if there is evidence of intestinal involvement, such as obstruction of the duodenum or colon.

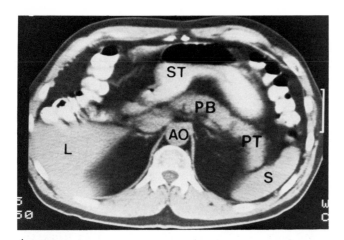

A

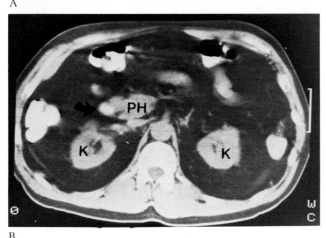

B

Fig. 1-79. A. CT scan through upper abdomen details the normal anatomy of the body (PB) and tail (PT) of the pancreas and surrounding structures. B. A lower scan shows the head of the pancreas (PH). L = liver, ST = stomach, S = spleen, AO = aorta, K = kidney. Arrow indicates duodenum.

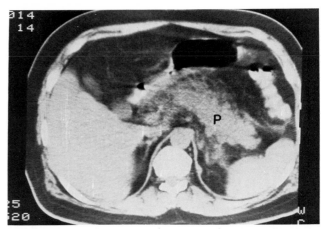

Fig. 1-80. Acute pancreatitis. CT scan shows enlarged pancreas (P) with irregular borders and inflammatory streaks into the surrounding fat.

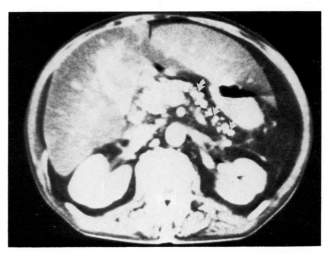

Fig. 1-81. Chronic pancreatitis (CT). In addition to fatty infiltration of the liver, which can be seen in chronic pancreatitis, there is marked atrophy and calcification of the pancreas (*arrows*).

INFLAMMATION. Acute Pancreatitis. The major causes of this entity are alcohol abuse, cholelithiasis, and trauma. Therefore, in addition to the clinical presentation, attention is directed toward evaluation of the biliary system. Use of ultrasound at this initial stage is recommended in order to detect the presence of gallstones. Mild to moderate uncomplicated pancreatitis does not require additional studies. If a CT scan is done in uncomplicated acute pancreatitis, a swollen gland with irregular edematous borders is identified (Fig. 1-80). A normal pancreas can also be seen in patients with mild pancreatitis.

Chronic Pancreatitis. This is most commonly seen in patients with chronic alcohol abuse. The gland becomes atrophic and fibrotic. Calculi can be seen on plain-film examination and CT (Fig. 1-81) and are due to concretions within the ducts. The pancreatic duct becomes dilated, due to glandular atrophy with or without stricture formation (Fig. 1-82). Endoscopic retrograde pancreatography (ERCP) is frequently done in patients with recurring pancreatitis in order to look for an anatomic defect (e.g., stricture or calculi) of the pancreatic duct. Surgical therapy can then be planned.

Complications of Pancreatitis. Severe pancreatitis is associated with outpouring of fluid or blood from the pancreas.

A noninfected, semisolid inflammatory mass may occur; this is called a *phlegmon* (Fig. 1-83). In contrast, fluid collections may become discrete and form within a fibrous capsule; this is called a *pseudocyst* (Fig. 1-84). Pseudocysts frequently are connected to the pancreatic ducts and are seen as pure pancreatic fluid collections, although debris, hemorrhage, and infection can occur. These complications of pseudocysts are seen as a change from a pure water density mass to one that has areas of increased density on CT or increased echoes on sonography. Pancreatic abscess is usually a more advanced complication of a phlegmon or pseudocyst. Unless air is identified within the lesion (Fig. 1-85), infection cannot be confirmed without needle aspiration.

Narrowing and obstruction of the common bile ducts can occur with acute pancreatitis or can become a chronic stricture with recurrent pancreatitis. Following the identification of bile duct obstruction by sonography, an endoscopic retrograde cholangiogram or percutaneous transhepatic cholangiogram is obtained for evaluation. Occasionally it is difficult to differentiate a benign stricture from a neoplastic process.

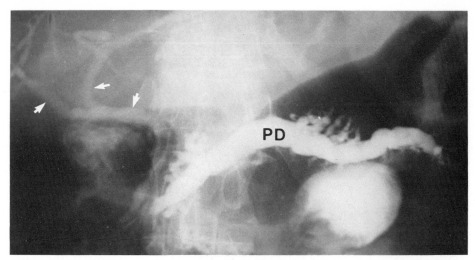

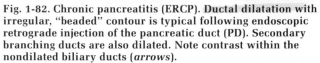

Fig. 1-82. Chronic pancreatitis (ERCP). Ductal dilatation with irregular, "beaded" contour is typical following endoscopic retrograde injection of the pancreatic duct (PD). Secondary branching ducts are also dilated. Note contrast within the nondilated biliary ducts (*arrows*).

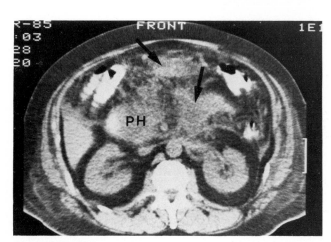

Fig. 1-83. Pancreatic Phlegmon. The head of the pancreas (PH) is enlarged and edematous. Two non-infected inflammatory masses (*arrows*) representing phlegmons are seen in the peripancreatic fat.

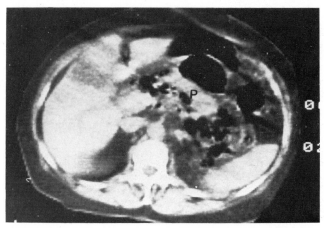

Fig. 1-85. Irregular, mottled collections of air in and around the pancreas (P) indicate pancreatic abscess in this patient who initially presented with severe acute pancreatitis and phlegmon.

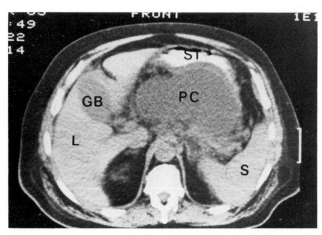

Fig. 1-84. A large, uncomplicated fluid-filled pancreatic pseudocyst (PC) is identified in the lesser sac, displacing the stomach (ST) anteriorly. L = liver, GB = gallbladder, S = spleen.

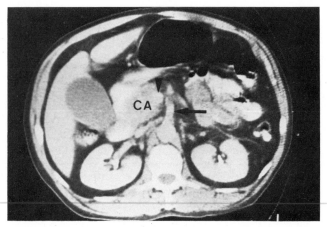

Fig. 1-86. CT scan shows carcinoma (CA) in the head of the pancreas invading the superior mesenteric vein (*arrowhead*). Arrow indicates superior mesenteric artery.

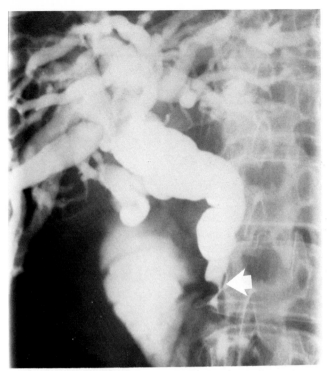

Fig. 1-87. Percutaneous cholangiogram shows abrupt narrowing (*arrow*) of the distal common bile duct, characteristic of carcinoma in the head of the pancreas.

NEOPLASMS. Exocrine Tumors. The most common neoplasm in this group is adenocarcinoma of the pancreatic ducts. Computed tomography scan of the pancreas is the procedure of choice when looking for the presence and staging of a primary pancreatic cancer. A rounded, irregular mass is usually seen (Fig. 1-86). Biliary obstruction, liver metastases, bowel invasion, or adenopathy can be associated with the tumor mass. If biliary obstruction is present, a percutaneous transhepatic cholangiogram (PTC) is performed (Fig. 1-87) and drainage provided. Angiography is rarely performed and, when done, is for preoperative evaluation. As with other neoplasms easily seen on CT, an

Fig. 1-88. Posttraumatic pseudocysts. This endoscopic pancreatogram shows a normal pancreatic duct proximally, but narrowing, irregularity, and multiple small pseudocysts (*arrows*) distally. This pattern was caused by blunt trauma to the part of the pancreas that overlies the spine.

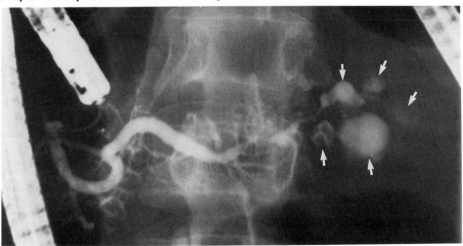

aspiration biopsy can be performed to help confirm the diagnosis.

Macrocystic and microcystic cystadenomas of the pancreas are rare. Macrocystic lesions are considered premalignant and are seen more commonly in the head or body of the pancreas. A large mass is identified, usually with cystic spaces that vary in size. Calcification is uncommon in this lesion. In contrast, microcystic cystadenomas are most commonly found in the body and tail of the pancreas and are not considered premalignant. Cystic spaces are rarely identified. However, calcification centrally within the tumor is frequently seen.

Endocrine Tumors. Endocrine tumors are very rare and include glucagonomas, insulinomas, gastrinomas (Zollinger-Ellison syndrome), vipomas, and somatostatinomas. Again, CT scan is the procedure of choice for initial evaluation. These tumors are found as discrete masses of soft-tissue density similar to that found in carcinoma.

MISCELLANEOUS DISORDERS. Trauma. The pancreas may be involved with blunt or penetrating trauma that may result in hemorrhage or pancreatitis. When caused by trauma, pancreatitis and its complications have the same appearance as described with other etiologies. This includes the development of posttraumatic pseudocysts (Fig. 1-88).

Annular Pancreas. Annular pancreas is a rare congenital abnormality in which portions of the pancreas surround the second portion of the duodenum. It is an incidental finding unless obstruction of the duodenum develops. Upper gastrointestinal series or endoscopy reveals a circumferential narrowing. Pancreatic tissue in this region can be identified on CT. The diagnosis is confirmed by an endoscopic retrograde pancreaticogram showing pancreatic ducts around the duodenum.

Diseases of the Peritoneum, Mesentery, and Omentum

From an imaging point of view, many of the abnormalities discussed in this section are uncommon. However, computed tomography has added a significant dimension to

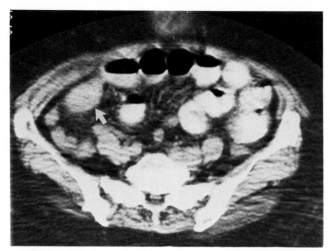

Fig. 1-89. Peritoneal metastasis. A soft tissue mass (*arrow*) is seen attached to the anterior surface of the peritoneum. This spread from an ovarian carcinoma.

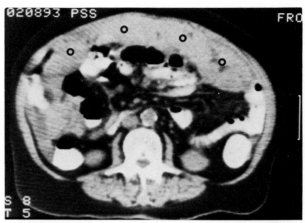

Fig. 1-90. Omental "cake". CT scan in this patient with ovarian carcinoma demonstrates tumor spread into the omentum (O), giving a "cake-like" appearance. (Photograph provided by Harvey M. Goldstein, M.D.)

the diagnosis and treatment of the various abnormalities described herein. It has also aided in the knowledge of the pathogenesis of these entities.

PERITONEUM. Peritonitis. Peritonitis is most definitely a clinical diagnosis. Imaging is rarely done and patients are usually explored surgically. If a radiologic study is obtained, it is usually computed tomography in order to search for the source of peritonitis.

Mesothelioma. This rare, primary tumor of the peritoneum is associated with asbestos exposure in approximately 65 percent of patients. Mesothelioma has also been linked to exposure to thorium dioxide (Thorotrast). Findings on CT or sonography include ascites and thickening of the peritoneal surface, which usually begins in one area and progresses to involve the abdomen in a circumferential fashion.

Carcinomatosis. Secondary involvement of the peritoneum by malignant neoplasm is common. The primary carcinomas are usually adenocarcinomas that arise from the gastrointestinal tract, pancreas, or ovary. Ascites is the usual finding. However, on occasion peritoneal masses can be demonstrated. (Fig. 1-89).

Pseudomyxoma Peritonei. This rare entity is a complication of mucoceles of the appendix or spread of mucinous cystadenocarcinoma of the ovary. A semisolid, gelatinous material is formed and deposited within the peritoneum. This material can become generalized, causing abdominal distention and crowding of the intraabdominal contents. These findings can be demonstrated on ultrasound or CT. Calcification of these gelatinous masses can be seen on plain abdominal films.

Retroperitoneal Fibrosis. This entity is characterized by a fibrotic plaque in the retroperitoneum adjacent to the aorta. The ureters are commonly involved, and on an intravenous pyelogram are seen to be deviated medially, with hydronephrosis proximally. The cause is usually idiopathic, although in a significant percentage of patients this fibrosis is associated with reticulum cell sarcoma, lymphoma, carcinoid tumors, and the administration of methysergide.

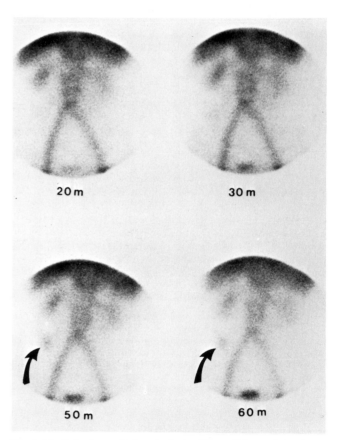

Fig. 1-91. Colonic angiodysplasia (radionuclide study). The anterior view of this ^{99m}Tc-tagged red blood cell scan identified the bleeding site in the right lower quadrant (*arrows*). This was caused by angiodysplasia of the ascending colon (see Fig. 1-94). (Photograph provided by Ralph Blumhardt, M.D.)

MESENTERY AND OMENTUM. Mesenteric Fibromatosis. Mesenteric fibromatosis has also been called a desmoid and is usually seen in association with Gardner's syndrome. This represents a very aggressive fibrosis within the mesentery that progresses to engulf the intestinal and vascular structures. Barium examinations show obstruction of the small bowel or colon as well as irregular out-

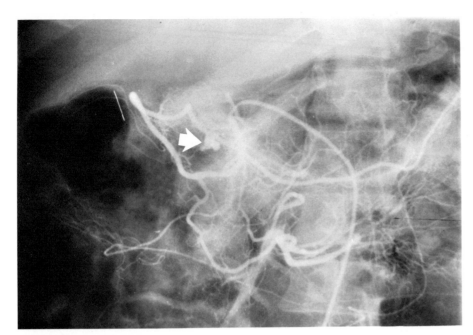

Fig. 1-92. Bleeding duodenal ulcer. A. A celiac arteriogram was performed in this patient with severe acute upper gastrointestinal bleeding. Extravasation (*arrow*) from the bleeding ulcer is easily seen. B. Subsequent arteriogram after embolization with antologous blood showed that the bleeding had stopped (*arrow*). (Photograph provided by Stewart R. Reuter, M.D.)

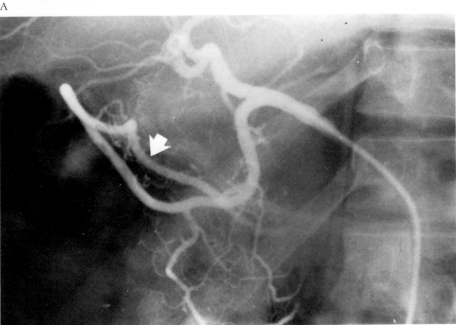

B

lines and sharply angulated kinking of the bowel. A soft-tissue mass similar to mesenteric metastasis is identified on CT scan, with its epicenter located in the mesentery.

Mesenteric Cysts. Etiology of these lesions is unknown. They may be secondary to trauma, surgery, or lymphatic obstruction. They present as a smooth, freely mobile mass. They cause a smooth, extrinsic mass effect on small or large bowel. On CT scan or ultrasound mesenteric cysts are found within the mesentery as well defined cystic masses with or without septations. Rarely, the cysts may rupture causing ascites or may contain hemorrhage or infection. These states obviously alter their normal, benign, fluid appearance. Intestinal duplications cannot be differentiated from these cysts unless there is communication with the bowel lumen on barium examination.

Mesenteric and Omental Tumors. Benign lesions include fibromas, lipomas, and myomas. The malignant category includes lymphoma and metastatic disease from the same primaries noted in carcinomatosis. Except for a lipoma, which is seen as a fatty density, the others are identified as rounded soft-tissue masses on CT scan. Metastatic lesions may form a large conglomeration of soft-tissue density and become attached to the anterior peritoneal surface or omentum (Fig. 1-90). This finding has been described as omental or mesenteric "cakes". On barium studies these masses are seen as extrinsic masses displacing bowel.

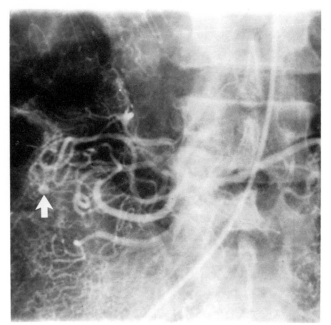

Fig. 1-93. This superior mesenteric arteriogram revealed a collection of extravasated contrast (*arrow*) in a right-sided bleeding colonic diverticulum. (Photograph provided by Stewart R. Reuter, M.D.)

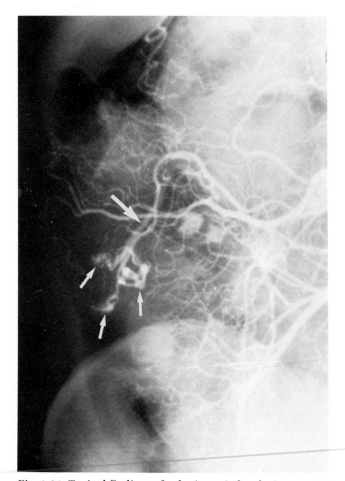

Fig. 1-94. Typical findings of colonic angiodysplasia are seen in this superior mesenteric arteriogram, where there are an irregular tangle of vessels (*small arrows*) and an early draining mesenteric vein (*large arrow*) in the right colon.

Gastrointestinal Bleeding

Because of imaging and technologic advances, radiologists have become more involved in diagnosis as well as treatment of gastrointestinal bleeding. The type of intervention varies with the clinical situation and etiology. The two major types of therapeutic maneuvers that can be done are intraarterial or intravenous infusion of a vasoconstrictor or direct embolization of a bleeding site.

The initial clinical evaluation as to whether bleeding is from an upper or lower gastrointestinal site determines the diagnostic procedures. For an acute upper gastrointestinal hemorrhage endoscopy is recommended. If bleeding is too brisk for diagnosis, then angiography should be considered. For lower gastrointestinal tract bleeding, the initial diagnostic procedure depends on the rate of bleeding. If bleeding is brisk (greater than 0.5 ml/min), then angiography should be performed. If bleeding is slow (0.1–0.5 ml/min) but steady, a radionuclide examination is preferred in order to identify a site for selective angiography. The latter is performed with either ^{99m}Tc sulphur colloid or ^{99m}Tc tagged red blood cells (Fig. 1-91). If the radionuclide study is normal, no bleeding is seen with arteriography.

ACUTE BLEEDING. Upper Gastrointestinal Tract. The common etiologies for acute hemorrhage include gastritis, duodenal ulcer, gastric ulcer, and gastroesophageal varices. Except for gastritis, in which a diffused blush is seen, a focal area of extravasation is seen at arteriography and embolectomy can be performed (Fig. 1-92). In most instances of variceal bleeding, only the varices are identified. In general if the bleeding site is diffuse or if selective catheterization for embolization cannot be performed, intraarterial infusion with a vasoconstrictor such as vasopressin is performed. For variceal bleeding the superior mesenteric artery is infused to decrease the blood flow through the esophageal varices.

Lower Gastrointestinal Tract. This includes all bleeding sites beyond the ligament of Treitz. However, bleeding sites from the small intestine are very uncommon. The common lesions in the colon are diverticulosis (Fig. 1-93), angiodysplasias (Fig. 1-94), ulcerations, carcinoma, and inflammatory bowel disease. These last two diseases rarely cause severe hemorrhage.

CHRONIC BLEEDING. Chronic bleeding is defined as slow or intermittent bleeding that is manifested by anemia, with or without occult blood in the stool. Most lesions that cause acute bleeding can also cause chronic bleeding. Such lesions include polyps, hemorrhoids, anal fissures, Meckel's diverticulum, regional enteritis, and small bowel tumors. Telangiectatic lesions anywhere within the gastrointestinal tract may cause chronic bleeding; these occur spontaneously or are associated with hereditary telangiectasia (Osler-Rendu-Weber disease).

The usual evaluation of gastrointestinal bleeding is with barium, and sometimes also endoscopic, studies of the upper and lower gastrointestinal tracts because these are the most frequent sites for chronic bleeding. If these parts of the anatomy are normal, the use of enteroclysis for evaluation of the small intestine is recommended. Even though the yield is still low, it has the best opportunity for identifying abnormalities. Arteriography is utilized only as a last resort or in a situation where angiodysplasia or arteriovenous malformation is suspected.

Bibliography

The abdominal plain film
Felson, B. (ed.). *The Acute Abdomen.* New York: Grune & Stratton, 1973.
Mindelyun, R. F., and McCort, J. J. Radiology of the Acute Abdomen. In A. R. Margulis and H. J. Burhenne (eds.), *Alimentary Tract Radiology* (3rd ed.). St. Louis: Mosby, 1983.

Diseases of the esophagus
Dodds, W. J. Radiology of the Esophagus. In A. R. Margulis and H. J. Burhenne (eds.), *Alimentary Tract Radiology* (3rd ed.). St. Louis: Mosby, 1983.
Levine, M. S., et al. Adenocarcinoma of the esophagus: Relationship to barrett mucosa. *Radiology* 150:305, 1984.
Ott, D. J., et al. Esophagogastric region and its rings. *A.J.R.* 142:281, 1984.

Diseases of the stomach and duodenum
Feczko, P. J., Halpert, R. D., and Ackerman, L. V. Gastric polyps: Radiological evaluation and clinical significance. *Radiology* 155:581, 1985.
Laufer, I. Stomach. In I. Laufer (ed.), *Double Contrast Gastrointestinal Radiology with Syndoscopic Correlation.* Philadelphia: Saunders, 1979.
Moss, A. A., and Margulis, A. R. Overview. In A. R. Margulis and H. J. Burhenne (eds.), *Alimentary Tract Radiology* (3rd ed.). St. Louis: Mosby, 1983.
Stevenson, G. W. and Laufer, I. Duodenum. In I. Laufer (ed.), *Double Contrast Gastrointestinal Radiology with Endoscopic Correlation.* Philadelphia: Saunders, 1979.

Diseases of the small bowel
Maglinte, D. D. T., et al. Meckel diverticulum: Radiologic demonstration by enteroclysis. *A.J.R.* 134:925, 1980.
Marshak, R. H., and Lindner, A. E. *Radiology of the Small Intestine* (2nd ed.). Philadelphia: Saunders, 1976.
Ott, D. J., et al. Detailed per-oral small bowel examination vs. enteroclysis. *Radiology* 155:29, 1985.
Sellink, J. L. Enteroclysis. In A. R. Margulis and H. J. Burhenne (eds.) *Alimentary Tract Radiology* (3rd ed.). St. Louis: Mosby, 1983.

Diseases of the colon
Dodd, G. D., and Zornoza, J. Colon Malignancies. In A. R. Margulis and H. J. Burhenne (eds.), *Alimentary Tract Radiology* (3rd ed.). St. Louis: Mosby, 1983.
Dodds, W. J., and Stewart, E. T. Colon Polyps. In A. R. Margulis and H. J. Burhenne (eds.), *Alimentary Tract Radiology* (3rd ed.). St. Louis: Mosby, 1983.
Marshak, R. H., Lindner, A. E., and Maklansky, D. *Radiology of the Colon.* Philadelphia: Saunders, 1980.

Idiopathic inflammatory bowel disease
Marshak, R. H., Lindner, A. E., and Maklansky, D. *Radiology of the Colon.* Philadelphia: Saunders, 1980.
Munyer, T. P., et al. Postinflammatory polyposis (PIP) of the colon: The radiologic pathologic spectrum. *Radiology* 145:607, 1982.

Diseases of the liver
Heiken, J. P., et al. Hepatic metastasis studied with MR and CT. *Radiology* 156:423, 1985.
Johnson, C. M. et al. Computed tomography and angiography of cavernous hemangiomas of the liver. *Radiology* 138:115, 1981.
Kunstlinger, F., et al. Computed tomography of hepatocellular carcinoma. *A.J.R.* 134:431, 1980.
Stanley, R. J. Liver and Biliary Tract. In J. K. T. Lee, S. S. Sagel, and R. J. Stanley (eds.), *Computed Body Tomography.* New York: Raven, 1983.
Stark, D. D. et al. Magnetic resonance imaging and spectroscopy of hepatic iron overload. *Radiology* 154:137, 1985.

Diseases of the gallbladder and bile ducts
Berk, R. N. Radiology of the Gallbladder. In A. R. Margulis and H. J. Burhenne (eds.), *Alimentary Tract Radiology* (3rd ed.). St. Louis: Mosby, 1983.
Cooperberg, P. L., and Burhenne H. J. Real-time ultrasonography: Diagnostic technique of choice in calculous gallbladder disease. *N. Engl. J. Med.* 302:1277, 1980.
Mauro, M. A., McCartney, W. H., and Melmed, J. R. Hepatobiliary scanning with ^{99m}Tc PIPIDA in acute cholecystitis. *Radiology* 142:193, 1982.
Ralls, P. W., et al. Real-time sonography in suspected acute cholecystitis. *Radiology* 155:767, 1985.

Diseases of the pancreas
Balthazar, E. J., et al. Acute pancreatitis: Prognostic value of CT. *Radiology* 156:767, 1985.
Mauro, M. A., and Stanley, R. J. Pancreas. In J. K. T. Lee, S. S. Sagel, and R. J. Stanley (eds.), *Computed Body Tomography.* New York: Raven, 1983.
van Sonnenberg, E., et al. Complicated pancreatic inflammatory disease: Diagnostic and therapeutic role of interventional radiology. *Radiology* 155:335, 1985.

Diseases of the peritoneum, mesentery, and omentum
Brun, B., et al. CT in retroperitoneal fibrosis. *A.J.R.* 137:535, 1981.
Levitt, R. G. Abdominal Wall and Peritoneal Cavity. In J. K. T. Lee, S. S. Sagel, and R. J. Stanley (eds.), *Computed Body Tomography.* New York: Raven, 1983.

Gastrointestinal bleeding
Baum, S. Angiography and the gastrointestinal bleeder. *Radiology* 143:569, 1982.
Rahn, N. H., et al. Diagnostic and interventional angiography in acute gastrointestinal hemorrhage. *Radiology* 143:361, 1982.

2. Cardiovascular Disease

Ina L. D. Tonkin

Imaging Tools

THORACIC RADIOGRAPHS. The chest radiograph is a readily available diagnostic tool. Considerable information can be obtained from a posterior-anterior (PA) and lateral chest radiograph with or without a barium esophagogram (Fig. 2-1A, B).

Normal Cardiac Anatomy. The anatomic structures comprising the cardiac silhouette in the PA or frontal view are defined best in the older child and young adult (Fig. 2-2A). In the middle-aged to elderly patient normal cardiac contour changes with time, due to the normal loss of elastic tissue within the aortic wall or vascular ectasia.

The appearance of the chest film evolves normally with age, as does the electrocardiogram (ECG). Owing to its large thymus, the healthy infant typically demonstrates a large cardiothymic silhouette. The ECG may show right ventricular hypertrophy and normally shifts to the left as the infant grows.

The teenager or young adult shows prominence of the main pulmonary artery segment or pulmonary trunk (Figs. 2-1A, 2-2A). The left atrial appendage may be inapparent normally or may be large in rheumatic mitral valve disease or mitral valve insufficiency. The left ventricle normally has a rounded contour (Fig. 2-2B).

In the healthy middle-aged to elderly adult, the normal aging process shows loss of elastic tissue. A prominent ascending aorta is seen as well as a prominent aortic arch and descending aorta.

Four views of the chest with barium may be helpful in defining cardiac anatomy. The frontal view with barium in the esophagus can show enlargement of the left atrium with deviation of the barium-filled esophagus to the right (Fig. 2-3A). The lateral radiograph can show an enlarged left atrium displacing the barium-filled esophagus posteriorly (Fig. 2-3B) and can demonstrate an enlarged left ventricle, as well as right ventricular enlargement in the retrosternal area. In addition, aortic valve calcification may be seen in the upper middle third of the cardiac silhouette on the lateral projection. The right anterior oblique (RAO) projection (a 45° rotation to the left) with barium in the esophagus can show left atrial enlargement (Fig. 2-3C). This view is helpful in demonstrating mitral and aortic calcifications as those valves are moved away from the spine. In addition, the RAO view is most useful in evaluating left ventricular function with a cine left ventriculogram, echocardiography, or radionuclide evaluation.

The left anterior oblique (LAO) projection (60° rotation to the right) does not generally require barium on the plain chest radiograph (Fig. 2-3D). This view demonstrates aortic arch anomalies such as nonobstructive coarctation or pseudocoarctation, and dilatation secondary to aneurysms. The LAO view helps differentiate between left ventricular enlargement and right ventricular enlargement, since the ventricular septum is in profile.

ECHOCARDIOGRAPHY. Echocardiography has emerged as an important method for making cardiovascular diagnoses,

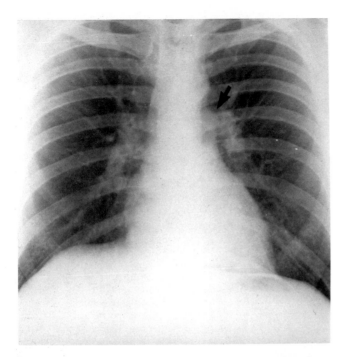

A

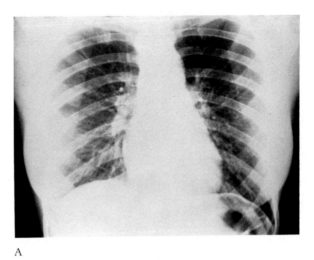

A

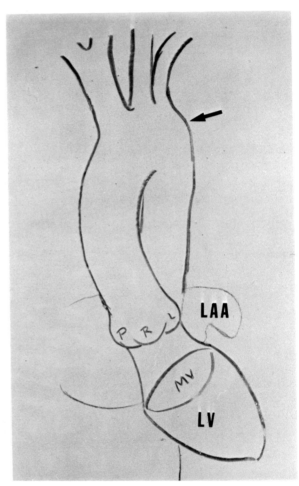

B

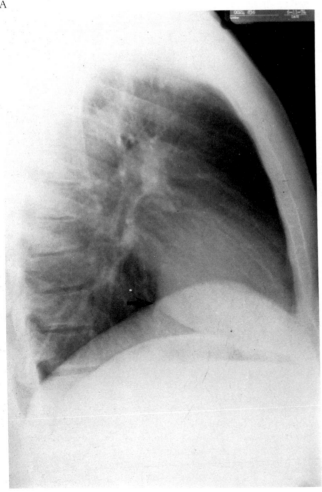

B

Fig. 2-1. A. The PA chest radiograph of this young adult shows normal pulmonary vascularity. Cardiac size and shape is normal with mild prominence of the main pulmonary artery segment (*arrow*). B. Normal lateral projection including normal inferior vena cava shadow (*arrow*).

Fig. 2-2. A. The PA chest radiograph of this 30-year-old woman shows normal vascularity and cardiac contour with a less apparent, but normal, pulmonary artery segment. B. The left heart border forming structures include the aortic arch (*arrow*), the main pulmonary artery, which was visualized on the previous figure, and the left atrial appendage (LAA), which is usually not a border forming structure unless the patient has mitral valve insufficiency or rheumatic heart disease. The left ventricle (LV) has a slightly rounded contour. The mitral valve (MV) is imaged on this overlay. The aortic sinuses are illustrated showing the posterior (P) or noncoronary sinus, the right (R) and the left (L) sinuses of Valsalva.

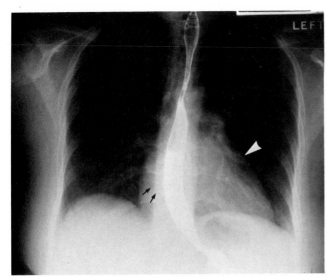

A

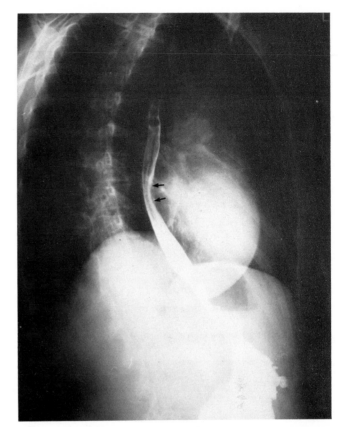

C

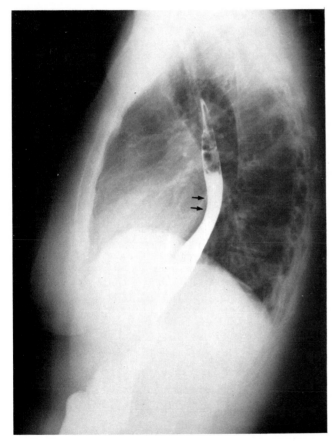

B

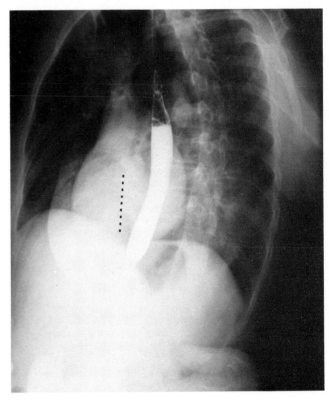

D

Fig. 2-3. A. PA with barium and overpenetration of the radiograph demonstrates left atrial enlargement (*white arrowhead*). The PA chest radiograph of this 30-year-old female with rheumatic mitral valve stenosis also shows left atrial enlargement with deviation of the barium-filled esophagus to the right, a double density along the right heart border (*arrows*), and elevation of the left main stem bronchus. B. The lateral projection shows left atrial enlargement with anterior impression on the barium-filled esophagus caused by the enlarged left atrium (*arrows*). C. The 45° right anterior oblique projection also demonstrates left atrial enlargement with deviation of the barium-filled esophagus posteriorly (*arrows*). D. The 60° left anterior oblique projection does not require barium in the esophagus as it may obscure cardiac anatomy and does not demonstrate left atrial enlargement. This view is helpful in evaluating right heart enlargement as well as left ventricular prominence since the ventricular septum (*dots*) is seen in profile.

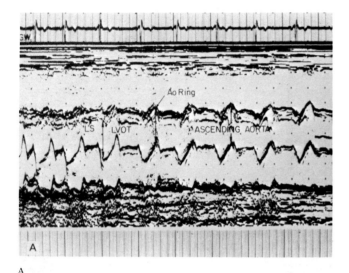

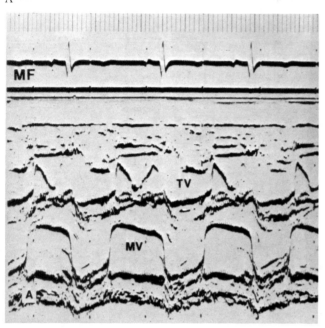

Fig. 2-4. A. This M-mode electrocardiogram demonstrates the anatomy from the ventricular septum with a sweep to the aortic valve and left ventricular outflow tract (LVOT). This represents a normal M-mode tracing showing the aortic valve or ring (Ao ring), and ascending aorta. B. An abnormal M-mode electrocardiogram demonstrating the squared appearance of the mitral valve (MV) compatible with the thickened anterior mitral valve leaflet and mitral valve stenosis. The tricuspid valve (TV) is within normal limits.

evaluating severity of cardiac disease, and following the course of a disease process. Two forms of echocardiography are widely used; these are M-mode and cross-sectional echocardiography.

M-Mode Echocardiography. In M-mode echocardiography, a sound wave is directed into the heart by a transducer, showing cardiac structures beneath the waveform; a relatively linear recording is made over time. A single area of interest can be observed over several cardiac cycles. The direction of the echo beam can be changed or swept from one area to another in order to view additional cardiovas-

cular structures (Fig. 2-4A). The relationship between structures and the continuity between cardiovascular structures can be observed. M-mode echocardiography is excellent for visualization of the mitral valve (Fig. 2-4B), the aortic root and valve, the pulmonary valve, the left ventricle, the intraventricular septum, and the left and right atrium. Cardiac tumors can also be observed with the use of M-mode echocardiography.

Two-Dimensional Echocardiography. In the cross-sectional form of echocardiography, the sonographic beam is quickly rotated through an arc of about 70° and a wedge-shaped section of the heart and adjacent structures is recorded. These recordings therefore represent a cross-section of the heart and great vessels. The cross-sectional area of the heart that is imaged depends on the direction of the sonographic beam. There are several conventional echocardiographic projections, which include the four planes that are commonly used for two-dimensional echocardiographic recording of the heart: (1) the *parasternal long axis view*, (2) the *parasternal short axis view* (perpendicular to the long axis), (3) the *oblique coronal view*, showing right-to-left relationships (often referred to as the *apical four chamber view*), and (4) the *suprasternal notch view*, for visualization of the great vessel anatomy. The first two planes are described with reference to the axis of the left ventricular outflow tract. The parasternal long axis view shows the left ventricular outflow tracts, the aortic sinuses, and movement of both the mitral and aortic valves. The apical long axis view shows the left ventricular apex, the papillary muscle structure, and the proximal portion of the left ventricular outflow tract as well as the aortic valve leaflets.

The parasternal short axis view demonstrates the plane at the level of the great arteries, showing the relationship of the pulmonary valve and aorta. In addition, views of the three sinuses of Valsalva of both the aortic and pulmonary valves can be obtained with this technique.

The four-chamber view demonstrates the atrial ventricular anatomy as well as the atrial and ventricular valves.

The suprasternal notch view is used for evaluation of the great vessels in patients with coarctation of the aorta (Fig. 2-5A) or patent ductus arteriosis (Fig. 2-5B), as well as in patients with thoracic aortic aneurysms.

COMPUTED TOMOGRAPHY. Computed tomography (CT) is a relatively new method for cardiac imaging. It can provide images with adequate spatial resolution for displaying anatomic structures in three dimensions and can provide unique physiologic data. The current limitations of CT imaging of the heart are primarily technical; the major problem is the relatively long exposure time of the whole body scanners compared with the cardiac cycle. The problem of cardiac motion, and to a lesser extent respiratory motion, is therefore significant, even more so in infants and children. However faster CT exposure times and even cine CT have made cardiovascular CT imaging feasible.

Contrast material in a bolus injection is required with CT methods. The cross-sectional imaging of the heart avoids the superimposition of cardiac structures (Fig. 2-6A, B). In addition, CT scanners have a high-density resolution and can evaluate contrast material density in smaller quantities (Fig. 2-7).

Gated CT scanning is necessary to evaluate the heart. To obtain an ECG-gated image, the ECG is recorded simultaneously with the CT scan and a fraction of the electrocardiographic R to R interval width of the ECG is monitored along with the CT images. Computed tomography has the advantage of being able to identify structural anomalies

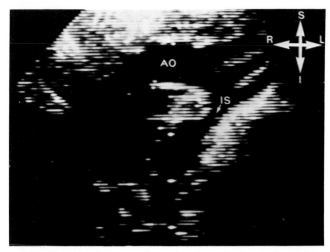

A

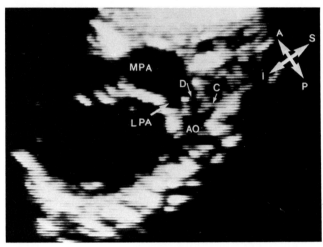

B

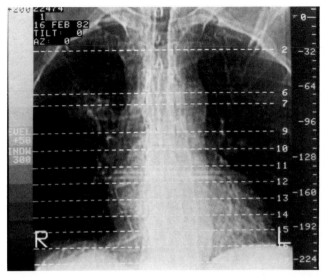

A

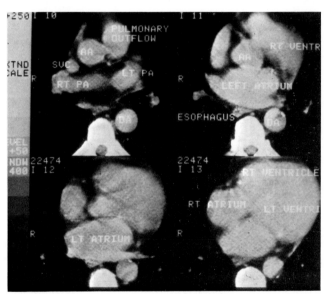

B

Fig. 2-5. A. Suprasternal notch, two-dimensional echocardiogram in a patient with a preductal coarctation shows narrowing of the aortic isthmus (IS, *arrow*). The ascending aorta (AO) is of normal size. B. An additional suprasternal notch view demonstrates a left patent ductus arteriosus (D) with imaging of the main pulmonary artery (MPA), left pulmonary artery (LPA), aorta (AO) and proximal coarctation (C). (Photographs provided by Jeffery F. Smallhorn, M.D., The Hospital for Sick Children, Toronto.)

Fig. 2-6. A. Computed tomography of the heart. The scout view, or topogram, of this 50-year-old patient shows the CT numbers of the horizontal cuts obtained in imaging the heart. B. A CT scan performed without contrast material shows the cardiac anatomy. The upper left image at level 10 demonstrates the superior vena cava (SVC), right pulmonary artery (RT-PA), and left pulmonary artery (LT-PA). In addition, the ascending aorta (AA) and descending aorta (DA) can be seen. The pulmonary outflow tract is also imaged. At upper right a slightly lower cut at level 11 demonstrates the left atrium with the right ventricular outflow tract and visualization of the esophagus. The lower left image at level 12 demonstrates the body of the left atrium (LT atrium). The lower right cut at level 13 shows the ventricular septum with imaging of the right ventricle (RT ventricle) and left ventricle (LT ventricle) as well as the right atrium (RT atrium). (Images provided by Allen K. Tonkin, M.D., Baptist Memorial Hospital, Memphis, TN.)

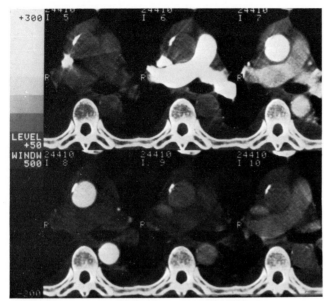

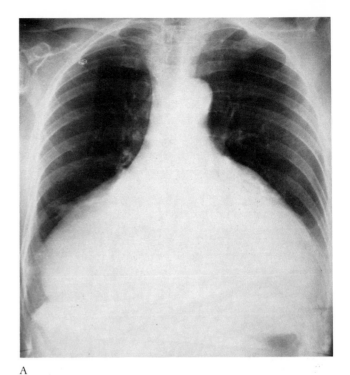

Fig. 2-7. A normal CT scan with dynamic contrast enhancement initially shows the superior vena cava on the top left image. The second image opacifies the right ventricular outflow tract and right and left pulmonary arteries with contrast material. In time, opacification of the ascending aorta with a small area of calcification as well as the descending thoracic aorta can be seen on the bottom left. The aorta is more densely opacified in the lower images and contrast material washes out normally.

A

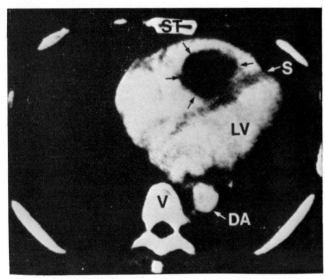

Fig. 2-8. CT scan with contrast material enhancement shows a low-density area in the right ventricle compatible with a cardiac tumor (*arrows*). In addition, the landmarks of the sternum (ST) and the vertebral column (V) and the ventricular septum (S) are seen as a relative lucency. There is contrast material in the left ventricle (LV) and in the descending thoracic aorta (DA). This image was obtained in a 59-year-old male with a metastatic soft tissue sarcoma (low density with arrows) to the right ventricle.

B

Fig. 2-9. A. The PA chest radiograph of this 55-year-old female shows marked enlargement of the pericardial-cardiac configuration with normal pulmonary vascularity. B. The CT scan with contrast material enhancement shows a massive pericardial effusion (E). This patient had a long standing chronic pericardial effusion with rheumatic mitral valve insufficiency.

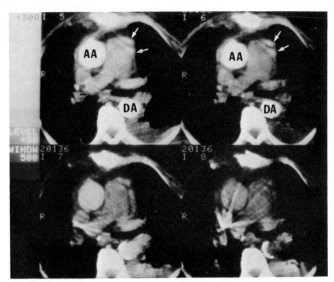

Fig. 2-10. Coronary artery bypass grafts in ischemic cardiovascular disease imaged with CT scanning and contrast enhancement. The contrast material opacifies the ascending aorta (AA) and descending aorta (DA). With dynamic scanning, one can see opacification of the left anterior descending sequential grafts (*arrows*) to the left ventricle. These grafts are open proximally with this noninvasive imaging technique. (Photographs provided by Allen K. Tonkin, M.D., Memphis, TN.)

while visualizing the endocardial wall and also the epicardial surface. The clinical applications of CT scanning include congenital anomalies involving the great vessels and venous structures, intracardiac shunts, cardiac tumors (Fig. 2-8), pericardial anomalies (Fig. 2-9A, B), and ischemic cardiovascular disease (Fig. 2-10).

MAGNETIC RESONANCE IMAGING. Moving blood, by virtue of its motion, produces little or no magnetic resonance imaging (MRI) signal. Thus ventricular cavities and great vessels appear dark on MRI (Fig. 2-11). Static blood or hemorrhage produces a bright density on MRI and may be indistinguishable from the ventricular wall. Gated magnetic resonance images have shown a clinical variation in the signal intensity of blood in the aorta and probably reflect changes in blood flow through the vessel. It may be possible to exploit the motion effect and use it to measure flow.

Indications for CT scanning of the heart are similar for MRI. Electrocardiogram-synchronized gating is extremely important for diagnostic images in the evaluation of congenital heart disease. This technique probably complements echocardiography, although it may allow physicians to see the myocardium and cardiac valves even better than does echocardiography. These techniques together should decrease the number of cardiac catheterizations done for diagnostic purposes.

RADIONUCLIDE EVALUATION. Radionuclide techniques for evaluating right and left heart hemodynamics have been used extensively in adults and have recently been applied to the pediatric population as well. Radionuclide angiography involves the injection of a radionuclide material which then flows through the heart. This is a simple and reasonable procedure that can be performed on outpatients. Left to right shunts, such as patent ductus arterio-

sus, ventricular septal defect, and atrial septal defects can be detected and quantitative ventricular function analysis in pre- and postoperative patients can be performed with this imaging technique.

The widest use of radionuclides has been for studies of ischemic cardiovascular disease and left ventricular function. Technetium-99m pyrophosphate is taken up by damaged muscle, and thus can be effective for detecting myocardial infarction (Fig. 2-12A). Electrocardiogram and enzyme studies are simpler and cheaper for studying infarcts, and so pyrophosphate scanning is normally reserved for patients in whom basic studies are equivocal.

Thallium-201 is a radionuclide that is a potassium analogue. Its myocardial uptake is a function of regional myocardial perfusion and metabolic activity. Intravenous injection during stress (activity) results in a "cold" area where myocardial perfusion is diminished. Reevaluation several hours after stress shows normal, uniform uptake (Fig. 2-12B).

Autologous red cells labelled with ^{99m}Tc can be used to evaluate ventricular wall function and determine the ventricular ejection fraction. Following tagging of the red cells, multiple ECG-gated images are acquired. From this acquisition, diastolic and systolic images can be generated and compared to evaluate wall motion and contractility (Fig. 2-12C).

Congestive Heart Failure

EVALUATION OF PULMONARY VASCULARITY. In a normal thoracic radiograph, the pulmonary vascular markings taper gradually toward the periphery of the lung fields (see Fig. 2-1A, B). The pulmonary vascular markings are composed of both pulmonary arteries and pulmonary veins and are more prominent in the lower lung fields. The vessels in the right hilum appear to be larger than those in the left, because the left hilum is partly covered by the cardiac silhouette. With pulmonary venous congestion, the chest radiograph shows a pattern of increased pulmonary venous vascularity, pulmonary venous hypertension, or obstruction that may occur with any condition that causes increased resistance distal to the pulmonary capillaries (Fig. 2-13). Mitral stenosis and acute left ventricular failure are two common causes of pulmonary venous hypertension.

In the early stages of pulmonary venous hypertension, there is a constriction of the lower lobe pulmonary veins. When pulmonary venous pressure or pulmonary arterial capillary pressure exceeds 12 mm Hg, there is redistribution of pulmonary vascularity. The type and severity of the vascular changes of pulmonary venous hypertension reflected in the chest film depend directly on the degree and duration of obstruction to pulmonary venous flow beyond the capillaries and not on the specific type of lesion. In the chest film, the physiologic and anatomic responses of the pulmonary vascularity are manifested by (1) redistribution of blood flow to the upper lobes and a corresponding decrease of blood flow to the lower lobes, and (2) edema forming around the bronchi and pulmonary vessels and in the intralobular septa and fissures, the pleural space, and finally within the alveoli (Fig. 2-13). When pulmonary venous pressure exceeds 25 mm Hg, fluid accumulates in the interstitial spaces, and Kerley B lines appear at approximately 22–25 mm Hg. At this point, the hilar vessels be-

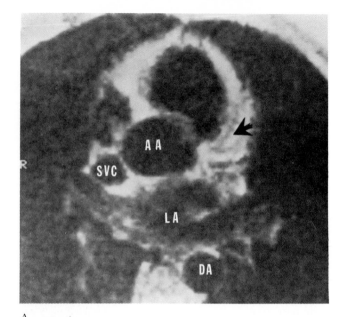

A

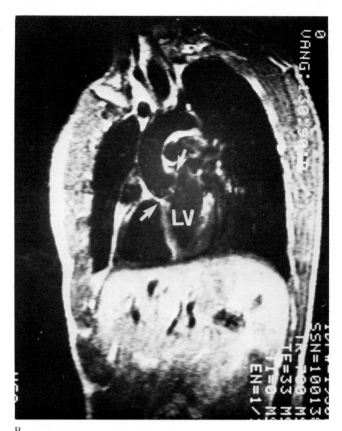

B

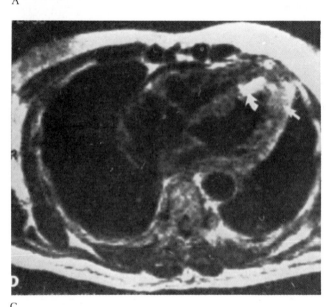

C

Fig. 2-11. A. Magnetic resonance imaging (MRI) with this cross-sectional view of the heart shows the left atrium (LA), superior vena cava (SVC), ascending aorta (AA), proximal left anterior descending coronary artery (*arrow*), and descending aorta (DA). The ventricular septum is well defined. B. The sagittal LAO image with ECG gating shows the left ventricle (LV) and left aortic arch anatomy well. Note the aortic valve (*arrows*). (Images provided by Robert Laster, M.D., and Leon Bell, M.D., Methodist Hospital, Memphis, TN.) C. Myocardial infarction can be detected with MRI without injection of contrast material or radiation. Note the high signal intensity of the anterior lateral wall of the left ventricle (*arrows*), which represents infarcted myocardium. Source: McNamara, M. T., Higgins, C. B., Schechtmann, N., et al. Detection and characterization of acute myocardial infarction in man with use of gated magnetic resonance. *Circulation* 71:717, 1985.

Large Anterior
Wall Infarction
TC PYP

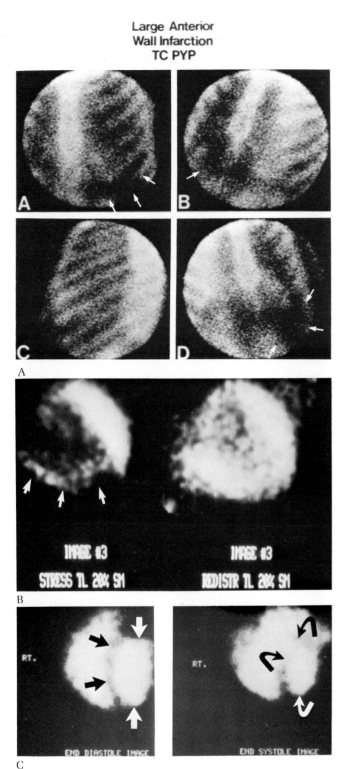

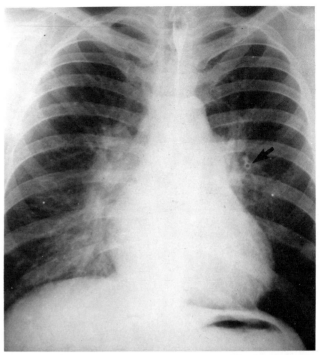

Fig. 2-13. The PA chest radiograph of this 51-year-old male in renal failure with barium in the esophagus shows interstitial edema of the right perihilar area and edema with cuffing of a left perihilar bronchus (*arrow*).

Fig. 2-12. A. Nuclear medicine scintigraphy with technetium pyrophosphate (TC-PYP) shows a massive myocardial infarction with increased uptake in the anterior lateral wall (*arrows*). Note images can be obtained in the anterior (A), lateral (B), LAO (C), and RAO (D) projections to define the portion of the myocardium involved and the probable distribution of the coronary artery anatomy. B. Thallium study in the anterior projection demonstrating diminished radioactivity (*arrows*) during the stress phase (left image) and normal radioactivity three hours later during redistribution phase (right image). Findings represent ischemia in the inferior wall of the left ventricle. C. Wall motion study showing difference between normal end-diastole (left) and normal end-systole (right).

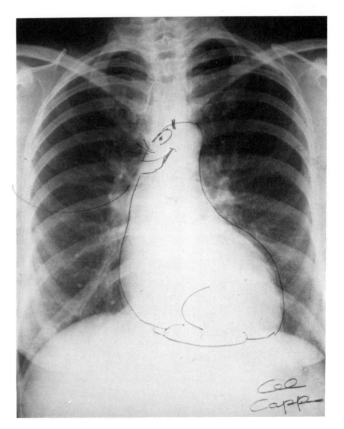

Fig. 2-14. "Shmoo-like" configuration is characteristic of left ventricular stress.
Source: Elliott, L. P., and Schiebler, G. L. *The X-Ray Diagnosis of Congenital Heart Disease in Infants, Children, and Adults: Pathologic, Hemodynamic, and Clinical Correlations As Related to Chest Film* (2nd ed.). Springfield, IL: Charles C. Thomas, 1979.

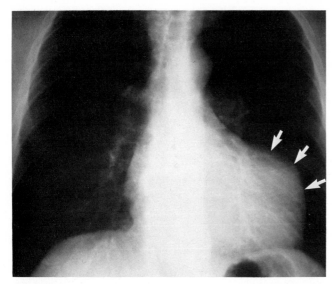

Fig. 2-15. The PA chest radiograph of a 65-year-old male shows an enlarged left ventricular configuration (*arrows*). This left ventricular bulge is secondary to an aneurysm of the left ventricle or area of akinesia with long-standing atherosclerotic cardiovascular disease and myocardial dysfunction.

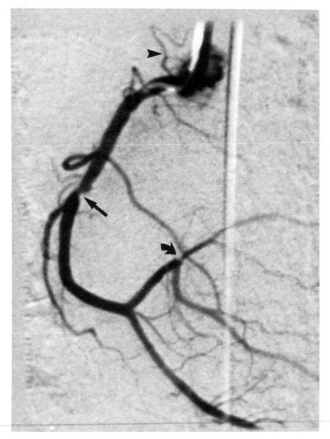

Fig. 2-16. Selective injection into the right coronary artery in the LAO projection with intraarterial digital subtraction angiographic technique. The first branch is the conus branch (*arrowhead*). In addition, there is 50 percent stenosis of the mid-right coronary artery (*arrow*). There is also 20 percent stenosis of the distal right coronary branch (*small arrow*).

come prominent and indistinct, and a cuff of edema may appear around the bronchi in the hilar region. As the venous pressure increases to more than 30–35 mm Hg, alveolar edema and pleural effusions occur.

LEFT VENTRICULAR CONTOUR. The most common configuration to the heart is a left ventricular contour that may be associated with left heart failure (Fig. 2-14). The most common causes of left-sided failure are (1) myocardial infarction, often with resulting aneurysm (Fig. 2-15), (2) hypertensive cardiovascular disease, and (3) aortic valve disease.

Ischemic Cardiovascular Disease. Atherosclerotic cardiovascular disease is extremely common and is the number one cause of death in the United States. The two major manifestations of atherosclerotic disease are ectasia and narrowing from plaques, either with or without complete obstruction in the coronary arteries (Fig. 2-16). The main objective of coronary arteriography is to demonstrate the vascular anatomy of both the proximal and distal areas of obstruction and the presence of collateral circulation.

Currently, coronary arteriography is used in the management of acute myocardial infarction to demonstrate the site of obstruction and to guide the infusion of thrombolytic therapy. Digital subtraction angiography may be used for the same purposes.

Left Ventricular Aneurysm. Left ventricular aneurysms are generally a complication of myocardial infarction and are acquired. Aneurysms of the left ventricle produce localized abnormalities of left ventricular wall motion. Hypokinesia, akinesia, or dyskinesia (paradoxical systolic motion of the aneurysm) can result from aneurysm formation.

There may be no abnormal radiographic findings or there may be a localized bulge of the left ventricle, abnormal pulsation, or intramyocardial calcification (see Fig. 2-15).

Left ventricular aneurysms can be demonstrated by radionuclide flow studies and more precisely by cine left ventriculography. In addition, digital subtraction angiography can be used in the evaluation of left ventricular function and can demonstrate aneurysm formation. Computed tomography and MRI can provide useful information regarding the location and extent of infarction (see Fig. 2-11C).

Hypertensive Cardiovascular Disease. Systemic hypertension is common and is a leading cause of death in the United States. Death results from the effects of hypertension on the cerebral, renal, and coronary arteries and from left ventricular failure due to the increased workload on the left ventricle. There are no radiographic features of mild hypertension. With moderate or long-standing hypertension, cardiac size is initially normal, with a left ventricular configuration. Later, cardiac enlargement develops and eventually pulmonary venous congestion or pulmonary venous hypertension.

Aortic Insufficiency. Aortic insufficiency is usually acquired and is generally the result of rheumatic heart disease. The aortic valve leaflets become inflamed and are scarred, with resultant aortic valve insufficiency. Aortic valve insufficiency can also be secondary to syphilitic aortitis and other forms of bacterial endocarditis. Rarely, aortic insufficiency results from direct trauma to the chest from an aortic aneurysm, Marfan's syndrome or other collagen disease, and particularly from ankylosing spondylitis.

Most patients are asymptomatic, but with progressive aortic valve insufficiency congestive heart failure occurs. The radiographic features vary with the amount of regurgitation. In mild aortic regurgitation, cardiac size is normal, as is the cardiac contour. In moderate and severe aortic regurgitation, cardiac enlargement is present with a left ventricular contour (Fig. 2-17A, B). With aortic valve insufficiency there is an enlarged left ventricular contour with downward pointing of the apex. On the LAO projection, the left ventricle projects behind the spine (Fig. 2-18A). Aortography in the left anterior oblique projection demonstrates the degree of aortic valve insufficiency (Fig. 2-18B).

Both aortography and left ventriculography should be performed to assess the degree of aortic regurgitation (from 1–5 or higher) and the status of left ventricular function and myocontractility. Hypokinesis is commonly observed in long-standing aortic valve insufficiency. In most instances, symptomatic aortic valve insufficiency must be treated by aortic valve replacement, which should be performed before significant and irreversible congestive heart failure occurs.

MITRAL CONTOUR. Rheumatic Heart Disease. Rheumatic fever is the primary cause of symptoms of mitral valve disease. During acute rheumatic fever, the inflammatory process may involve the heart. The patient may present with myocarditis, and children frequently present with a systolic murmur from rheumatic mitral valve insufficiency. Over a period of years, chronic thickening and fibrosis of the mitral valve leaflets with fusion and shortening of the chordae tendineae may occur. Mitral valve damage due to rheumatic fever is much more prevalent in females than in males.

Radiographic findings on the PA and lateral radiograph show pulmonary venous hypertension and a four-bump left heart border (Fig. 2-19). The four-bump includes the aortic knob, the main pulmonary artery (due to pulmonary arterial hypertension and/or venous hypertension), the left atrial appendage (which is the hallmark of rheumatic mitral valve disease), and a left ventricular bulge. The left atrium enlarges, as well as the left atrial appendage, due to the inflammatory process. With rheumatic mitral valve stenosis, physicians may see calcification of the mitral valve and severe pulmonary venous hypertension. With rheumatic mitral valve insufficiency, the most common features are cardiac enlargement, which is marked due to the volume overload of the left heart, and radiographic findings of mild pulmonary venous hypertension. The presence of Kerley B lines indicates significant mitral valve stenosis with pulmonary venous hypertension and possibly right heart hypertrophy as well (Fig. 2-20A, B). Following treatment of congestive heart failure, the Kerley B lines may disappear, leaving only mild to moderate residual pulmonary venous hypertension (Fig. 2-20C).

The echocardiographic features of rheumatic heart disease with M-mode echocardiogram may include a low E to F slope during diastole and a squared appearance of the mitral valve tracing (see Fig. 2-4B). The angiogram shows a thickened mitral valve that is best demonstrated in the RAO projection, with a left ventricular injection.

Prolapse of the Mitral Valve. Prolapse of the mitral valve (Barlow's syndrome) is a congenital myxomatous abnormality of the mitral valve. Mitral valve prolapse (MVP), defined as echocardiographic, angiographic, and pathologic protrusion of the mitral leaflets into the left atrium

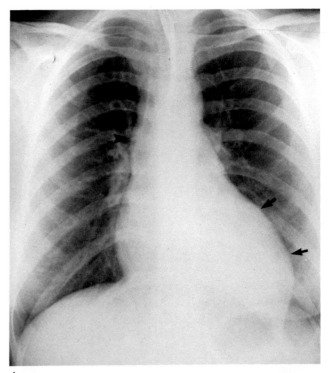

A

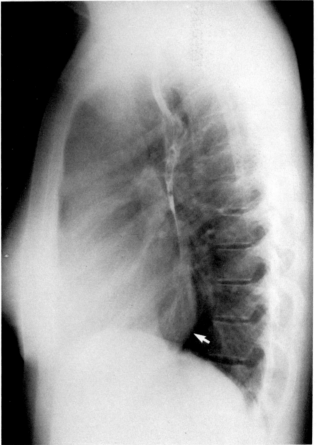

B

Fig. 2-17. A. The PA chest radiograph of this 50-year-old female shows normal vascularity with an enlarged heart. There is an enlarged left ventricular configuration (*arrows*) and prominence of the ascending thoracic aorta (*arrowhead*). B. On the lateral projection, left ventricular prominence with a normal right heart (*arrow*) is seen.

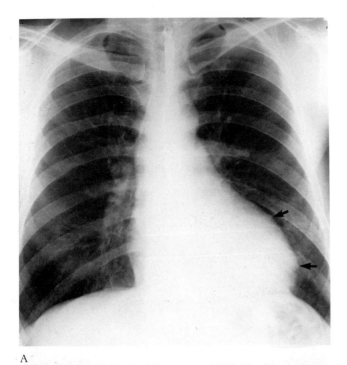

A

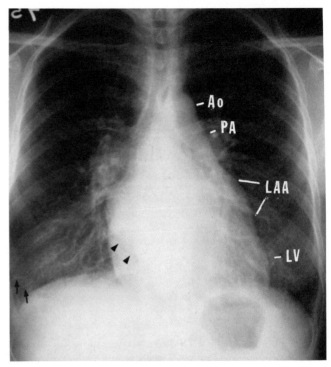

Fig. 2-19. The PA chest radiograph of a 28-year-old female with rheumatic mitral valve disease. The pulmonary vascularity is increased showing redistribution of flow and indistinctness. In addition, there are small bilateral pleural effusions. Kerley B lines are noted along the right costophrenic margin (*arrows*). The cardiac anatomy shows the four bump heart border compatible with rheumatic mitral valve disease. The first bump is the aorta (Ao) followed by the pulmonary artery segment (PA) and the left atrial appendage (LAA). The last border forming structure is the left ventricle (LV). In addition, one can see enlargement of the body of the left atrium with a double density (*arrowheads*) and some elevation of the left main stem bronchus.

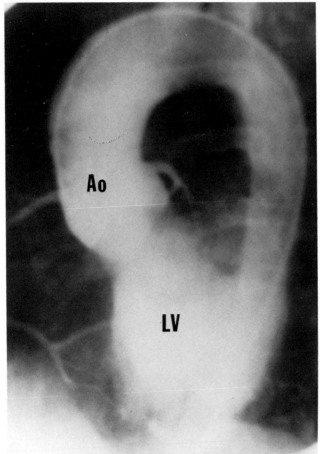

B

Fig. 2-18. A. The PA chest radiograph of a 21-year-old male shows normal vascularity and no evidence of congestive heart failure. This patient has an enlarged heart with a left ventricular configuration (*arrows*). B. At catheterization, this patient had an abnormal aortic valve with severe aortic valve insufficiency. The injection was made in the ascending aorta (AO) with regurgitation into the left ventricle (LV). The left ventricle is more densely opacified than the aorta.

during systole, may affect 5 percent of the population. With this congenital abnormality, the patient may present with an audible click and an abnormal ECG. The patient is also at risk for cardiac arrhythmias and sudden death.

The radiographic findings may show a normal chest radiograph or occasionally narrow anterior-posterior diameters, the so-called "straight back" configuration. Occasionally, physicians may see pulmonary venous hypertension and left atrial enlargement as well as enlargement of the body of the left atrial appendage, with severe mitral valve insufficiency and prolapse.

The diagnosis can be made with echocardiography. The abnormal valve can be seen with either M-mode or 2-D echocardiography; cardiac catheterization is needed only for pressure measurement or evaluation of other lesions. There is an approximately 15 to 20 percent incidence of prolapse of the mitral valve associated with atrial septal defect.

CARDIOMYOPATHY. Cardiomyopathies have multiple origins, including (1) infection, particularly viral (i.e., with Coxsackie B virus), causing myocarditis, (2) metabolic diseases involving storage of abnormal materials such as glycogen, (3) skeletal muscle diseases—many patients with cardiomyopathy may have histologic abnormalities that are also present in skeletal muscles, (4) cardiotoxic (i.e.,

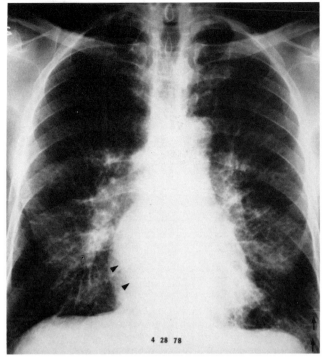

A

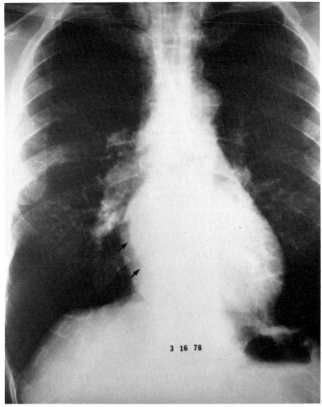

C

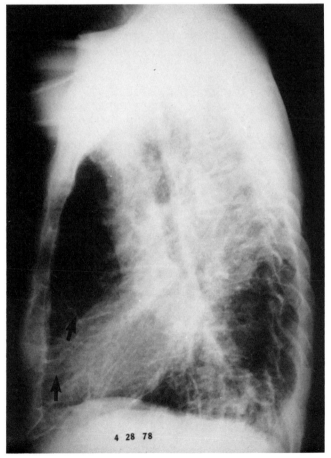

B

Fig. 2-20. A. The PA chest radiograph of this 63-year-old female shows severe pulmonary venous hypertension with Kerley B lines (*arrows*) as well as Kerley A lines or thickened interlobular septa. The double density of left atrial enlargement is evident (*small arrowheads*). B. The lateral projection again shows Kerley B lines and Kerley A lines (*arrows*). C. Following treatment of acute congestive heart failure, there is marked improvement in fluid within the fissures and in the interstitium. The pulmonary vascularity remains abnormal with mild redistribution of flow but shows improvement in edema. Note continued left atrial enlargement (*arrows*).

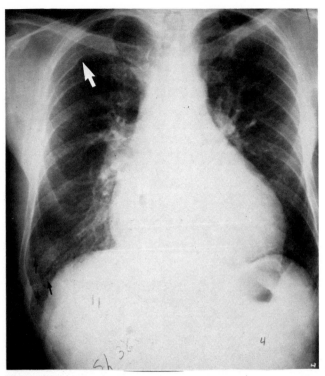

Fig. 2-21. The PA chest radiograph of a 50-year-old male with alcoholic cardiomyopathy. In evaluating the bones, note that there is a fracture of the right fourth rib (*arrow*). This is secondary to previous trauma. In addition, Kerley B lines are noted in the costophrenic angle (*arrows*). There is generalized cardiac enlargement.

used for treatment of malignancies) agents, and (5) family histories of syndromes associated with cardiomyopathies.

The radiographic features of cardiomyopathies show an abnormal congestive pulmonary vascular pattern with redistribution of pulmonary vascularity (Fig. 2-21). In addition, the heart may have a globular appearance and pericardial effusion should be excluded with echocardiography. All chambers may be involved or only the left ventricular and left atrium, due to left pump failure and mitral valve insufficiency. With alcoholic cardiomyopathy, physicians may see evidence of trauma, such as rib fractures (Fig. 2-21). Echocardiography and chest radiography are frequently diagnostic, but catheterization may be indicated to evaluate associated anomalies. Management is frequently with medical therapy; however, occasionally patients may require prosthetic valve replacement.

Prosthetic Cardiac Valves

Prosthetic cardiac valves can be identified easily from the chest radiograph as to both their location and type (Fig. 2-22A). Their function can be evaluated with fluoroscopic visualization and recording with video tape, cine filming, or digital subtraction angiography.

One of the most commonly used valves is the Bjork-Shiley prosthetic valve, which is a low profile valve. The disk can be measured in both systole and diastole to evaluate valve malfunction. A rocking motion of the valve base may indicate a perivalvular leak and decreased excursion of the disk may imply thrombosis.

The St. Jude's valve prosthesis is barely radiopaque. The two valve disks must be on end to be seen on a chest radiograph. Digital subtraction angiography or echocardiography may be helpful in evaluating abnormal valve motions (Fig. 22B, C). Once the type of valve is identified, its function is evaluated under fluoroscopic observation. The movement of the disk is extremely important, as the development of thrombosis is the most common cause of valve malfunction.

Uncommon in today's practice but still seen in some patients is the Starr-Edwards valve. This was one of the early successful cardiac prostheses, and is a classic ball valve (Fig. 2-22D). Porcine valves are also in use but are not radiopaque.

Cardiac Calcifications and Diseases of the Pericardium

Cardiac calcifications frequently imply degenerative disease. Calcifications may be visualized on the PA and lateral chest radiograph, with fluoroscopy, video tape, cine filming at cardiac catheterization, echocardiography, computed tomography, and occasionally with MRI.

Coronary artery calcification can be seen normally in the elderly patient. If calcification of the coronary arteries is visualized before age 50, the patient may have an early degenerative disease, such as hyperlipidemia, or an atherosclerotic syndrome (Fig. 2-23A, B). In addition, valvular heart disease implies a degenerative process. If the physician detects valvular calcification in the aortic position before age 40, the patient may have congenitally bicuspid aortic valve disease, which occurs in 2 percent of the population. If the physician observes mitral valve calcification, this may imply rheumatic mitral valve disease, which is the most frequent cause of rheumatic heart disease.

Mitral annular calcification frequently occurs in the elderly female patient (Fig. 2-23B). This is a C-shaped or comma-shaped annular calcification that does not necessarily imply abnormal mitral valve leaflets. However, these patients are at risk for cardiac arrhythmias.

Calcification may be visualized in the endocardium with aneurysm formation after myocardial infarction. In addition, calcification of the pericardium may imply an inflammatory disease, such as tuberculosis pericarditis.

The normal pericardium cannot be seen as a separate entity on the PA and lateral chest radiograph. Diseases of the pericardium can be imaged with the PA and lateral chest radiograph, echocardiography, computed tomography, and magnetic resonance imaging.

Acute pericarditis has a number of causes, which are (1) infection—viral, pyogenic, or tuberculous, (2) collagen vascular disease—rheumatoid arthritis and rheumatic fever, (3) atherosclerotic disease—myocardial infarction, (4) trauma, (5) metabolic causes (e.g., uremia), (6) neoplastic involvement of the pericardium, (7) postcardiovascular surgery, and (8) idiopathic.

The radiographic features of pericardial effusion include loss of the main pulmonary artery segment border and a globular configuration to the heart. The lateral projection may show a radiolucent line (epicardial fat) separating the cardiac silhouette into two parts, with the pericardial effusion anterior and the water density of the cardiac shadow posterior. Calcification of the pericardium is frequently seen in postinflammatory or posttraumatic conditions (Fig. 2-24A, B). Calcification may also occur with

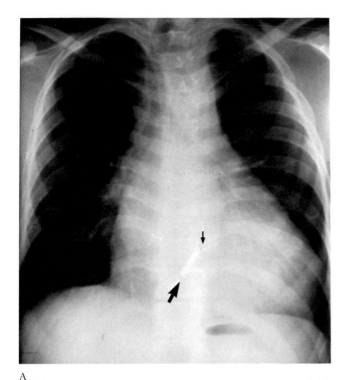

A

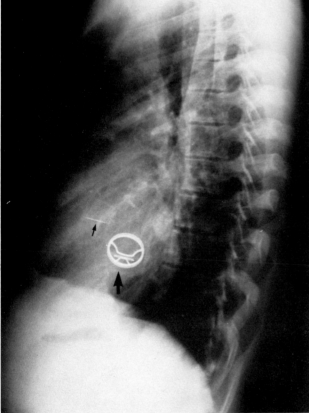

B

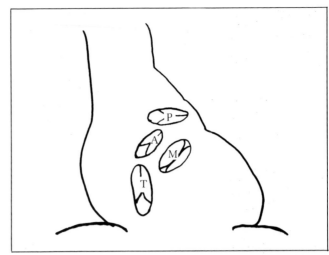

C

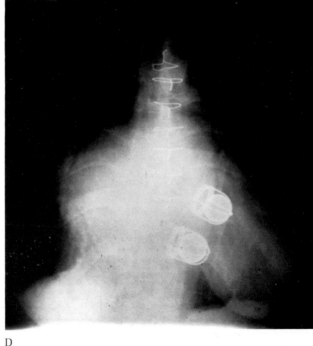

D

Fig. 2-22. A. Prosthetic cardiac valves. The PA chest radiograph of a 16-year-old male with replacement of the aortic valve with the St. Jude's prosthesis (*small arrow*). The valve is barely radiopaque and must be seen in profile to be visible. In addition, the Bjork-Shiley valve prosthesis is in the mitral position (*large arrow*). B. The lateral projection of the same patient shows the Bjork-Shiley valve in the mitral position (*arrow*) with visualization of the disk and two U-shaped retainers. Again, the St. Jude's prosthetic valve is visualized (*small arrow*) in the upper middle third of the cardiac silhouette. C. Frontal view of the heart shows the relative positions of the four cardiac valves. These are the pulmonary (P) valve, aortic (A) valve, mitral (M) valve and tricuspid (T) valve. The aortic and mitral valves are in fibrous continuity in the normal heart. D. Overpenetrated film demonstrating Starr-Edwards prosthetic valves in both the mitral and tricuspid positions.

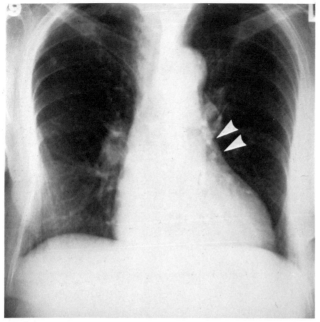

A

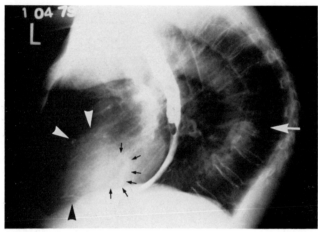

B

Fig. 2-23. A. The PA chest radiograph of an 82-year-old female shows normal vascularity with a slight left ventricular contour. There is calcification in the left upper heart border secondary to coronary artery disease (*arrowheads*). B. The lateral projection shows extensive kyphotic changes and osteopenia of the spine (*arrow*). In addition, one can see extensive calcification of the coronary arteries (*arrowheads*) and the C-shaped calcification of coronary annular calcium (*small arrows*).

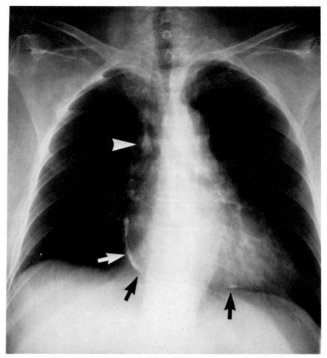

A

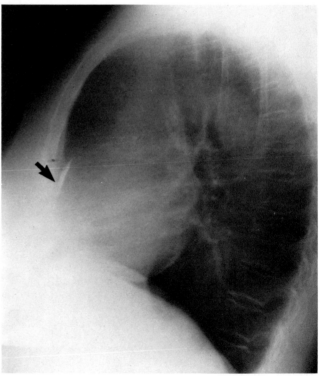

B

Fig. 2-24. A. The PA chest radiograph shows curvilinear calcification around the pericardium compatible with previous tuberculous pericarditis (*arrows*). In addition, this patient has a calcified right perihilar node (*arrowhead*). B. The lateral projection of this same patient again shows curvilinear calcification secondary to inflammatory pericarditis (*arrow*).

chronic constrictive pericarditis. Tuberculosis was formerly the most common cause of constrictive pericarditis. Currently, constrictive pericarditis may occur as a late complication of acute pericarditis, which may be infectious, neoplastic, or even associated with hemorrhage secondary to cardiac surgery or trauma. Echocardiography is diagnostic of pericardial effusion and calcifications (Fig. 2-25).

Computed tomography and MRI are excellent cross-sectional methods that can be used to evaluate the pericardium with or without contrast enhancement (see Figs. 2-9A, B, and Fig. 2-26). Contrast enhancement may be necessary to image the pericardium with computed tomography and in the case of significant pericardial effusions.

Pulmonary Hypertensive Heart Disease and Pulmonary Embolism

In pulmonary heart disease, hypertrophy and dilatation of the right ventricle result from pulmonary abnormalities. Causes of pulmonary hypertensive heart disease, or cor pulmonale, include primary hypertension, pulmonary embolism (which may be chronic), chronic infection, chronic obstructive pulmonary disease, cystic fibrosis, or musculoskeletal disease.

The radiographic findings frequently include right heart enlargement with prominence of the main pulmonary arteries and decreased peripheral pulmonary vascularity (Fig. 2-27A). The diagnosis can be made by echocardiography or angiocardiography (Fig. 2-27B).

Primary pulmonary hypertension is a rare condition seen in females 15 to 40 years of age. The pulmonary artery pressure may equal systemic pressures and injections of contrast material into the main pulmonary artery may be dangerous. Therefore, radionuclide imaging may be helpful, as well as echocardiography. Digital subtraction angiography can safely image the pulmonary vascularity without a central pulmonary artery injection, which may cause acute right heart failure with elevated pulmonary artery pressures.

Pulmonary embolism or thrombosis may develop either acutely or chronically, or may be associated with a variety of conditions including long-term immobility, childbirth, rheumatic heart disease, fractures (especially fat embolism), iatrogenic injury, and blood dyscrasias. The embolic material may be blood clot, fat (usually associated with fractures), erythrocytes (as in sickle cell anemia), air (an iatrogenic injury), or amniotic fluid (as in childbirth). The blockage of the pulmonary capillaries by the embolic material leads to hypoxia, which leads in time to pulmonary arterial hypertension.

A diagnosis can be made by radionuclide imaging with ventilation-perfusion studies involving the lungs and pulmonary vasculature. In addition, the diagnosis can be made with digital subtraction angiography (Fig. 2-28A). Therapy includes streptokinase infusion or removal of the clot material. In addition, the placement of an umbrella filter in the inferior vena cava may prevent recurrent thrombosis from the lower extremities or pelvic disease (Fig. 2-28B). In addition, the patient may remain on medical therapy with long-term anticoagulation. Surgical em-

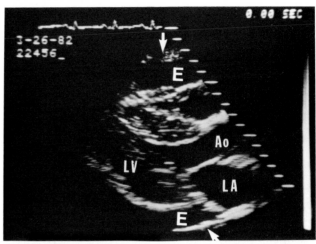

Fig. 2-25. Pericardial effusion demonstrated by echocardiography in the long axial oblique projection. The long axial view shows a sector scan with increased echo areas anteriorly (*top arrow*) as well as posteriorly (*lower arrow*) compatible with pericardial effusion (E). In addition, one can see the left ventricle (LV) and aorta (Ao). (Photograph provided by Thomas Ratts, M.D., University of Tennessee, Memphis.)

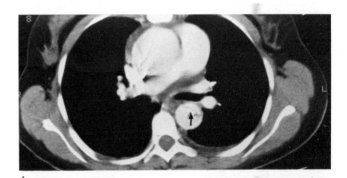

A

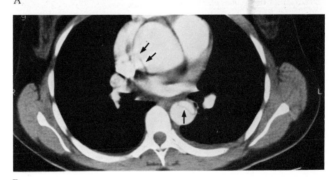

B

Fig. 2-26. A. The CT scan with contrast enhancement in this 40-year-old patient with acute back pain shows enlargement of the ascending aorta with a linear flap in the descending aorta (*arrow*). B. In addition, there is a low CT area representing dissection involving the ascending and descending thoracic aorta (*arrows*). This is compatible with type A of Stanford or I of DeBakey aortic dissection. This patient underwent successful surgical repair following this emergency CT scan without aortography. (Photographs provided by Wesley Atwood, M.D., BMH, Memphis, TN.)

62

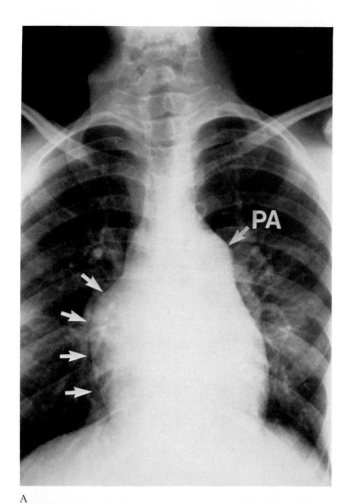

A

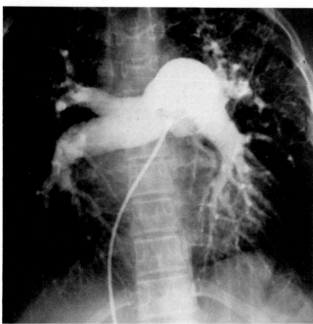

B

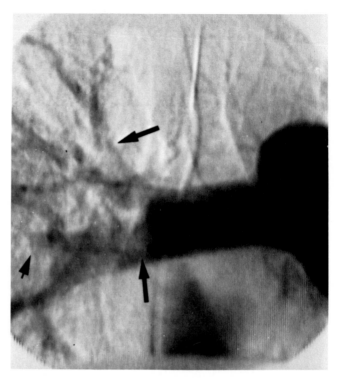

A

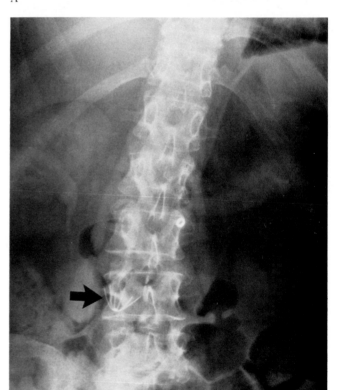

B

Fig. 2-27. A. Patient with dyspnea on exertion shows mild prominence of the central pulmonary arteries with peripheral vascular tapering. There is right heart enlargement (*arrows*) and prominence of the main pulmonary artery segment (PA). B. Pulmonary angiography in the PA projection shows marked central pulmonary artery prominence in this patient with idiopathic pulmonary hypertension.

Fig. 2-28. A. Intravenous digital subtraction angiography in a 52-year-old woman with dyspnea and calf tenderness shows filling defects within the proximal right pulmonary artery (*arrows*). The filling defects represent pulmonary emboli. B. One method of preventative therapy for pulmonary emboli is placement of an umbrella filter (*arrow*) in the inferior vena cava. This is a detachable device placed from a jugular venous cutdown approach. The device should be placed below L-3 (i.e., below the origin of the renal veins).

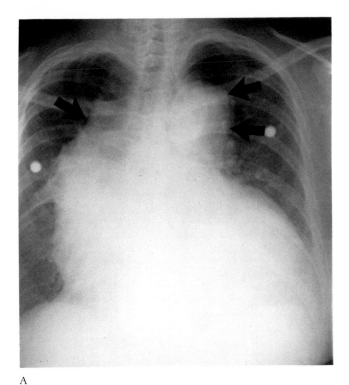

A

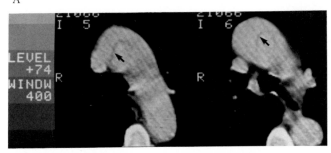

C

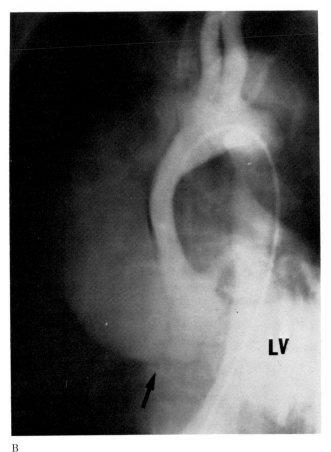

B

Fig. 2-29. A. The PA chest radiograph of a 60-year-old female with longstanding hypertension. Note the irregular and shaggy ascending and descending aorta (*arrows*). These findings are compatible with a chronic dissecting aneurysm. **B.** An aortogram demonstrates the liner flap in the ascending aorta (*arrow*) with dense opacification of the true channel supplying the left carotid and left subclavian arteries. The innominate artery arises from the false channel, which is less densely opacified. In addition, there is aortic valve insufficiency with opacification of the left ventricle (LV). **C.** A CT scan of the aortic arch without contrast enhancement in a 55-year-old female with hypertension and chest pain shows the linear flaps (*arrows*) of a type A aortic dissection. (Photographs provided by Allen K. Tonkin, M.D., BMH, Memphis, TN.)

bolectomy may be performed in patients who have extremely large clots within the lungs.

The echocardiographic features include a thickened anterior wall of the right ventricle, with the pulmonary valve showing a diminishing A wave and a flat E-F slope. Echocardiography is especially helpful in distinguishing primary pulmonary hypertension from hypertension associated with congenital heart disease or mitral stenosis.

The management of pulmonary-induced heart disease is difficult. Infections may be difficult to eradicate, and digitalis and diuretics often have little effect. Efforts to improve pulmonary function often have little effect as well. Pulmonary damage may be irreversible.

Diseases of the Aorta

AORTIC ANEURYSMS. Aortic aneurysms are localized bulges of the aorta that may be either fusiform, involving the entire aortic circumference, or saccular, involving only a portion of the aortic circumference. Fusiform aneurysms are often the result of syphilis. Patients with aneurysms often have other serious conditions, such as hypertension, ischemia, or cerebral vascular disease.

A dissecting aneurysm results from the entry of blood into the aortic media, usually through a tear in the intima. Dissection usually occurs in an abnormal media, such as one with atherosclerosis, or in patients with Marfan's syndrome, who frequently have cystic medial necrosis. The dissection generally begins at the ascending aorta immediately above the aortic valve and extends all the way into the abdomen in the so-called type I of DeBakey or type A of the Stanford classification. In type III of DeBakey (or in type B according to Stanford) the dissection occurs distal to the left subclavian artery and extends into the abdominal aorta. The PA chest radiograph frequently shows an abnormal mediastinal contour (Fig. 2-29A). The diagnosis can be made by aortography, echocardiography, CT scanning, or MRI (Fig. 2-29B, C). Angiography shows the true channel as well as the false channel, with contrast material and blood on either side of the intimal flap.

Management of aneurysms and dissections includes surgical therapy with graft replacement of the area of aneurysm and occlusion or oversewing of the intimal flaps, so that recurrent dissection will not occur. In addition, control of hypertension is essential. Atherosclerotic cardio-

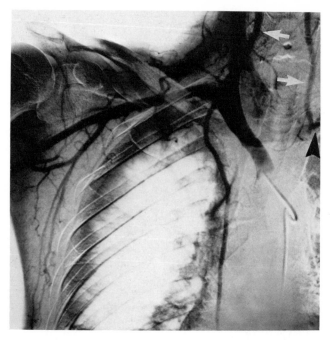

Fig. 2-30. An injection into the right innominate artery shows atherosclerosis with a subclavian steal. Contrast material extends through the right vertebral artery (*lower arrow*) to the left vertebral artery (*top arrow*) to the left subclavian artery (*arrowhead*). Angioplasty with a balloon dilatation catheter can be performed in this patient if a wire can be passed across the stenotic lesion.

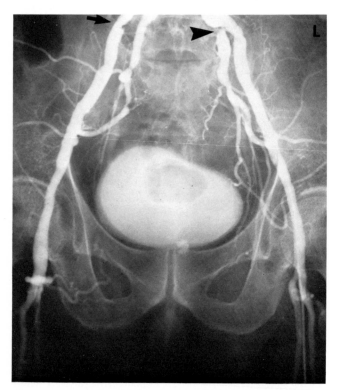

Fig. 2-31. A 60-year-old female presented with claudication and severe atherosclerotic stenosis involving the origin of the left hypogastric artery (*arrowhead*) as well as a stenosis of the right iliac artery (*arrow*).

vascular disease and bypass procedures can be imaged with CT scanning with contrast enhancement (see Fig. 2-10). Computed tomography scanning is extremely helpful to visualize graft abnormalities in postoperative patients.

Peripheral Atherosclerotic Disease and Treatment

Peripheral atherosclerotic disease is extremely common; atherosclerosis is a normal aging process. Angiography shows areas of atherosclerotic narrowing (Figs. 2-30, 2-31). Angioplasty can open atherosclerotic vascular lesions in the pelvis, extremities, in the great vessels, in the coronaries or in the renal arteries. Repeat angioplasties may be necessary.

Peripheral Venous Thrombosis

Venous thrombosis has many causes including trauma, immobility, and chronic infection. The diagnosis of peripheral thrombosis can be made by venography, with the injection of contrast material into an antecubital or dorsal foot vein (Fig. 2-32A, B). In addition, radionuclide studies have been used to image peripheral thrombosis. Following injection of the radionuclide material, imaging of the lungs can be performed to detect or exclude pulmonary emboli as well. Central thrombosis, such as superior vena caval thrombosis, may be caused by malignancies with metastatic disease and by fibrosing mediastinitis, as with histoplasmosis. Radiation therapy can also damage vessels in this region. The therapy for peripheral venous thromboembolic disease includes heparin, aspirin, and coumadin for long-term therapy and streptokinase for lysis of acute thromboses.

Cardiac Tumors

Primary cardiac tumors are rare, with atrial myxoma being the most common. Atrial myxoma occurs most often in the left atrium and along the atrial septum within the right atrium secondarily.

Breast and lung tumors are the most common primary tumors metastasizing to the heart, and frequently to the right atrium and pericardium specifically.

The radiographic findings of cardiac tumors may be generalized or localized. The tumor may simulate cardiac chamber enlargement. For example, a tumor of the right ventricle may mimic right ventricular enlargement. If a patient has left atrial myxoma, it may obstruct the mitral valve and cause a presentation similar to mitral valve stenosis or cor triatriatum, with pulmonary venous hypertension and enlargement of the left atrium. An atrial myxoma may calcify. Pericardial effusions may occur and may be the only radiographic abnormality.

Additional cardiac tumors include the rhabdomyomas associated with tuberous sclerosis and fibromas. These tumors may also calcify. The diagnosis of cardiac tumor may

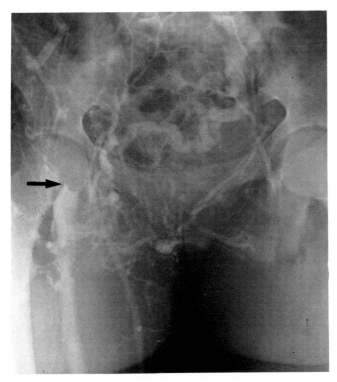

A

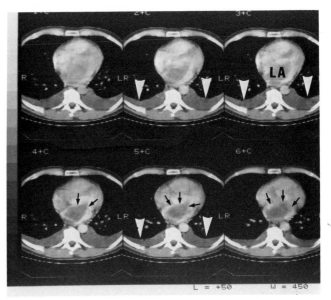

Fig. 2-33. Dynamic CT scanning with contrast enhancement shows a low-density area posteriorly in the region of the left atrium (LA) (*arrows*). This was a left atrial myxoma. In addition, there are bilateral pleural effusions (*arrowheads*). (Photographs provided by William Lankford, M.D., BMH, Memphis, TN.)

be made on plain film, echocardiography, CT scanning, or MRI (Fig. 2-33). Tumors may also be diagnosed with injection of contrast material at catheterization.

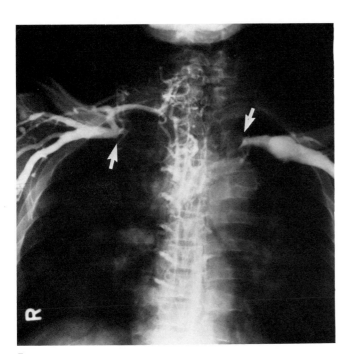

B

Fig. 2-32. A. A peripheral venogram in a 17-year-old patient with lupus erythematosus demonstrated total occlusion of the right common femoral vein (*arrow*) with a filling defect secondary to clot. Multiple collaterals are imaged with late opacification of the left iliac vein and inferior vena cava. B. Bilateral antecubital venous injections were performed in this 54-year-old male with metastatic squamous cell carcinoma in the mediastinum. There is total occlusion of the subclavian veins (*arrows*) and superior vena cava with collateral flow into the hemiazygous system.

Bibliography

Imaging tools in cardiovascular disease

Brundage, B. H., et al. Detection of patent coronary bypass grafts by computed tomography. *Circulation* 61:826, 1980.

Elliott, L. P., and Schiebler, G. L. *The X-ray Diagnosis of Congenital Heart Disease in Infants, Children, and Adults: Pathologic, Hemodynamic, and Clinical Correlations as Related to the Chest Film* (2nd ed.). Springfield, Ill. Thomas, 1979.

Gedgaudas, E., et al. *Cardiovascular Radiology.* Philadelphia: Saunders, 1985.

Lipton, M. J., and Higgins, C. B. Computed Tomography. In W. F. Friedman and C. B. Higgins (eds.), *Pediatric Cardiac Imaging.* Philadelphia: Saunders, 1984. P. 120.

Slutsky, R. Response of the left ventricle to stress: Effects of exercise, atrial pacing, afterload stress and drugs. *Am. J. Cardiol.* 47:357, 1981.

Tajik, A. J., et al. Two-dimensional real-time ultrasonic imaging of the heart and great vessels. *Mayo Clin. Proc.* 53:271, 1978.

Tonkin, I. L. D., and Tonkin, A. K. Viscero-arterial situs abnormalities: Sonographic and computed tomographic appearance. *A.J.R.* 138:509, 1982.

Turi, Z. G., et al. Electrocardiographic, enzymatic, and scintigraphic criteria of acute myocardial infarction as determined from study of 726 patients. *Am. J. Cardiol.* 55:1463, 1985.

Vlietstra, R. E., et al. Balloon angioplasty in multivessel coronary artery disease. *Mayo Clin. Proc.* 58:563, 1983.

Congestive heart failure

Artman, M., Parish, M. D., and Graham, T. Recognition of heart failure in childhood and adolescence. *Am. Heart J.* 105:471, 1978.

Baltax, H. A., Amplatz, K., and Levine, D. C. *Coronary Arteriography* (2nd ed.). Springfield, Ill.: Thomas, 1975.

Cooley, R. N., and Schreiber, M. H. *Radiology of the Heart and Great Vessels* (3rd ed.). Williams & Wilkins, 1978.

Daves, M. L. *Cardiac Roentgenology.* Chicago: Year Book, 1981.

Elliott, L. P., and Schiebler, G. L. *The X-Ray Diagnosis of Congenital Heart Disease in Infants, Children, and Adults: Pathologic, Hemodynamic, and Clinical Correlations as Related to the Chest Film* (2nd ed.). Springfield, Ill.: Thomas, 1979.

Klatte, E. C., et al. The roentgenographic manifestations of aortic stenosis and aortic valvular insufficiency. *A.J.R.* 88:57, 1962.

Mendlowitz, M. Fundamentals of clinical cardiology: The hypertensive complex. *Am. Heart J.* 95:389, 1978.

Tonkin, I. L. D. Radiology of Diseases Involving the Aortic Valve and Thoracic Aorta. In M. J. Kelley (ed.), *Cardiology Clinics.* Philadelphia: Saunders, 1983. Vol. 1, p. 625.

Rheumatic Heart Disease and Cardiomyopathy

Cooley, R. N., and Schreiber, M. H. *Radiology of the Heart and Great Vessels* (3rd Ed.). Williams & Wilkins, 1978.

Elliott, L. P., and Schiebler, G. L. *The X-Ray Diagnosis of Congenital Heart Disease in Infants, Children, and Adults: Pathologic, Hemodynamic, and Clinical Correlations as Related to the Chest Film* (2nd ed.). Springfield, Ill.: Thomas, 1979.

Jeresaty, R. M. Mitral valve prolapse. *J.A.M.A.* 254:793, 1985.

Perloff, J. K. The cardiomyopathies: Dilated and restrictive. *Circulation* 63:1189, 1981.

Prosthetic cardiac valves

Castaneda-Zuniga, W. R., et al. In vivo radiographic appearance of the St. Jude valve prosthesis. *Radiology* 134:775, 1980.

Gedgaudas, E., et al. *Cardiovascular Radiology.* Philadelphia: Saunders, 1985. P. 212.

Gross, B. H., Shirazi, K. K., and Slater, D. A. Differentiation of aortic and mitral valve prosthesis based on postoperative frontal chest radiographs. *Radiology* 149:389, 1983.

Mehlman, D. J., and Resnekov, L. A guide to the identification of prosthetic heart valves. *Circulation* 57:613, 1978.

Cardiac calcifications and diseases of the pericardium

Carsky, E. W., Azimi, F., and Mauceri, R. Epicardial fat sign in the diagnosis of pericardial effusion. *J.A.M.A.* 244:2762, 1980.

Freundlich, I. M., and Lind, T. A. Calcification of the heart and great vessels. *CRC Crit. Rev. Clin. Radiol. Nucl. Med.,* 6:171, 1975.

Moss, A. J., and Bruhn, F. The echocardium: An ultrasound technique for the detection of pericardial effusion. *N. Engl. J. Med.* 274:380, 1966.

Soulen, R. L., Stark, D. D., and Higgins, C. B. Magnetic resonance imaging of constrictive pericardial disease. *Am. J. Cardiol.* 55:480, 1985.

Souza, A. S., Bream, P. R., and Elliott, L. P. Chest film of coronary artery calcification: The value of the CAC triangle. *Radiology* 129:7, 1978.

Pulmonary hypertensive heart disease and pulmonary embolism

Bettman, M. A., and Salzman, E. W. Current concepts in the diagnosis of pulmonary embolism. *Mod. Concepts Cardiovasc. Dis.* 53:1, 1984.

Grollman, J. H., and Reaner, J. W. Transfemoral pulmonary angiography: Update in technique. *A.J.R.* 136:624, 1981.

Harrison, D. A. Diagnosing pulmonary thromboembolic disease. *Postgrad. Med.* 59:89, 1976.

Kelley, M. J., and Elliott, L. P. The radiologic evaluation of the patient with suspected pulmonary thromboembolism disease. *Med. Clin. North Am.* 59:3, 1974.

Moses, D. C., Silver, T. M., and Bookstein, J. J. The complementary roles of chest radiography, lung scanning, and selective pulmonary angiography in the diagnosis of pulmonary embolism. *Circulation* 49:179, 1974.

Diseases of the aorta

Castaneda-Zuniga, W., et al. Hemodynamic assessment of obstructive aortoiliac disease. *Am. J. Roentgenol.* 127:559, 1976.

Dailey, P. O., Trueblood, H. W., and Stinson, E. B. Management of acute aortic dissections. *Ann. Thorac. Surg.* 10:237, 1970.

DeBakey, M. E., Henley, W. S., and Cooley, D. A. Surgical management of dissecting aneurysms of the aorta. *J. Thorac. Cardiovasc. Surg.* 49:130, 1965.

Godwin, J. D., et al. Computed tomography for follow-up of chronic aortic dissections. *Radiology* 139:655, 1981.

Rosch, J., et al. Healing of deep venous thrombosis venographic findings in a randomized study comparing streptokinase and heparin. *Am. J. Roentgenol.* 127:553, 1976.

Soto, B., et al. Angiographic diagnosis of dissecting aneurysm of the aorta. *Am. J. Roentgenol.* 116:146, 1972.

Tonkin, I. L. D. Congenital vascular compression of the trachea and esophagus. *Contemp. Diagn. Radiol.* 5:1, 1982.

Tonkin, I. L. D. The Thoracic Aorta and Its Branches. In P. Stanley and J. H. Miller (eds.), *Pediatric Angiography.* Baltimore: Williams & Wilkins, 1982. P. 47.

Tonkin, I. L. D. Radiology of diseases involving the aortic valve and thoracic aorta. *Cardiol. Clin.* 1:625, 1983.

Tonkin, I. L. D., et al. Evaluation of vascular rings with digital subtraction angiography. *A.J.R.* 142:1287, 1984.

Webber, M. M., et al. Thrombosis detection by radionuclide particle (MAA) entrapment: Correlation with fibrinogen uptake and venography. *Radiology* 111:645, 1974.

Cardiac tumors

Bogren, H. G., DeMaria, A. N., and Mason, D. T. Imaging in the detection of cardiac tumors, with emphasis on echocardiography: A review. *Cardiovasc. Intervent. Radiol.* 3:107, 1980.

DeMaria, A. N., et al. Unusual echocardiographic manifestations of right and left heart myxomas. *Am. J. Med.* 59:713, 1975.

Edwards, J. Cardiac Tumors. In A. J. Moss, F. H. Adams, and G. C. Emmanouilides (eds.), *Heart Disease in Infants, Children and Adolescents* (3rd ed.). Baltimore: Williams and Wilkins, 1980. P. 694–699.

3. Respiratory Tract Disease

Robert L. Siegle

Basic Principles of Pulmonary Disease

Certain definitions and understandings provide a base on which to facilitate a discussion of pulmonary disease. The subjects discussed in this chapter include alveolar and interstitial patterns, and atelectasis. Some of their features overlap and can cause confusion.

CONSOLIDATION. Air space or alveolar filling plays a key role in pulmonary radiology. The alveoli may fill with edema, pus, blood, or hyaline. These different air space fillers result in the same radiographic characteristic, which is relatively uniform opacification of an area of lung with virtually no volume loss. The consequence on the chest radiograph is essentially the same—lung consolidation. Since the bronchi often remain patent while the alveoli opacify, lung consolidation provides clinicians with a unique opportunity to see these bronchi radiographically. Dr. Benjamin Felson coined the term *air bronchogram* to describe this feature (Fig. 3-1). Air-filled bronchi are not seen on normal chest radiographs because the bronchi are surrounded by air-filled alveoli. Lung consolidation provides the contrast necessary for bronchial visualization. Air bronchograms often accompany lung consolidation, but they are not a sine qua non for the diagnosis.

There are other radiographic features of air space filling in addition to air bronchograms, uniform opacification, and no volume loss. For instance, the shape and extent of involvement is important; consolidated lung often has a segmental or lobar distribution. In other circumstances it may assume a fluffy, coalescent appearance, resembling absorbent cotton. Pulmonary edema often develops a unique bat wing or butterfly pattern or perihilar alveolar filling (Fig. 3-2). Some of the medical problems that can generate a pattern of consolidation on the chest radiograph include bacterial pneumonia, infarct, contusion, hemorrhage, edema, shock lung, alveolar cell carcinoma, and sarcoid. The specific radiographic patterns for each entity are discussed in the sections devoted to the specific diseases.

Silhouette Sign. A unique feature of lung consolidation allows clinicians to readily determine the lobe and segment involved. Consolidation of lung adjacent to a soft-tissue density obliterates the edge or silhouette of that soft tissue. Dr. Felson coined the term *silhouette sign* for this very useful phenomenon. (The term is not quite accurate since it more properly describes the *loss* of the silhouette, but a name usually creates a more lasting impact if it is short and expressive even if not completely accurate.) There is really no magic involved in the loss of the silhouette. The silhouette of a soft-tissue density, such as a right or left heart border, is only evident because it is contiguous with the less dense, air-filled lung adjacent to it. If the lung becomes consolidated it develops a radiographic density similar to the heart, and the density interface between them is lost. The lung and the heart each would now absorb the same proportion of the photon beam from the

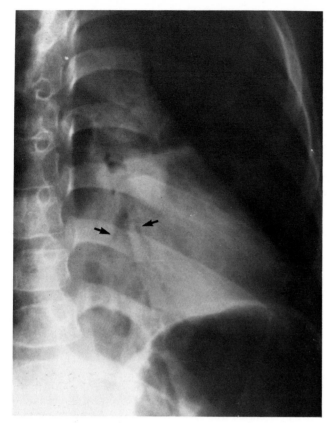

Fig. 3-1. Air bronchograms (*arrows*) in consolidated left lower lobe behind the heart.

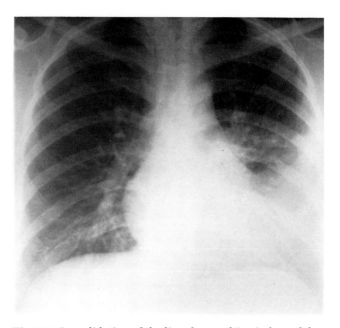

Fig. 3-3. Consolidation of the lingula, resulting in loss of the left cardiac border. Note that the left hemidiaphragm remains visible because the left lower lobe is not consolidated.

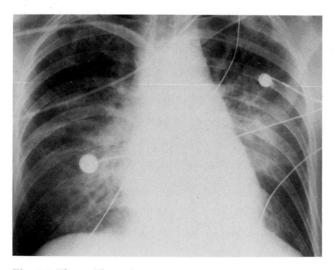

Fig. 3-2. The confluent bat wing pattern of perihilar pulmonary edema. The small disks represent cardiac monitoring leads.

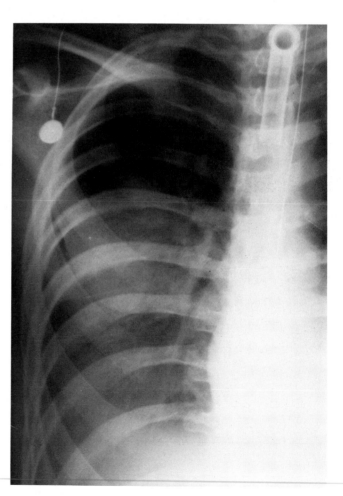

Fig. 3-4. Right lower lobe consolidation, resulting in loss of the right hemidiaphragm silhouette and preservation of the right heart border. Incidental findings include the disk of a cardiac monitoring lead and a tracheostomy tube.

x-ray tube and so create the same shadow on the radiographic film. Patchy consolidation does not obliterate a silhouette.

The following lobes and segments can often be identified by the loss of the adjacent silhouette.

1. The right middle lobe affects the right heart border, and the lingula affects the left heart border (Fig. 3-3).
2. The apical posterior segment of the left upper lobe affects the aortic knob, and the anterior segment of the right upper lobe affects the ascending aorta.
3. Diaphragm silhouettes are affected by consolidation of adjacent segments of the lower lobes (Fig. 3-4). This may be more evident on the lateral than on the PA projection.

Bacterial Pneumonia Patterns. Because classical bacterial pneumonia is so fundamental to chest radiology, its patterns deserve discussion in this section on basic principles. The accepted model is pneumococcal pneumonia, which characteristically involves anatomically defined areas, segments, or lobes, whose air spaces rapidly fill with pus. Air bronchograms commonly occur. Usually no change in volume occurs, although small degrees of atelectasis may develop during resolution as bronchi become transiently blocked by mobilized secretions. Pleural effusions are uncommon, and with appropriate treatment clinical resolution is rapid and complete. The radiographic pattern clears just as rapidly. Any underlying respiratory disease, such as emphysema, modifies the classic pattern.

Staphylococcal pneumonia often has features on x-ray that help to separate it from pneumonia caused by pneumococci. Staphylococcal pneumonia creates fewer air bronchograms and more atelectasis because it usually generates more exudate than pneumococcal pneumonia. Abscesses and pleural effusions are fairly common complications, occurring in about half of all staphylococcal pneumonias. *Pseudomonas* pneumonia, most commonly hospital acquired in debilitated patients, is much like staphylococcal pneumonia in radiographic appearance and incidence of abscess formation. *Klebsiella* sp. generates such an exuberant reaction when it causes pneumonia that the affected lung expands (Fig. 3-5). This is apparent on x-ray, as the fissures around the pneumonia bulge outward and areas of adjacent lung are often compressed.

INTERSTITIAL DISEASE. By definition lung pathology that does not involve alveolar spaces must be interstitial. Therefore, lung patterns other than consolidation on x-ray reflect interstitial disease. There is no consensus on what represents interstitial disease radiographically, but some of the accepted patterns are multiple small nodules, as in miliary tuberculosis (Fig. 3-6), honeycombing, the end stage of extensive interstitial fibrosis (Fig. 3-7), Kerley A and B lines, perivascular and peribronchial thickening, and almost any other small irregular shadows. Fairly extensive pathologic correlation has been shown for Kerley lines. Kerley B lines, the more commonly observed set, are short, horizontal lines at the periphery near the costophrenic angles, while Kerley A lines are longer lines in the upper lobes that all seem to be aimed toward the hilar regions (Fig. 3-8). Both sets of lines prove to be thickened interlobular septa.

Discussions have often centered on the fact that disease is infrequently purely alveolar or purely interstitial and that radiographic distinctions based on these features are often artificial. In one sense the proponents of this argument are correct, as distinctions between interstitial and

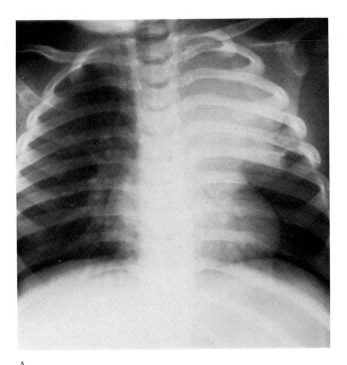

A

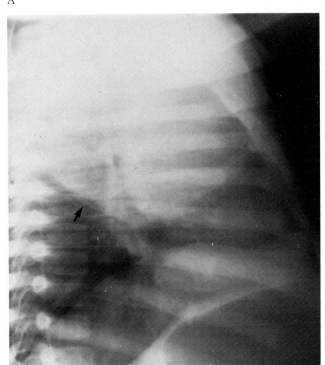

B

Fig. 3-5. *Klebsiella* **pneumonia. A. PA projection demonstrating complete consolidation of the left upper lobe. B. Lateral projection showing pneumonia causing bulging of the major fissure (*arrow*).**

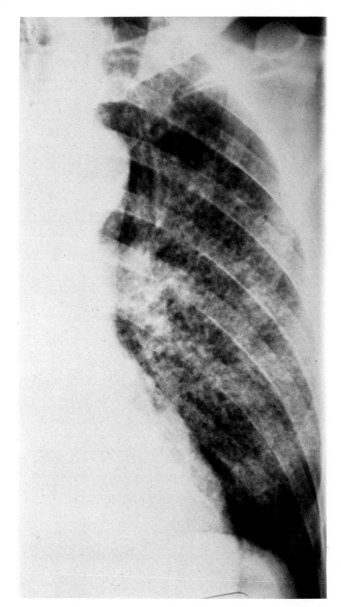

Fig. 3-6. Miliary pattern. Note multiple small nodules filling up the lung.

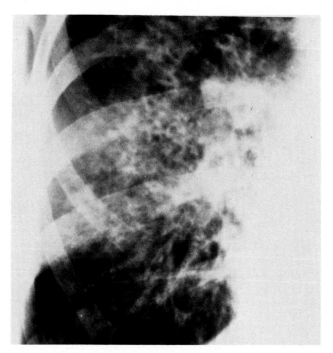

Fig. 3-7. Honeycombing in perihilar distribution.

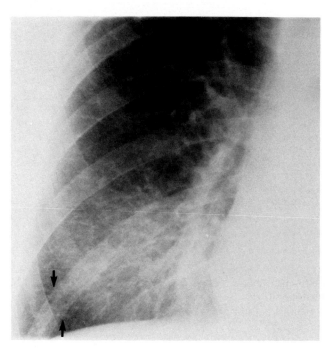

Fig. 3-8. Kerley B lines seen near the right base peripherally as horizontal linear densities (*arrows*).

alveolar may not conform to pathologic fact. In another sense they are wrong, because radiologists are usually adept at diagnosing diseases using these criteria. Because of its successful application to radiologic diagnosis, pattern reading based on the interpretation of interstitial and alveolar shadows remains an accepted procedure.

ATELECTASIS. Atelectasis refers to an airless portion of lung with significant associated volume loss. Radiographic density is increased just as in consolidation, although in consolidation no volume loss occurs. Many people use the terms *atelectasis* and *collapse* interchangeably. This seems reasonable, but collapse is also frequently used to refer to a pneumothorax. Collapse needs to be distinguished under these two sets of circumstances; collapse associated with atelectasis implies an unviolated pleural space with normal negative pressure, while collapse associated with pneumothorax denotes air in the pleural space with resultant loss of physiologic negative pressure.

Bronchial obstruction results in atelectasis. Aspiration of a foreign body and postoperative mucous plugging rank high as causes. The air is gradually absorbed by the circulatory system, and volume loss ensues. Air bronchograms do not normally appear, since the obstructed bronchi as well as the alveoli are airless. Volume loss and the absence of air bronchograms are features that separate atelectasis from lung consolidation. Atelectasis may be partial or complete and may involve a segment, lobe, or whole lung. Endobronchial tumors may also cause atelectasis.

Radiographic Appearance. The features of atelectasis depend on the lobe affected.

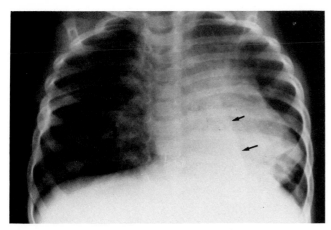

Fig. 3-9. Left lower lobe atelectasis. The lateral margin of the collapsed lobe is seen as a thin, oblique line (*arrows*).

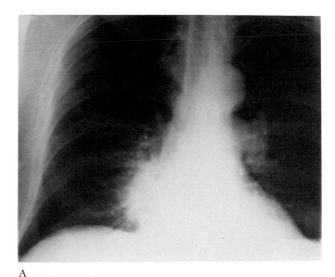

A

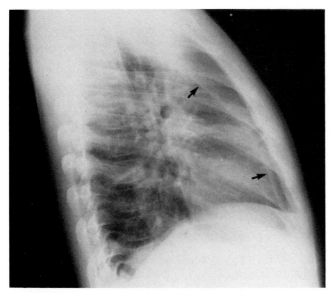

Fig. 3-11. Lateral projection demonstrating left upper lobe (including the lingula) collapse. The line behind the sternum (*arrows*) represents the displaced major fissure.

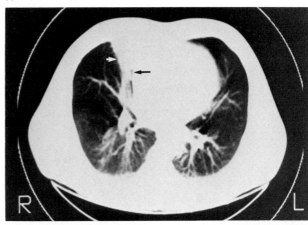

B

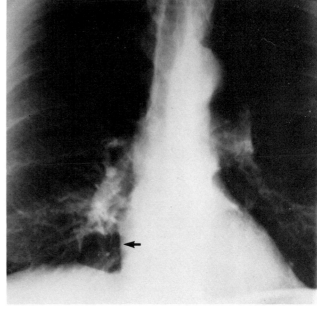

C

Fig. 3-10. Right middle lobe atelectasis. A. PA projection of middle lobe atelectasis obliterating the right heart border. B. CT section demonstrating the anteriorly collapsed right middle lobe (*white arrow*) adjacent to the right cardiac border (*black arrow*). C. Resolution of middle lobe atelectasis, with reappearance of right heart border (*arrow*).

Left Lower Lobe. This is the lobe most commonly involved postoperatively, for several reasons. The patient often finds it painful to breathe deeply and to cough, because mucous occludes the bronchi. In the supine position the lower lobe bronchi are almost all dependent, and the heart compounds the felony by lying on the left lower lobe. Complete atelectasis results in a triangular density behind the heart, obliterating the medial portion of the silhouette of the left hemidiaphragm (Fig. 3-9).

Right Lower Lobe. Collapse here results in a posterior density on the lateral projection, giving a silhouette sign with the right hemidiaphragm.

Right Middle Lobe. Atelectasis of this lobe is often associated with extrinsic pressure from enlarged lymph nodes on the middle lobe bronchus. The result is intermittent or partial atelectasis, often with concurrent pneumonia. The complex is known as *middle lobe syndrome.* Atelectasis here results in obliteration of the right heart border (Fig. 3-10).

Fig. 3-12. Linear densities (*arrows*) above both hemidiaphragms representing discoid atelectasis.

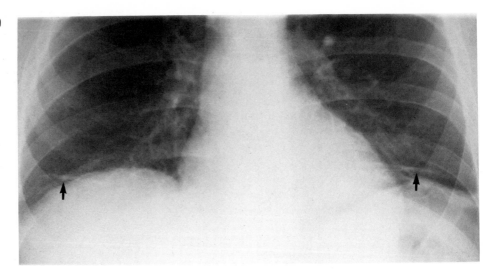

Lingula. Atelectasis of the lingula is not a common isolated finding. It manifests as density along the left heart border.

Upper Lobes. The upper lobes are anterior structures, and collapse causes them to be plastered against the anterior chest walls. On the PA projection this might only appear as a slight increase in density over the involved hemithorax, while on the lateral projection the collapsed lobe is apparent behind the sternum (Fig. 3-11).

Atelectasis has other radiographic features independent of the specific anatomy involved. When volume loss is extensive, compensatory hyperaeration of the uninvolved portion makes the remainder of that lung hyperlucent. There may even be mediastinal shift toward the affected side and diaphragmatic elevation, all to compensate for volume loss. Partial volume loss closely resembles consolidation.

Subsegmental Atelectasis. Atelectasis involving very small bronchi or bronchioles results in subsegmental atelectasis and may be identical radiographically to patchy pneumonia. An important subcategory, plate-like or discoid atelectasis (Fig. 3-12) appears as horizontal linear densities near the diaphragms and usually extends over several centimeters. It customarily occurs in bedridden patients and usually disappears on resumption of activity and deep breathing. Parenchymal scars look similar but do not disappear.

Lung Neoplasms

BRONCHOGENIC CARCINOMA. Lung cancer continues to play its ominous role in modern medicine. For males, the lung cancer death rate is the highest for all malignancies, and for females its incidence continues to climb alarmingly. Few doubt the strong association between lung cancer and cigarette smoking. Despite the certainty of cause, sophisticated diagnostic procedures, and modern treatment regimens, the outlook is grim. The recovery rate remains only about 10 percent. There are other lung carcinogens, especially in industrial environments; these include organic solvents and uranium, but statistically

such agents play a minor role in lung cancer. Other factors, such as asbestos, may work synergistically with smoking to increase the risk of lung cancer even further. The practical conclusion is that a smoker over the age of 45 with a new density on his chest radiograph has bronchogenic carcinoma until proved otherwise.

Radiographic Appearance. Some features of bronchogenic carcinomas on x-ray are characteristic of the cell type involved; therefore a description of the common cell types is useful.

Squamous or Epidermoid Carcinoma. At least one-third and as many as one-half of lung cancers in most series belong in this category. When the cells are very poorly differentiated, it may be very difficult to distinguish squamous from large cell undifferentiated carcinoma. Squamous cell carcinomas demonstrate central cavitation more frequently than do other forms of lung cancer, but any cell type can cavitate, especially during chemotherapy (Fig. 3-13).

Large Cell Undifferentiated Carcinoma. This cell type usually makes up less than 15 percent of lung cancers. Tumors of this cell type tend to be larger at initial presentation than squamous cell tumors and may appear anywhere in the lung.

Small Cell Undifferentiated (Oat Cell) Carcinoma. This cell type has several features that make it distinctive. Small cell tumors account for most of the lung cancers with hormonal activity. They make up about 15 percent of all lung cancers, and along with squamous cell carcinomas are the malignancies most clearly related to cigarette smoking. Small cell tumors metastasize so early in their course that the primary malignancies are often not apparent on chest radiographs. Hilar or mediastinal adenopathy may be the presenting feature on the initial chest radiograph. If the primary tumor is evident, it is rarely large in comparison to subsequent nodal involvement.

Adenocarcinoma. This cell type also accounts for about 15 percent of lung cancers. Adenocarcinoma is also the cell type associated with scar carcinomas. Just as the name implies, the scar carcinoma develops in close proximity to a parenchymal scar, such as occurs in the lung apex adjacent to old tuberculous disease. Any change in the radiographic

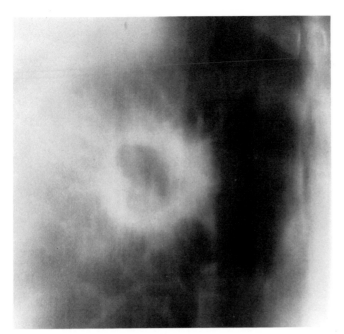

Fig. 3-13. Squamous cell carcinoma. Tomographic section of an irregular, spiculated, right upper lobe mass with central cavitation.

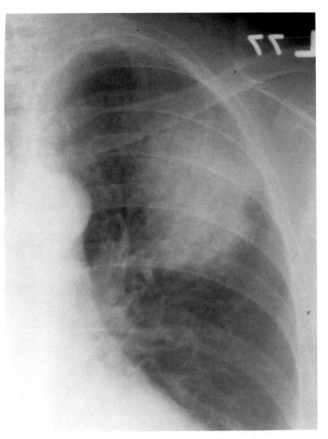

Fig. 3-14. Alveolar cell carcinoma resembling pneumonia with poorly defined borders and faintly seen air bronchograms.

appearance of old fibrocalcific disease raises the possibility of a scar carcinoma.

Bronchioloalveolar (Alveolar Cell) Carcinoma. This is a distinct variant of adenocarcinoma and makes up about 5 percent of lung cancers. Like other adenocarcinomas, these tumors are peripheral and are unrelated to smoking. Radiographically some tend to be nodular and are indistinguishable from other lung cancers, but others have a feature that gives them the following characteristic radiographic appearance. Bronchioloalveolar tumor cells live and grow on the normal lung architecture rather than destroy it, and consequently may present as segmental or lobar consolidation, even traversed by air bronchograms on occasion (Fig. 3-14). As a result these tumors often resemble pneumonias, albeit pneumonias that fail to respond to antibiotics. If appropriate treatment is delayed, bronchioloalveolar tumors often spread extensively throughout the lungs with the development of many poorly defined masses, occasionally even mimicking miliary tuberculosis.

The statement is often made that two-thirds of lung cancers on x-rays are medial and one-third peripheral. The relative frequencies of the different cell types give substance to this statement, which roughly reflects the frequency of squamous and small cell carcinomas versus the frequency of adenocarcinoma.

Many bronchogenic carcinomas have certain radiographic features that are not dependent on the cell type but are simply a function of the cells' malignancy. When one or more of these features appear on a radiograph, the physician's suspicion of malignancy should increase. Like most other signs in medicine these radiographic findings are not pathognomonic, but they do tilt the balance in favor of malignancy.

Primary lung cancers tend to have irregular, spiculated margins. Benign lesions commonly have smoother, more rounded borders. The periphery of lung cancer often resembles a sunburst, with various densities radiating out from the central mass (Fig. 3-15); desmoplasia, a feature of

many tumors, may cause this appearance. Desmoplasia may result from lymphatic obstruction or small areas of atelectasis adjacent to the tumor. One or more satellite lesions may also exist. All such features are a function of the unbridled growth of the tumor, and this uncontrolled growth alone constitutes a key radiographic feature. Any small shadow that changes in size or shape over several months must be considered a malignancy. Similarly, the small shadow that has had a constant appearance over years, has rightly been considered an old granuloma, and now changes in size or shape strongly suggests a scar carcinoma.

Some fairly peripheral pulmonary malignancies extend their fibrotic reactions to the adjacent pleural surface and may even create a pleural dimple. This connection is often called a *pleural tail* and should be considered additional circumstantial evidence for lung cancer. However, it is not an absolute sign, and some granulomas also demonstrate it. Tumors frequently cause atelectasis of the lung peripheral to tumors or hilar nodes if they become bulky enough to compress and obstruct bronchi.

Some lung cancers cavitate, but so do many other disease entities, such as tuberculosis and fungal diseases. Smooth, very thin-walled cavities (1–2 mm) are rarely malignant; tumor walls tend to be thicker and lumpier. One report (Woodring, 1982) in the radiographic literature indicates that virtually all cavitating masses are malignant if the thickest part of the wall is at least 15 mm. A cavitating mass with walls between 1 mm and 15 mm falls in an indeterminate zone.

The superior sulcus tumor (Pancoast's tumor) is a unique class of lung cancer. It occurs in about 5 percent of lung cancers, may be of any cell type (although squamous

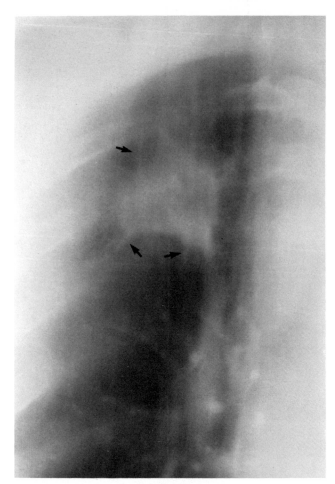

Fig. 3-15. Characteristic appearance of primary lung neoplasm. Tomographic section demonstrates an irregular shape and multiple spiculations (*arrows*).

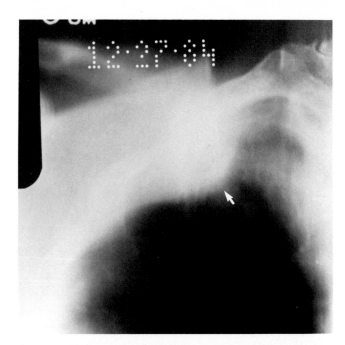

A

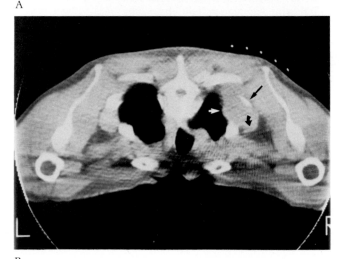

B

Fig. 3-16. Pancoast's tumor. A. Tomographic section demonstrating soft-tissue density in the right apex (*white arrow*) involving the pleura and possibly the ribs. B. Tomographic section with the patient prone (preparing for biopsy), showing Pancoast's tumor (*white arrow*) involving the rib (*black arrow*) and extending farther into the axilla (*curved arrow*).

is the most common), and tends to metastasize late. Radiographically, the tumor is easy to miss as it is hidden among the ribs, clavicle, and mediastinal shadows near the lung apex. Tomography or CT is often necessary to delineate a superior sulcus tumor, and at times it may appear early in its course as only local pleural thickening. The symptoms often suggest the diagnosis; these include arm or shoulder pain or weakness and Horner's syndrome (Fig. 3-16). A more advanced stage of disease results in striking radiographic features, including adjacent rib and vertebral body destruction as well as the tumor mass itself.

Certain lung cancers have a pronounced effect on pulmonary perfusion to the affected side. These tumors are usually medial and often have extensive adenopathy. A perfusion lung scan is useful to confirm these findings. The tumor or nodes may invade or encase and compress the pulmonary artery. In other situations there is no direct vascular involvement; some theories maintain that poor ventilation distal to the tumor causes a reflex vasoconstriction and redistribution of flow. Consequently, the radiographic pattern of unilateral decrease in vascular markings suggests a medial bronchogenic carcinoma.

Radiographic Contribution to Staging. Radiology can make significant contributions to the work-up of a bronchogenic carcinoma, but there are limitations. If fine detail of the mass is necessary, conventional tomographic sections are useful; they may confirm pleural or rib involvement. Such findings indicate reduced chances for cure. Computed

tomography in the staging of lung cancer raises as many questions as it provides answers. Computed tomography demonstrates enlarged nodes, but the correlation between size and malignant infiltration varies in the published studies from different institutions. A large node may not always be tumor-ridden nor may a normal-sized node be tumor-free. Our own experience as well as published reports from MD Anderson Hospital indicate that both sensitivity and specificity of CT evaluation of the mediastinum and proximal bronchi are less than those necessary for the study to replace more invasive staging procedures such as mediastinoscopy and nodal biopsy. As a consequence, CT tends to be additive rather than substitutive and may contribute more to patient expense than to patient care.

Despite all the sophisticated diagnostic machinery available, the biggest problem facing radiologists today is that lung cancer is still difficult to find on a chest x-ray. Studies from several groups have shown that routine screening chest x-rays do not materially affect the survival rate in lung cancer. A study from Johns Hopkins (Muhm, 1983) of chest x-rays at four-month intervals on men at high risk for lung cancer emphasized this point. When the diagnosis of lung cancer was finally made, half the patients had the tumor visible in retrospect five to eight months before it was detected.

BRONCHIAL ADENOMAS. Benign tumors of the lung are infrequent, accounting for less than 10 percent of all lung neoplasms. More than half are adenomas, and they occur earlier than bronchogenic carcinomas, usually before age 50. The cell type of most adenomas is carcinoid. They are likely related to oat cell tumors, and those that are not are mostly cylindromas.

Radiographic Appearance. Adenomas are endobronchial masses that may arise in any part of the lung. They frequently appear smooth and round on conventional radiographs or tomograms. If the affected bronchus is occluded, distal atelectasis results. This atelectasis may be contiguous to the tumor and thus obscure its margin. Although these tumors are usually classified as benign, up to 10 percent have potential for malignancy and metastasize to regional nodes and beyond if they are observed for several years and not removed.

METASTASES TO LUNG. Metastases to the lungs from primary malignancies in other organs are very common. This high degree of involvement should be expected, since the entire circulation is filtered by the lungs on every pass. The most common primary malignancies are also the most common metastases to the lungs. Most metastases are multiple, but several notable exceptions exist. Squamous cell, transitional cell, kidney, and colon malignancies present more frequently than those with solitary metastases in the lungs.

Radiographic Appearance. Metastases most often appear radiographically as smooth, round, and multiple (Fig. 3-17). Desmoplastic reaction and local atelectasis are very uncommon. These features are significant when viewing a single new lung shadow and suggest a solitary metastasis instead of a primary lung cancer. Multiple metastases usually involve both lungs, demonstrate different diameters for each metastasis, and rarely cause hilar adenopathy. Cavitating metastases most commonly occur when the primary tumor is squamous cell from the head, neck, or genitourinary tract. Any cell type can cavitate during chemotherapy.

Certain tumors have very characteristic appearances upon spread to the lungs. Thyroid carcinoma sometimes appears as a "snowstorm" of tiny densities throughout the lungs, resembling miliary tuberculosis (nodules less than 5 mm in diameter) (Fig. 3-18). Metastases of choriocarcinoma and lymphoma at times have poorly defined edges representing adjacent infiltration or hemorrhage. An occasional metastatic malignancy, usually renal cell or melanoma, may present as an endobronchial mass indistinguishable from a primary bronchogenic tumor.

Occult Primary Tumors. Some tumors present initially as metastases to the lungs. If the primary tumor is not readily found through simple diagnostic procedures, a long, ex-

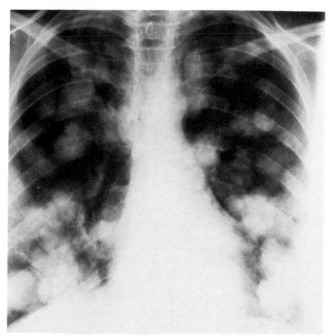

Fig. 3-17. Metastases to the lung from primary breast cancer showing well-defined, rounded densities of multiple sizes.

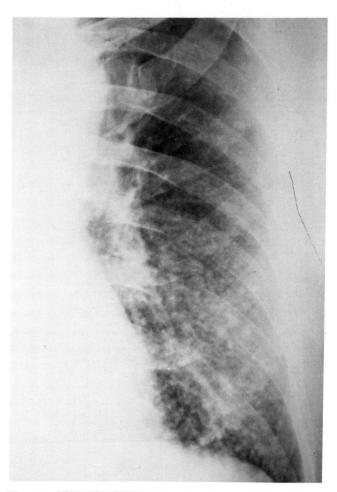

Fig. 3-18. Thyroid metastases. Multiple tiny nodules dot the entire lung field giving the characteristic snowstorm appearance.

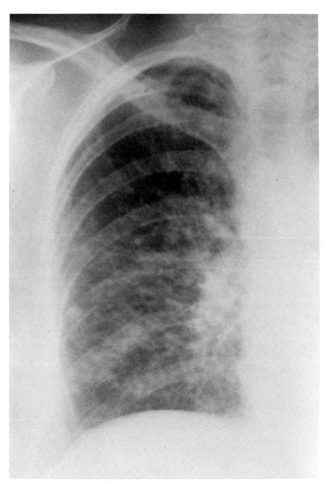

Fig. 3-19. Lymphangitic spread. Metastases from primary renal carcinoma have resulted in lymphangitic obstruction, with numerous streaked densities pointing toward the hilum.

Table 3-1. Causes of the Solitary Nodule

Cancer—primary lung, metastasis, lymphoma
Granuloma—tuberculous or fungal
Hamartoma
Arteriovenous malformation
Loculated pleural fluid
Round pneumonia
Artifact
Extrapulmonary mass—nipple or skin tumor
20–30 Esoteric entities

ease. Further complicating the problem of lymphangitic spread is the fact that a significant proportion of patients with lymphangitic spread proved by biopsy have no radiographic evidence of it.

The Solitary Pulmonary Nodule

Solitary pulmonary nodule sounds stilted as an expression describing a small, isolated shadow on a lung. *Coin lesion* has much greater acceptance, probably because it is concise and graphic, but it is unfortunately rather inaccurate as well. Such a shadow is more accurately referred to as a *marble lesion.*

Whether described as a coin or a marble, the lesion has round, sharply defined edges and may or may not demonstrate calcium within it. Approximately ten entities occur frequently enough that they should be considered common causes of coin lesions (Table 3-1).

pensive, fruitless diagnostic evaluation may ensue. If the cell type proves to be squamous on biopsy of a pulmonary metastasis, the primary tumor usually resides in the head or neck. It may be a very small mass, but thin-section CT of the head and neck often reveals it. If the cell type is adenocarcinoma, there is less hope for recovery. The primary tumor is often unrevealed; in one study (Steckel, 1980) the primary tumor was not even found at autopsy in half the cases. Another study (Stewart, 1979) concluded that finding the primary tumor had no effect on the survival rate in this special category of metastatic cancer.

Lymphangitic Metastases. Tumors may spread through the lungs via pulmonary lymphatic channels. To a large extent these originate as blood-borne metastases to the lung periphery that secondarily invade lung lymphatics. Alternately, there may be lymphatic invasion from affected hilar lymph nodes, creating retrograde spread. The common tumors cause lymphangitic metastases; these include primaries from lung, gut, breast, and cervix.

The radiographic appearance includes coarse linear markings converging on the hilar regions that primarily involve the lower half of the lungs (Fig. 3-19). Kerley B lines commonly appear, and occasionally small nodules also develop. The radiographic appearance of lymphangitic spread is not unique and may be confused with interstitial pulmonary edema or almost any other interstitial lung dis-

DIFFERENTIAL DIAGNOSIS. Some features on the chest film help to distinguish among the possible entities. Tuberculous and fungal granulomas often calcify. If the calcifications appear central, smoothly laminated, or spherical at the periphery, a granuloma can be diagnosed with a high degree of confidence (Fig. 3-20). Eccentric calcifications do not conclusively prove a granuloma. A cancer may develop at the edge of a granuloma or calcified scar, subsequently engulf it, and give the appearance of a mass with eccentric calcifications.

Hamartomas frequently have multiple stippled or popcorn-like calcifications (Fig. 3-21). If a hamartoma is without calcification, it lacks any distinguishing features on conventional radiographs.

An arteriovenous malformation has prominent afferent and efferent vessels serving the vascular tangle, which appears as a soft-tissue mass. These feeders can often be seen on the conventional chest radiograph. Tomography or CT demonstrates them more clearly if necessary. If surgery is contemplated to remove this vascular shunt, a pulmonary arteriogram is necessary to ensure that all feeders are identified (Fig. 3-22).

Pleural fluid occasionally becomes loculated within a major fissure and may appear as a lung mass on a frontal chest film. The lateral projection should display its association with the major fissure and also its characteristic disk-like configuration.

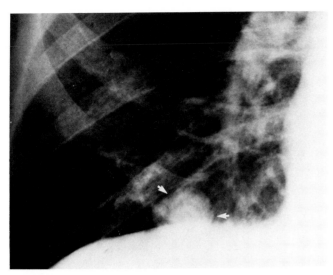

Fig. 3-20. Circular calcified laminations in this sharply marginated coin lesion near the diaphragm strongly indicate its benign, probably granulomatous, origin.

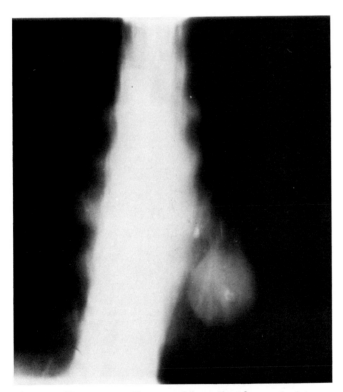

Fig. 3-21. Hamartoma. Tomographic section demonstrates rounded, soft-tissue mass adjacent to the vertebral column with a single calcification.

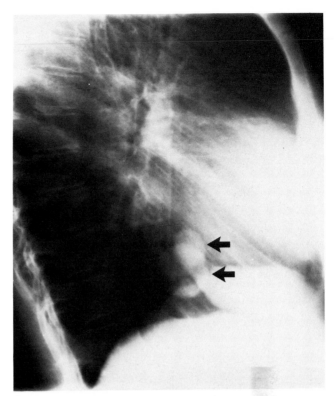

A

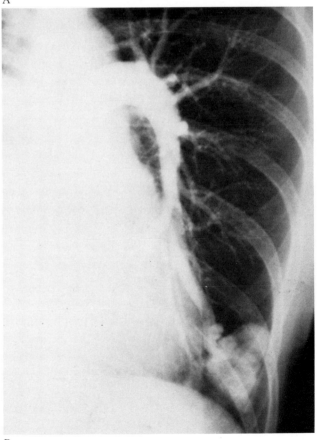

B

The term *round pneumonia* speaks for itself. Children are more susceptible to this unusual presentation of pneumonia than are adults. A repeat film in 24 hours virtually always shows progression to the expected segmental consolidation (Fig. 3-23).

Extrapulmonary densities may also cause coin lesions. These densities include nipples, other cutaneous tumors, and film-cassette artifacts. The lateral projection often identifies cutaneous tumors in profile. A repeat frontal film with metallic markers over the nipples should clarify whether or not a shadow is a nipple. A radiologist can usu-

Fig. 3-22. Arteriovenous malformation. A. Lateral chest radiograph demonstrating two soft-tissue masses (*arrows*) superimposed on the cardiac silhouette. B. Pulmonary arterial injection with contrast material demonstrating a large feeder and a tangle of opacified vessels characteristic of an arteriovenous malformation.

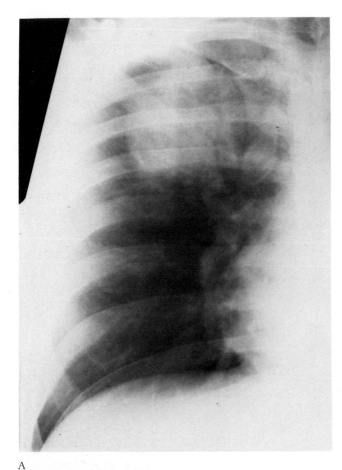

A

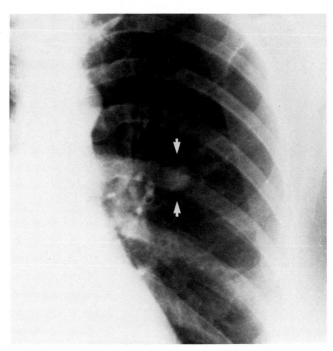

Fig. 3-24. Typical appearance of a solitary pulmonary nodule (*arrows*) with no distinguishing characteristics. This example proved to be a primary small cell carcinoma that had already metastasized to the brain.

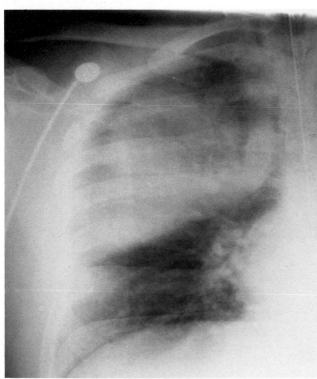

B

Fig. 3-23. Round pneumonia. A. Rounded, soft-tissue mass in right upper lung field. B. Progression to extensive lobar consolidation within 24 hours.

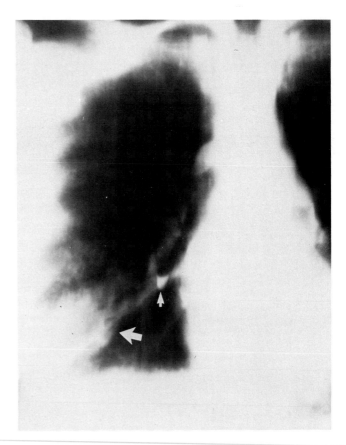

Fig. 3-25. Tomographic section through the right lung demonstrating an aspirated tooth (*small arrow*) wedged in the right lower lobe bronchus with distal atelectasis and pneumonia (*large arrow*).

ally recognize an artifact. The disappearance of an artifact on a repeat film confirms the diagnosis.

Many solitary pulmonary nodules have no distinguishing traits, however (Fig. 3-24). In no way does this mean that entities like hamartoma or granuloma can be eliminated from the differential list, but it does mean that malignancy must be considered. The tumor may be primary lung cancer, if age and history are appropriate, or a metastatic tumor if a primary tumor already exists.

The principal effort must be directed at proving the benignancy or malignancy of the identified mass in the absence of the characteristic features described above. Results from other diagnostic studies, such as negative sputum cytology and positive skin tests, provide only circumstantial evidence that a lesion is benign. Old chest films showing no change in the size and shape of the nodule over at least a year provide the only proof, short of excision or bronchoscopic biopsy, that the mass is benign.

The advent of CT has raised the possibility that its precise, computerized, numerical reading of radiographic density might facilitate differentiating benign from malignant lesions. Studies reported in the radiologic literature indicate that densely calcified lesions have characteristically high CT numbers, and some radiologists feel that such determinations can be definitive in diagnosing benignancy. Others feel that the same information is present on conventional chest films or tomography and that only rarely does CT provide additional information significant for evaluating a coin lesion.

Upper Airway Disease

Upper airway disease includes problems encountered between the epiglottis and the bronchi. The most acute problems in respiratory disease present in this area, and radiography often provides the opportunity for rapid diagnosis in an atraumatic manner.

ASPIRATION. Aspiration of a foreign body is usually considered a childhood occurrence, and often it is. But adults are also subject to such problems, especially if under the influence of drugs or alcohol. For an erect person, a discrete foreign body of appropriate size commonly falls into the most direct downward extension of the trachea, the right mainstem bronchus, then into the bronchus intermedius, and finally into the right lower lobe bronchus. The foreign body wedges itself into the first of these structures that has a diameter less than its own (Fig. 3-25).

Distal atelectasis may ensue, but a ball-valve effect with distal air-trapping more commonly occurs as an immediate effect. If a whole lobe is involved, there is increased lucency on the chest film and frequently diminished excursion of the affected hemidiaphragm as it appears fixed in an inspiratory phase of respiration. A comparison of inspiratory and expiratory phase films provides the best evidence for the limited diaphragmatic motion on the affected side (Fig. 3-26).

TUBE PLACEMENT. Endotracheal tubes can obstruct lobes and even whole lungs. The placement of an endotracheal tube is at best difficult, and the risks are even greater when done on an emergency basis. If accidentally placed beyond

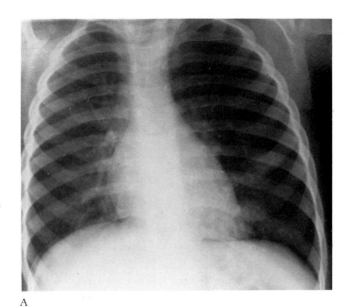

A

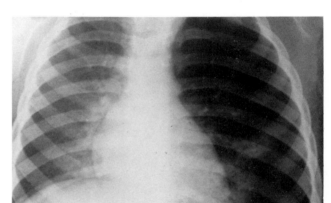

B

Fig. 3-26. Ball-valve effect demonstrated on inspiratory and expiratory phase films of a patient with a radiolucent foreign body in the left main bronchus. A. Inspiratory phase film showing slightly increased volume to the left hemithorax and slight increased lucency. B. Expiratory phase film showing no volume loss in the left and accentuating the difference between the two sides.

the carina, the tube tends to follow the same path as the aspirated foreign body, that is, right main bronchus to bronchus intermedius to lower lobe bronchus. If the cuff is inflated with the end in the right main bronchus, atelectasis of the left lobe likely occurs. Even without a cuff, wedging the tube in the bronchus intermedius obstructs the right upper lobe bronchus and causes atelectasis (Fig. 3-27). A portable chest film done after tube placement should show its end 2 to 4 cm above the carina if properly placed.

ACUTE UPPER AIRWAY OBSTRUCTION. Epiglottitis causes rapid respiratory embarrassment. The acute attack, normally caused by *Haemophilus influenzae,* is usually a disease of children, but adults can also be afflicted. Radio-

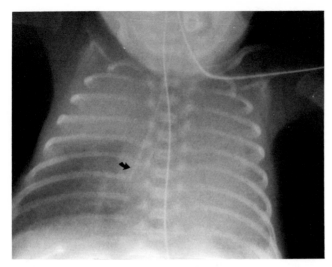

Fig. 3-27. A neonate with endotracheal tube (*arrow*) wedged in the bronchus intermedius, resulting in atelectasis of the entire left lung and right upper lobe.

graphs provide an excellent atraumatic means of making the diagnosis. Direct visualization of the inflamed epiglottis is ideal, but the patient may be in considerable respiratory distress and attempts at direct visualization may precipitate further occlusion. A lateral radiograph of the neck with soft-tissue technique clearly and rapidly delineates the size of the epiglottis without provoking added respiratory distress (Fig. 3-28).

Several other causes for acute respiratory embarrassment occur in the same area and require the same radiographic technique for evaluation of size and extent. These include retropharyngeal abscess and retropharyngeal hematoma as complications of surgery, trauma, or anticoagulation. Laryngeal edema does not need radiologic confirmation since there is usually a clear association with an anaphylactic reaction.

TRACHEAL STENOSIS. Endotracheal tubes also have lasting effects long after they have been removed. Most problems occur at tracheostomy stoma sites. Cicatrization develops over the course of months to years, resulting in local encroachment upon the tracheal air column. A soft-tissue lateral radiograph of the neck demonstrates the abnormality.

If a cuffed tube has been in place, the balloon may have caused superficial ulceration and subsequent circumferential scarring. Thus, narrowing should be apparent on chest radiographs. On occasion the balloon damages the tracheal cartilage; the resulting localized malacia causes a segment of floppy trachea and consequent dyspnea on exertion, and stridor. Fluoroscopy may be adequate to define the abnormal segment of trachea, but a contrast study may be necessary to reduce the effect of overlying shadows.

The tube tip may also cause complications. The tip may chronically rub against the mucosa and denude it, again setting the stage for long-term scarring and tracheomalacia. If tracheal narrowing is evident on chest radiographs just proximal to the carina, the tube tip likely caused the problem.

TRACHEOBRONCHOMEGALY. Tracheobronchomegaly, also known as Mounier-Kuhn syndrome, appears to be a congenital connective tissue disorder resulting in marked

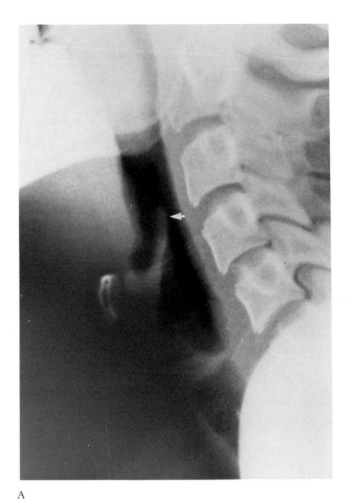

A

B

Fig. 3-28. The normal and abnormal epiglottis. A. Lateral view of the neck demonstrating a normal, thin epiglottis (*arrow*). B. View demonstrating an enlarged edematous epiglottis (*arrow*) and associated inflamed ariepiglottic folds (*curved arrow*). Note marked narrowing of the infraepiglottic space (*arrowhead*).

widening and flexibility of the cartilaginous rings of the trachea and the bronchi. Additional ectasia and sacculation of the mucosa between the rings also occurs. Clinically, patients develop chronic bronchitis and bronchiectasis as a result of the diminished ability to remove secretions.

Radiographically, the PA chest film shows what appears to be a mediastinal mass but is in fact a trachea 30 to 40 mm in diameter. Bronchography demonstrates the widening and sacculation of the trachea and large bronchi.

SABER SHEATH TRACHEA. Quite often an abnormality is identified without really knowing its significance; the *saber sheath trachea* is such an example. We and other radiologists have identified patients whose chest films demonstrate a trachea significantly wider on the lateral projection than on the PA projection by at least a factor of two (Fig. 3-29). This abnormal configuration is limited to the intrathoracic trachea. Virtually all the patients are males with emphysema and long histories of smoking. No one knows if the emphysema causes the unusually configurated trachea or the abnormal trachea contributes to the emphysema.

Chronic Obstructive Pulmonary Disease

With the aging of our population and the advances in treating infectious respiratory disease, chronic obstructive pulmonary disease (COPD) has become the most significant noncancerous pulmonary affliction. Environmental pollution and occupational exposure play a role in causation, but for the vast majority of the population cigarette smoking causes COPD. Chest radiographs are important for following the course of the disease and evaluating complications, but they have not been valuable for initial diagnosis. By the time the disease has progressed far enough for the radiologist to be unequivocal in the diagnosis, the patient can usually say, "Doctor, I have emphysema."

The two predominant forms are emphysema and chronic bronchitis. They are represented by the so-called "pink puffer" and "blue bloater", respectively. These terms portray clinical extremes, and in their pure forms are fairly easy to separate radiographically; however, many patients lie at other points along the clinical spectrum and so their radiographic features may be less than characteristic.

EMPHYSEMA. The radiographic changes in emphysema relate to both the lung parenchyma and the musculoskeletal thorax (Fig. 3-30). The lungs appear hyperlucent as a result of both their increased volume and the reduction of the bronchovascular markings due to the encroachment of emphysematous disease upon the interstitium. Hyperlucency alone, however, is inadequate for making the diagnosis of emphysema. Changes in radiographic technique, specifically over-exposing the film, may simulate hyperlucency of the lungs by blackening the entire image.

While the peripheral vessels tend to disappear on the emphysematous chest film, the perihilar arteries are often more prominent. This "pruned tree" appearance results from the pulmonary arterial hypertension secondary to the chronic lung changes and rising alveolar PCO_2. Even in

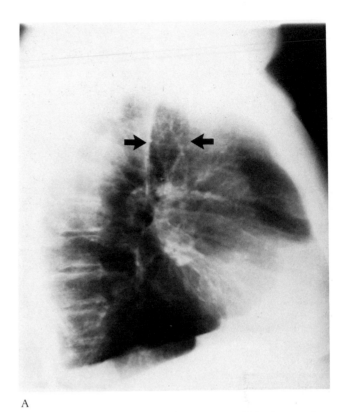

A

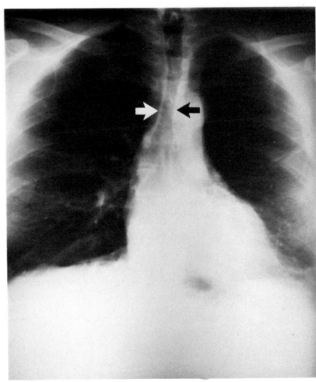

B

Fig. 3-29. Saber sheath trachea. A. Widened intrathoracic trachea (*arrows*) on lateral projection. B. Narrowed intrathoracic trachea (*arrows*) on PA projection.

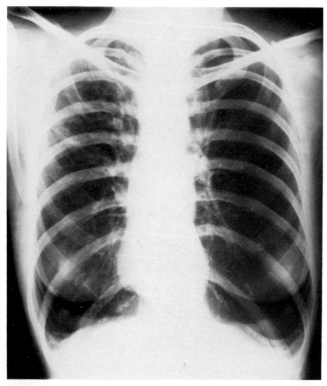

A

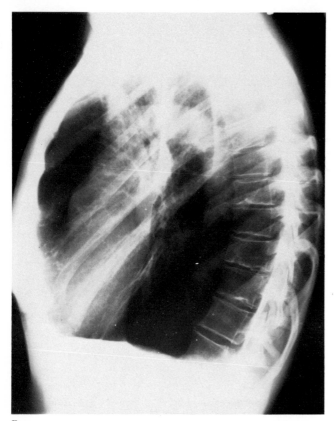

B

Fig. 3-30. Emphysema. A. PA projection demonstrating hyperlucent lungs, diminished bronchovascular markings, flattened diaphragms, and a vertical heart. B. Lateral projection demonstrating a barrel chest and prominent lucent space behind the bowed sternum.

patients where pulmonary hypertension is not yet significant, the generalized reduction in bronchovascular markings makes the remaining markings appear more prominent.

The changes in the thorax result in development of a barrel chest. The anterior-posterior dimension of the thorax increases, with development of a lucent space behind the sternum as it bows forward. The diaphragms also flatten. These thoracic changes combine to give the heart a vertical configuration; it appears to hang from its base rather than rest on the left hemidiaphragm.

CHRONIC BRONCHITIS. The chest film of a patient with long-standing emphysema looks pathologic, but the film of the blue bloater with chronic bronchitis does not look like much of anything. The chronic bronchitic may show increased bronchovascular markings, especially toward the lung bases, but so do many interstitial pulmonary diseases. Increased markings are likely the result of peribronchial thickening and inflammation from the basic disease process. They are the radiographic manifestations of the chronic bronchitic's classic clinical features, the hacking, smoker's cough, and the expectoration of much sputum. There are no emphysematous changes, and the heart can be either normal or enlarged.

Both these varieties of COPD, despite their radiographic differences, have the same pattern on a nuclear medicine ventilation lung scan. On single breath inhalation the uptake of radioactivity is patchy, and on the washout phase the clearance of radioactivity is delayed from the diseased segments (Fig. 3-31). Ventilation lung scans are usually not performed to make the diagnosis of COPD, since pulmonary function and blood gas studies are more sensitive. Lung scans are usually used to diagnose other problems, such as pulmonary embolus, and then the underlying pattern of COPD emerges, complicating the interpretation of the study.

OTHER OBSTRUCTIVE DISEASES. Alpha$_1$ antitrypsin deficiency is an autosomal recessive trait that has a high association with emphysema in young adults, starting in the third decade. The radiographic pattern of emphysema at a young age is conclusive for this inherited disease. The pattern usually shows a slight but recognizable difference from that of conventional emphysema. In conventional emphysema the upper lobes display the most severe disease and complicating blebs and bullae. In alpha$_1$ antitrypsin deficiency these same findings are most pronounced at the bases.

Asthma is more common in children than adults, and it is simpler to identify radiographically in children than adults. In a child the chest film demonstrates peribronchial thickening radiating from both hilar regions, along with flattened diaphragms and hyperlucent lungs characteristic of diffuse air-trapping. The peribronchial thickening creates "tram lines" if the bronchi are viewed in their long axis and "donuts" if they are seen axially (Fig. 3-32). In theory the same findings exist on the film of an adult asthmatic during an acute episode. In practice the findings are often not very impressive. Most impressive is the lack of diaphragmatic excursion as a result of the air-trapping, but limited excursion is a fluoroscopic finding, and there is normally no reason to fluoroscope these patients. Most radiographs of asthmatics are requested to evaluate the lungs for possible pneumonia, which is occasionally the insult that triggered the asthmatic episode.

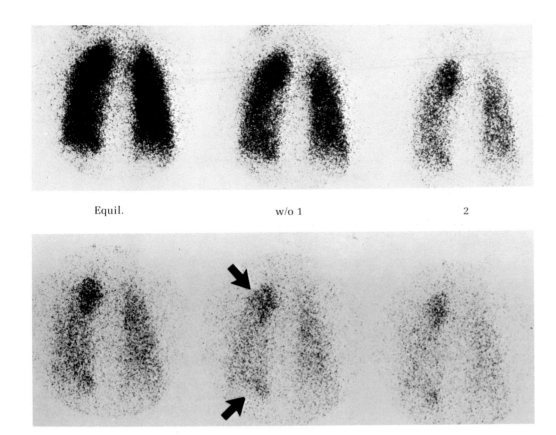

Equil.   w/o 1   2

3   4   5

Fig. 3-31. Ventilation lung scan demonstrating equilibration phase. Five images during washout show delayed clearance of radioactivity in diseased areas (*arrows*).

upper

Lower in α-1 antitryp

COMPLICATIONS. Blebs and bullae are abnormal cystic accumulations of air that occur secondary to emphysema. Precise definitions exist to separate blebs and bullae. In general, blebs are cystic accumulations contiguous with the visceral pleura, while bullae are intraparenchymal cystic changes from the panacinar destructive process. Practically, the distinctions are insignificant since there may be no radiographic way to prove that an air-filled cyst truly abuts the pleura. Blebs and bullae most often affect the apices of emphysematous upper lobes (Fig. 3-33).

Should one of the cystic accumulations of air rupture through the visceral pleura, a pneumothorax occurs. In patients with COPD, a pneumothorax usually results in only partial lung collapse because the underlying obstructive disease tends to keep much of the lung expanded. Previous pleuritis and resulting adhesions also hold the lung in place (Fig. 3-34).

An acute asthmatic attack produces a pneumomediastinum more commonly than a pneumothorax. The bronchial spasm most prominent in the expiratory phase of respiration causes increased bronchial and alveolar pressure, raising the risk of dissection of air into the lung interstitium. The air tracks centripetally to the hilum, resulting in a pneumomediastinum. On the PA chest film the air creates a lucent band or halo just lateral to the upper cardiac silhouette (Fig. 3-35). On the lateral projection the lucency is just above or anterior to the heart. If the patient still has a thymus that has not involuted, the pneumomediastinum lifts the thymus off the heart, thereby making the diagnosis of mediastinal air more evident.

Cor pulmonale results from the persistent stress of pulmonary arterial hypertension on the heart. Resulting right heart failure may complicate any form of COPD, but tends to occur earlier in the course of chronic bronchitis than in the course of emphysema. There is often no significant radiographic change beyond the previously described pulmonary arterial hypertension, despite right ventricular failure.

Pneumoconioses

The pneumoconioses are diseases that result from inhalation and deposition of inorganic materials that are at best merely lung irritants. Such exposures are usually work-related, and often take 10 to 20 years to become debilitating. The more common entities have certain characteristic radiographic features.

SILICOSIS AND COAL WORKER'S PNEUMOCONIOSIS. Significant similarities exist between silicosis and coal worker's pneumoconiosis (CWP), both in the clinical picture and the x-ray findings. For each, the classic appearance of uncomplicated disease is a pattern of small soft-tissue nodules (3 to 8 mm) spread evenly throughout the lungs but tending to predominate in the upper lobes. On occasion calcification occurs, but it tends to be a central nidus in each nodule. Variations include associated reticular patterns such as Kerley lines. Hilar adenopathy may also occur. Peripheral calcifications of hilar nodes, known as egg-

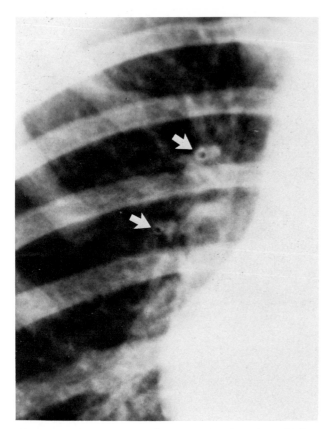

Fig. 3-32. Donuts (*arrows*) characteristic of peribronchial thickening in asthma.

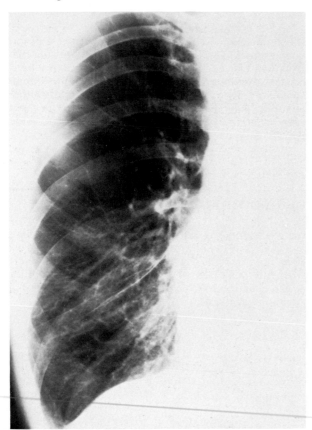

Fig. 3-33. Blebs and bullae in a patient with severe emphysema, resulting in loss of lung markings in the upper half of the right lung and compression of the remaining lung markings in the lower half.

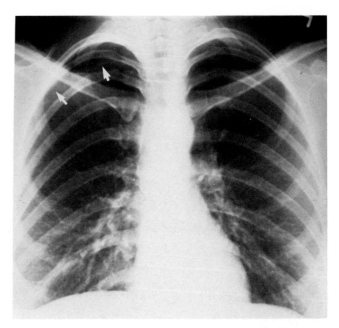

A

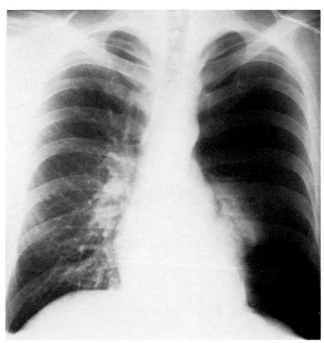

B

Fig. 3-34. Pneumothorax. A. Small pneumothorax at the right apex, with the pleural line (*arrows*) barely visible. B. Complete left-sided pneumothorax with lung collapsed down on the left hilum.

shell calcifications, are almost pathognomonic for silicosis (Fig. 3-36).

Confusion exists because experts have not agreed whether CWP is different from silicosis. Some authorities maintain that CWP develops in the absence of silica, but there appears to be a much higher incidence of CWP in anthracite regions where considerable silica is present in the coal. Other authors refer to the disease as anthracosilicosis, intentionally blurring the distinction.

Both diseases have an advanced form with the same basic radiographic appearance; however, there are slight

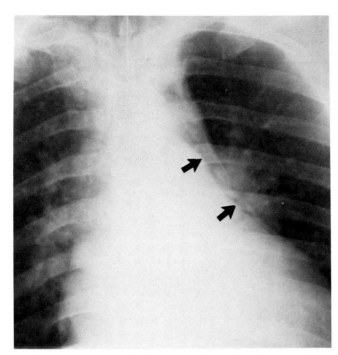

Fig. 3-35. Pneumomediastinum. Note lucent band (*arrows*) along the left cardiac border.

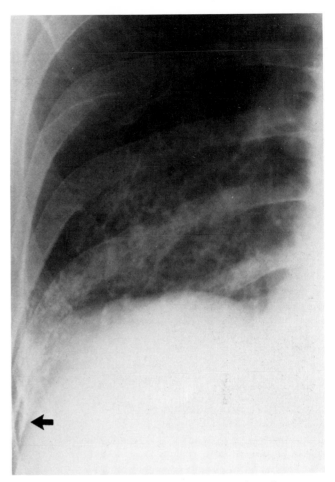

Fig. 3-37. Asbestosis with increased interstitial markings at the lung base and calcified pleural plaque (*arrow*).

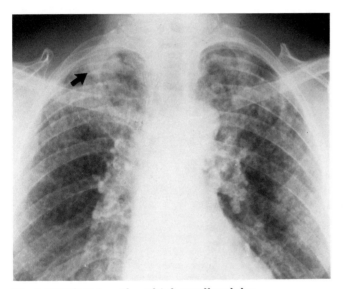

Fig. 3-36. Silicosis with multiple small nodules predominating in the upper lobes and peripheral eggshell calcifications in perihilar and paratracheal lymph nodes. Note conglomerate mass (*arrow*) near right apex.

differences in the terminology used to describe them. Complicated or advanced silicosis is characterized by the confluence of silicotic nodules into conglomerate masses that reside in the upper lobes and are pulled toward the hilar regions by cicatrization (see Fig. 3-36). The peripheral portions of the lungs often suffer severe emphysematous changes.

Complicated CWP develops virtually the same features that advanced silicosis does, but in CWP these are termed *progressive massive fibrosis* (PMF). If any radiographic distinctions are to be made, conglomerate masses tend to have irregular, fuzzy borders, while the densities of PMF are more likely to be discoid and smooth. Respiratory dis-

ability results from secondary emphysema more than from the centripedally moving masses, which cavitate on occasion. Difficulties may also arise in distinguishing one of these masses from bronchogenic carcinoma or tuberculosis, which have formerly had a strong association with these pneumoconioses. An additional association exists between CWP and rheumatoid arthritis. Caplan's syndrome includes large necrobiotic nodules, 1 to 3 cm nonmigratory peripheral masses, in conjunction with rheumatoid arthritis and silicosis or CWP.

ASBESTOSIS. Among inhaled particles asbestos is unique for the variety of damage it can cause. It is responsible for direct pleural and parenchymal damage as well as for inducing pleural malignancy, mesothelioma, and acting synergistically with cigarette smoking to generate bronchogenic carcinomas. (The cancers are discussed in detail in the sections on pleural disease and lung cancer).

Asbestos particles produce a pattern of lung disease that differs very little from many other causes of interstitial fibrosis. After many years of exposure the principal radiographic manifestation is a fine, reticular pattern predominantly involving the lower half of the lungs (Fig. 3-37). Over a span of years the pattern progresses to the more coarse appearance of honeycombing. Upper lobe involvement follows lower lobe involvement at a slower pace.

Asbestos has a high incidence of pleural disease. The characteristic lesion is the parietal pleura-based plaque, which appears as a small, soft-tissue density between lung

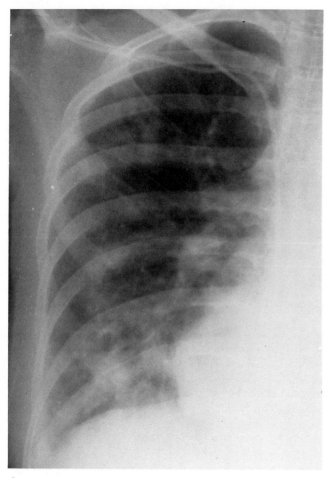

A

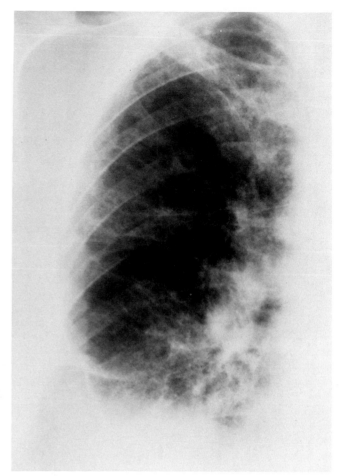

B

Fig. 3-38. Hypersensitivity pneumonitis. A. Acute exposure in a sensitized pidgeon breeder showing hazy, confluent densities. B. Same patient 15 years later with extensive nonspecific fibrosis.

and ribs tending to follow the rib contour. On a PA chest film such a plaque is only visible along the lateral chest wall. Plaques often appear in the absence of parenchymal disease. Some patients demonstrate a more diffusely thickened pleura that may extend for multiple interspaces, and a small percentage of patients may also have pleural effusions. Computed tomography provides more complete evaluation of pleural surfaces and usually demonstrates more extensive pleural involvement than is apparent on plain films.

Pleural plaques often develop linear calcifications (Fig. 3-37). Calcified plaques are especially common along the diaphragm and are almost pathognomonic for asbestos exposure. The incidence of pleural calcifications has been reported variously to be from 20 to 60 percent in patients with plaques, the higher frequency resulting from CT studies, which are more sensitive for detecting calcium than are conventional films.

BERYLLIOSIS. Beryllium exposure is one of the more esoteric occupational inhalation diseases. At one time beryllium had fairly wide usage, including incorporation in fluorescent light bulbs. Currently its use appears limited to the aero-space industry and nuclear reactor work. Overwhelming exposure to beryllium fumes results in acute pulmonary edema similar to that resulting from acute exposure to large doses of many other toxic gases.

Long-term exposure to small quantities of beryllium results in chronic lung disease. The radiographic pattern is less distinctive than that of asbestosis or silicosis. Berylliosis causes a reticular pattern with superimposed, small,

irregular nodules diffusely involving the entire lung. These features progress to extensive debilitating fibrosis and honeycombing. Hilar adenopathy may also develop. The general lung pattern suggests sarcoidosis (see Fig. 3-54).

HYPERSENSITIVITY PNEUMONITIS. Another whole set of inhalational lung diseases results from exposure to antigenic material. Most of these diseases result from occupational hazards, and so they also belong in the category of pneumoconiosis. The prototype is farmer's lung caused by exposure to stored, moldy hay; the disease process has both an acute and chronic phase. Other relevant diseases are bagassosis, mushroom worker's lung, pigeon-breeder's lung (bird-fancier's lung), and humidifier lung. In most of these conditions the offending antigens are contaminating thermophilic actinomycetes, although other antigens are responsible for pigeon-breeder's lung. The disease process has also been known by other names, most commonly allergic alveolitis, but hypersensitivity pneumonitis is actually a more appropriate term since these conditions have both alveolar and interstitial components. The radiographic pattern is a function of the predominant component.

In a sensitized person acute exposure to an overwhelming concentration of antigen generates an alveolar response, with fluffy or hazy consolidation appearing predominantly in the mid-lungs and sparing the apices and bases. This bat wing pattern of edema is not different from that of noncardiogenic pulmonary edema or adult respiratory distress syndrome (Fig. 3-38A).

More chronic involvement results from years of low-grade exposure resulting in a gradual impairment of respiratory function and a concomitant increase in interstitial disease. Early radiographic manifestation is a nonspecific increase in reticular-nodular markings. Over 10 to 20 years markings become more coarse, representing extensive fibrosis and honeycombing (Fig. 3-38B). History is essential for making the diagnosis, because nothing in the radiographic appearance separates the fibrosis of long-standing hypersensitivity pneumonitis from the same pattern produced by a multitude of other causes.

Tuberculosis and Fungal Diseases

These infections have many similar characteristics, the most significant of which is the extended time frame for interaction between microorganism and host. The infectious process, its treatment, and its radiographic changes are measured in months to years. Often, little separates the radiographic appearance of any one of these infections from the rest.

TUBERCULOSIS. Although the incidence of infection has dropped dramatically over the past 50 years in the United States, there are still 25,000 new cases per year. These infections do not distribute evenly through the population; most occur in the poor and the elderly in high-density population areas, patients who are most likely to make use of teaching medical centers. The disease process can be roughly divided into primary infection and reactivation phases.

Primary Infection. Primary infection refers to the interaction between host and bacteria during the first exposure of the host to the tuberculosis bacillus. The responses include parenchymal disease, adenopathy, or pleural effusion. The mid-lung is an especially frequent site for this pneumonic process. Regional adenopathy frequently appears in conjunction with the pneumonia (Fig. 3-39). Routine pyogenic pneumonias rarely generate enlarged nodes, so adenopathy and pneumonia that are prolonged despite antibiotics are circumstantial evidence for primary tuberculous infection. This is the usual appearance in children, who typically get primary tuberculosis: however, adults are now also at risk for developing primary tuberculosis because many were not exposed to the disease as children, due to improved tuberculosis control in our society. Adults present radiographically with the same basic patterns as children. Other, less distinctive findings may also occur with primary tuberculosis in children or adults. There may be adenopathy without pneumonia or even just an isolated pleural effusion. Other patients remain asymptomatic with primary exposure and may have no radiographic findings to go with the conversion to a positive PPD.

Most patients resolve this primary infection uneventfully. Frequently all that remains is a small parenchymal scar (often called a Ghon lesion) and a prominent, partly calcified, regional lymph node. The combination of scar

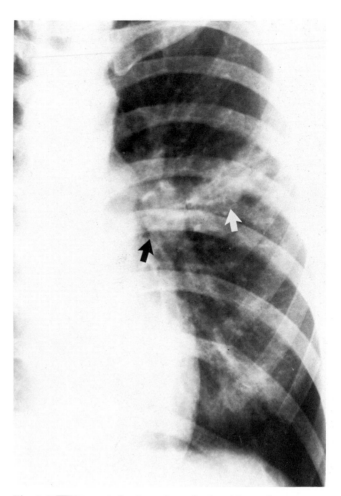

Fig. 3-39. Primary infection tuberculosis with patchy pneumonia (*white arrow*) and hilar adenopathy (*black arrow*).

and node is sometimes known as the Ranke complex, although this term is less common today (Fig. 3-40).

A granuloma or tuberculoma may also develop at the site of primary infection. This generally round, soft-tissue, 0.5 to 3 cm density probably represents a partially healed, partially walled-off primary infection that never resolved to a simple scar. If calcification is present, either circumferentially or in a laminated pattern, the diagnosis of granuloma can be quite certain, but asymmetric or irregular calcifications may appear in granulomas or malignancies (Fig. 3-41). Multiple granulomas may exist in the same patient, since the primary air-borne infection may have lodged at multiple foci.

Not all primary infections disappear harmlessly and leave only a scar, a granuloma, and a converted skin test as a souvenir; complications can occur. On occasion, for reasons that may not be clear, the primary infection erupts from confinement and spreads endobronchially, resulting in a virulent, aggressive pneumonia. Another uncommon complication is breakthrough of the infection into the vascular system, resulting in tuberculous septicemia. The shower of bacteria creates a characteristic lung pattern, miliary tuberculosis, which resembles a smooth carpet of 2 to 4 mm soft-tissue densities distributed uniformly throughout both lungs (Fig. 3-42). The uniformity of size and distribution is really only characteristic of tuberculosis, fungal diseases, and a few estoeric entities like alveolar microlithiasis and chickenpox pneumonia. Emboli of

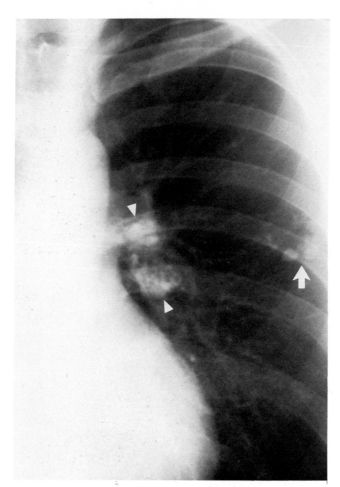

Fig. 3-40. Ranke complex, including calcified peripheral scar (*arrow*) and calcified hilar lymph nodes (*arrowheads*).

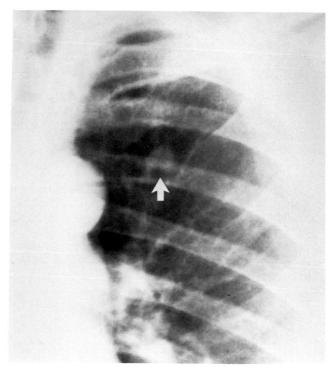

A

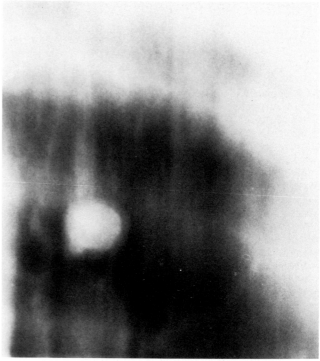

B

Fig. 3-41. Granuloma. A. Left upper lobe nodules (*arrow*) poorly defined on chest film. B. Circumferential calcification on tomographic section establishing its benign nature.

other bacteria usually distribute unevenly and appear in an array of sizes.

Reactivation. This phase of the disease, also known as secondary tuberculosis, may occur months to years following the primary infection. The consensus is that secondary tuberculosis almost always results from breakdown of the previously contained primary infection rather than from a new exogenous insult; hence the name reactivation.

The infection settles in the lung apices in at least two-thirds of patients and is frequently bilateral. The initial radiographic appearance is that of a poorly-defined, hazy density often partly concealed under the medial third of the clavicle. Small nodular and linear densities develop, with stranding extending down toward the hilum. These features result from the progression of the infection along with partial healing, all occurring simultaneously.

Cavitation commonly occurs in the area of reactivated infection. The radiographic features of this breakdown vary. Cavities may be single, multiple, air-filled, fluid-filled, thin-walled, thick-walled, smooth, or irregular. Bilateral apical disease occurs commonly, and the two sides are often at different stages of progression. The disease course runs over months to years, ultimately creating extensive, fibrocalcific scarring extending from the apex to the hilum, with marked parenchymal distortion and hilar elevation. Cavities may persist despite clearing of infection. Complications include hemoptysis, endobronchial spread with pneumonia, and miliary spread.

Conventional PA and lateral chest films are often inadequate for evaluating apical tuberculosis. Too much overlying bone detail from ribs and clavicle may obscure the shadows of early disease and the cavitary changes in later disease. Historically the apical lordotic projection was the alternate choice for viewing the lung apices with a minimum of overlying shadows. Conventional tomography

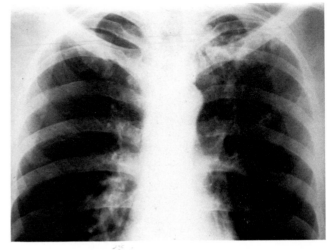

A

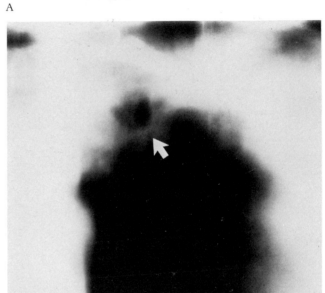

B

Fig. 3-43. Reactivation tuberculosis. A. PA chest film demonstrating poorly defined, increased density near the left apex behind the clavicle. B. Tomographic section clearly defining apical consolidation with cavitation (*arrow*).

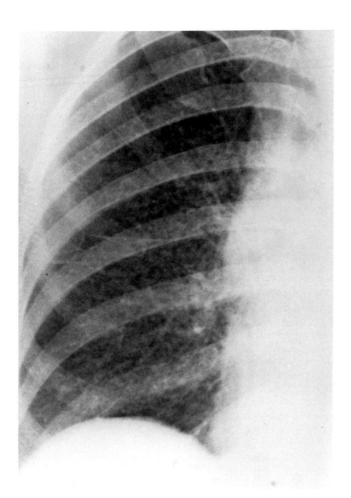

Fig. 3-42. Miliary tuberculosis characterized by uniform distribution of tiny nodules throughout the lung.

provides much fine detail and eliminates the complexities of positioning needed for the apical lordotic projection (Fig. 3-43).

Atypical tuberculosis. The radiographic findings of reactivation apical tuberculosis with negative tuberculin and fungal skin tests strongly suggest infection by an atypical mycobacterium, which can then be proved on culture. The two pathogenic strains are *Mycobacterium kansasii* and *M. intracellularis,* also known as the Battey bacilli. Both pathogens have radiographic features that are inseparable from those of *M. tuberculosis.* The bacterial type must be identified since treatment regimens differ.

HISTOPLASMOSIS. Few radiographic features separate tuberculosis from histoplasmosis. The concepts of primary infection and reactivation apply to both diseases.

Several differences are significant and should be mentioned. Histoplasmosis is endemic in the Ohio and Mississippi River valleys, and so chest films with granulomas from these areas are likely to show histoplasmosis. On occasion the patient's primary exposure to histoplasmosis is very great, and small foci of reactivity develop throughout the lungs. If these become granulomas, the radiograph demonstrates multiple 2 to 4 mm nodules spread diffusely throughout the lungs. In size these nodules resemble those of miliary spread, but usually number less than 100. If the granulomas calcify, the x-ray appearance is characteristic of histoplasmosis. The calcified granulomas loosely re-

semble multiple shotgun pellets (Fig. 3-44). Multiple calcified nodules of this size in the liver and spleen are also characteristic of histoplasmosis.

Another uncommon but notable complication of histoplasmosis is fibrosing mediastinitis as a result of cicatrization about involved nodes. Fibrosing mediastinitis has no specific radiographic appearance but its complications include superior vena cava syndrome, pulmonary artery obstruction, and bronchial occlusion. Malignancy is the more common cause of each of these problems, but histoplasmosis must be considered.

COCCIDIOIDOMYCOSIS. In the United States, coccidioidomycosis inhabits the arid environment ranging from west Texas to the San Joaquin Valley. Its radiographic appearance is similar to tuberculosis and histoplasmosis. Its cavitary form tends to have thinner walls than the other fungal diseases, but in any one patient wall thickness cannot be a critical factor in differential diagnosis (Fig. 3-45).

histo: shotgun pellets

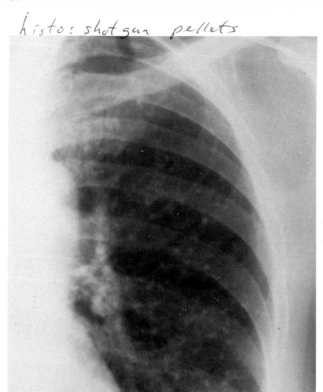

Fig. 3-44. Multiple, small calcified nodules throughout the lung characteristic of histoplasmosis.

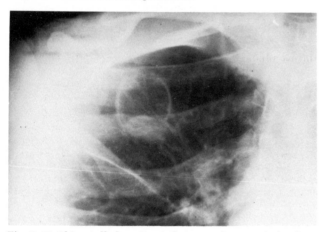

Fig. 3-45. Thin-walled cavity at the apex characteristic of coccidioidomycosis.

BLASTOMYCOSIS. Blastomycosis has a geographic distribution similar to histoplasmosis, but is far less common than histoplasmosis. Both primary and reactivation phases of the disease exist, but some patients have a subacute phase that tends to blur the distinctions between primary and reactivation phases. Primary infection tends to the lower lobes and chronic disease tends to the upper lobes, but the radiographic distinctions are not as clear as with tuberculosis and histoplasmosis.

ASPERGILLOSIS. Aspergillosis afflicts humans in multiple ways, and the immune competency of the host appears to be the key factor in determining the type of infection.

Allergic bronchopulmonary aspergillosis is characterized by asthma and positive skin testing to the antigen. The radiographic appearance of this hypersensitivity state includes air-trapping and mucous plugging, which may

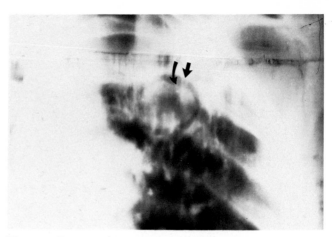

Fig. 3-46. Tomographic section showing a fungus ball (*curved arrow*) within an apical cavity (*arrow*).

progress to chronic fibrotic changes and bronchiectasis. Some patients also develop peripheral patchy areas of consolidation with eosinophilia (see the section on pulmonary infiltrates with eosinophilia).

Pulmonary aspergilloma is a fungus ball that may thrive wherever there is a preexisting lung cavity (Fig. 3-46). Tuberculous cavities appear to be the commonest sites. The radiographic appearance is that of a discrete, soft-tissue mass in a lung cavity. If the mass changes position on x-rays made in different patient positions, such as both decubitus projections, the diagnosis is a certainty. Should the mass be fixed to one wall, intracavitary clot or tumor is also a possibility. The aspergilloma may appear quite irregular and mimic thickening of a cavity wall, and then the diagnosis may be completely overlooked.

Invasive aspergillosis is the opposite extreme of allergic aspergillosis. The invasive form depends on immune incompetence and thrives in the same milieu as any other opportunistic invader. It proliferates in the terminally ill and immune-suppressed and is often fatal. Radiographically, invasive aspergillosis demonstrates progressive consolidation and may cavitate. Nothing in its appearance serves to distinguish it from any other fulminant infection under the same circumstances.

Bronchiectasis

Bronchiectasis is abnormal dilatation of bronchi, and is not a disease but rather the result of an assortment of problems affecting bronchi. These problems range from inherited diseases to overwhelming infection to damage behind a local obstructing mass. Overwhelming infection as a cause is very uncommon in this era of antibiotics, although such patients from third-world countries are still occasionally seen.

The appearance of bronchiectasis on chest x-ray is usually not definitive, and there may only be an increase in interstitial markings in the bronchiectatic region. On occasion tubular shadows are prominent as a result of peribronchial thickening; these appear as the tram lines and donuts seen more commonly in juvenile asthmatics (see section on chronic obstructive lung disease). The ectatic bronchi lose their ability to clear mucus. Mucoid plugs in such bronchi may appear as flame-shaped densities, or if these impactions occur at bronchial bifurcations they may result in V- or Y-shaped densities.

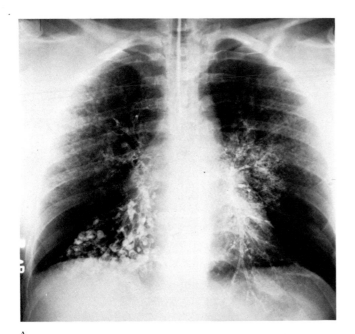

A

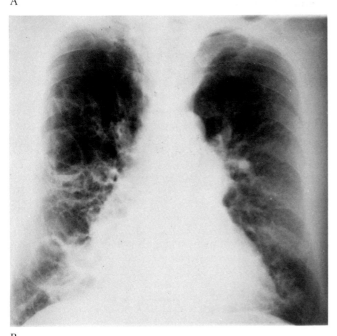

B

Fig. 3-47. Bronchiectasis. A. Cystic bronchiectasis at the right base. B. Saccular bronchiectasis involving the entire right lung.

The precise appearance of the bronchiectatic segment can only be established via bronchography. Descriptive terms include cylindrical, saccular, cystic, and varicose bronchiectasis (these descriptions arose in an era when bronchography was an art form). Cylindrical bronchiectasis shows no appropriate decrease in bronchial diameter with branching. Varicose bronchiectasis is a variant, with beading along the course of the affected bronchi. Saccular bronchiectasis is a more severe form, with pooling of contrast at the terminations of the bronchi. Cystic bronchiectasis demonstrates sacculations so extensive that they appear as bullae on plain films (Fig. 3-47).

Opportunities for performing bronchography are now limited, since bronchiectasis has become uncommon. In

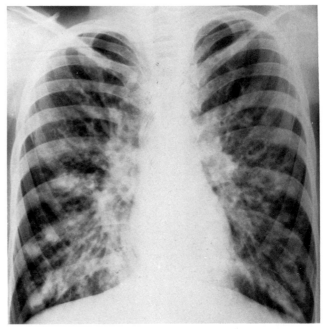

Fig. 3-48. Cystic fibrosis characterized by extensive bilateral air trapping, bronchiectasis, and fibrosis.

situations where the diseased portion of lung must be removed, surgeons may request bronchography to be certain that the remaining lung is normal. Other surgeons may be satisfied with a ventilation-perfusion lung scan to evaluate the remaining lung.

Diffuse bilateral bronchiectasis has only a limited number of causes. Cystic fibrosis produces extensive bronchiectasis because the viscous secretions plug the bronchi, creating ideal culture media for recurrent infection. The radiographic appearance of long-standing cystic fibrosis is a combination of air-trapping and extensive fibrosis in a young person (Fig. 3-48). There is, however, variable penetrance in cystic fibrosis, and many patients have only minimal x-ray findings. Recurrent aspiration and immune deficiency are other causes of repeated severe infection in the young that may produce x-ray findings similar to those of cystic fibrosis.

Most closely resembling cystic fibrosis in both development and radiographic appearance is the immotile cilia syndrome. Like cystic fibrosis, it has an autosomal recessive transmission and variable penetrance. Cilial inaction results in failure to mobilize bronchial secretions, which sets the stage for recurrent infection and bronchiectasis. Both cystic fibrosis and immotile cilia syndrome also develop associated pansinusitis.

Aspiration Pneumonia

Aspiration pneumonia often identifies itself by its tell-tale distribution. The bronchi to the lower lobes are the most dependent, and so aspiration pneumonia involves the lower lobes predominantly. Of course, if the patient has just tripped over his own feet and is now lying head down at the bottom of a short flight of stairs, the upper lobes may be preferentially affected. Significant radiographic differences exist between acute, fulminant aspiration pneumonia and chronic aspiration.

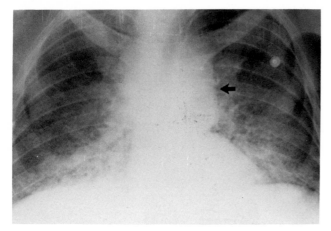

Fig. 3-49. Shock lung. Note the diffuse, ground-glass appearance of both lungs that developed following aspiration during unsuccessful surgery on an anterior mediastinal mass (*arrow*).

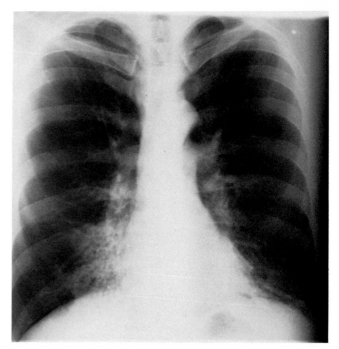

Fig. 3-51. Chronic aspiration. Fibrotic changes in both bases (partially obscured behind the heart) as a result of long-term abuse of oily nosedrops.

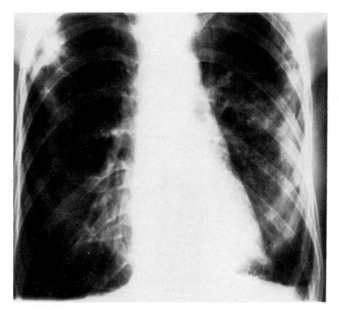

Fig. 3-50. Aspiration. Patchy pneumonia secondary to aspiration in both the right upper lobe and the periphery of the left lung.

ACUTE ASPIRATION. Acute aspiration most commonly occurs in the unresponsive person. Causes of the unresponsiveness include anesthesia, cerebrovascular accident, and drug or alcohol overdose. The worst possible scenario involves extensive aspiration of gastric contents with a low pH (<2.5). This material sets off both an inflammatory reaction and pulmonary edema, which may progress to adult respiratory distress syndrome (ARDS) in a matter of several days. Radiographically the early pattern of lower lobe, patchy consolidation progresses to the diffuse, ground-glass appearance of shock lung (Fig. 3-49). Alternately the chemical pneumonitis may be complicated by bacterial infection and even cavitation. Esophageal abnormalities, including achalasia and Zenker's diverticulum, predispose to aspiration (Fig. 3-50).

Hydrocarbon aspiration in small children is a special example. These aromatic materials (e.g., liquid furniture polish), are very attractive to youngsters and aspiration commonly occurs during drinking. Aspiration of aromatics even occurs in the absence of vomiting, possibly because the material with its very low surface tension is able to seep around the epiglottis and into the trachea. The pattern of pneumonia is usually basilar. Up to 24 hours may elapse between the time of ingestion and the radiographic evidence of consolidation.

CHRONIC ASPIRATION. The long-term ingestion of mineral oil and the use of oily nosedrops are the prime culprits for causing chronic aspiration. Neither occurs commonly anymore, but the sequelae persist. Restrictive lung changes occur at the bases, with fibrosis and scarring (Fig. 3-51). The radiographic pattern is indistinguishable from the basilar fibrosis of other disease entities, including asbestosis and collagen vascular disease. Without a high index of suspicion, it might be very difficult to identify aspirated oils as a cause of pulmonary fibrosis.

Somewhere between overwhelming, acute aspiration pneumonia and chronic aspiration lies a middle ground of intermittent low-grade aspiration. Causes include pharyngeal incoordination and epiglottic scarring. A special situation is the H-type tracheoesophageal fistula in the small child. This fistula is usually small enough that it is missed in the neonatal period. Recurrent pneumonia during early childhood should raise the possibility of aspiration through such a fistula.

ASPIRATION OF RADIOGRAPHIC CONTRAST. Standard, water-soluble, iodinated contrast material, the radiographic "dye" that is used for intravenous urography, CT enhancement, and arteriography, creates a real hazard in the lungs. Just as low pH gastric contents produce an inflammatory reaction and pulmonary edema, so does hypertonic (1600 mosm) contrast material. Hypertonicity is as deleterious as low pH.

Other radiographic contrast agents are significantly

safer. Iodized oils have a long, safe history in bronchography. Barium sulfate, despite its ugly appearance and uglier taste, is relatively harmless if aspirated. The new nonionic, low-osmolality, water-soluble contrast agents are the least harmful if aspirated. Consequently any radiographic procedure with an attendant risk of aspiration of the contrast should be performed with either barium sulfate or a nonionic iodinated agent.

Pulmonary Eosinophilia

A significant number of diseases with pulmonary involvement and eosinophilia exist. They have been loosely combined under the title pulmonary infiltrates with eosinophilia (PIE). The spectrum runs from the most benign Loeffler's syndrome through moderately severe chronic pulmonary eosinophilia to life-threatening Wegener's granulomatosis and polyarteritis. Problems exist with the PIE classification because some patients lack eosinophilia and others lack pulmonary infiltrates. Polyarteritis uncommonly affects the lungs and Wegener's granulomatosis usually demonstrates lumpy nodules that often cavitate (see the section on other interstitial lung diseases). The remaining eosinophilic lung diseases have a radiographic appearance that is often characteristic.

Benign pulmonary eosinophilia, or Loeffler's syndrome, is clinically characterized by its mild symptoms and transient nature. Radiographically there are patchy, cloud-like densities on the periphery of the lungs that result in a configuration that is the opposite of the bat wing pattern of pulmonary edema. At times the pattern is unilateral. Densities appear fluffy and alveolar and seem to overlap pulmonary segmental boundaries. They may also move over the course of days.

Chronic eosinophilic pneumonia is a protracted disease with the same radiographic appearance as Loeffler's syndrome (Fig. 3-52). The peripheral densities may change their configuration over the course of the disease, and asymmetry is quite common. The patients often suffer from atopy, and if an offending agent (pollen, drug, parasite, bronchopulmonary aspergillosis, etc.) can be identified and removed, the symptoms and peripheral densities resolve. For other patients the causes remain obscure, but steroids provide significant symptomatic and radiographic improvement.

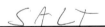

Sarcoidosis

Much mystery surrounds sarcoidosis. It can affect many systems, but the cause remains unknown and diagnosis remains difficult. About 80 percent of patients afflicted with sarcoidosis have thoracic involvement, and so the chest radiograph is very important. Radiographic findings in sarcoidosis can be divided on the bases of nodal and parenchymal involvement.

ADENOPATHY. Most patients with sarcoidosis exhibit hilar adenopathy, but many are asymptomatic. Thus, the disease is commonly identified on chest films sought for another purpose. Black females between the ages of 20 and 40 constitute the group at highest risk. Other disease pro-

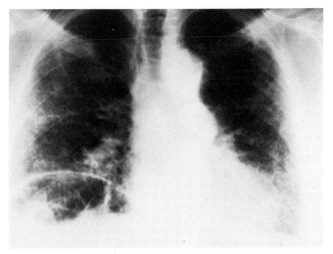

Fig. 3-52. Chronic eosinophilic pneumonia characterized by bilateral, patchy interstitial densities that are primarily peripheral.

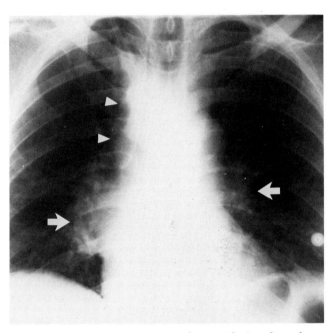

Fig. 3-53. Asymptomatic patient with sarcoidosis, where the chest film demonstrates large hilar lymph nodes (*arrows*) and enlarged although less apparent right paratracheal nodes (*arrowheads*).

cesses that might present in the same fashion include lymphoma, tuberculosis, and AIDS.

The most common radiographic appearance includes adenopathy in a triangular distribution, bilateral hilar adenopathy, and right paratracheal adenopathy (Fig. 3-53). The hilar nodes have been called "potato" nodes because of their lumpy, bumpy configuration. The lack of parenchymal involvement around them makes these lymph nodes all the more prominent. Less commonly, nodes in only two of these three sites are involved, and in about 5 percent of patients only one group of nodes is affected. Normally the nodes remain noncalcified, but in some patients they develop dense calcifications reminiscent of the healed granulomas of tuberculosis or histoplasmosis. Occasionally the nodes develop only peripheral calcifications, easily confused with the egg-shell calcifications of silicosis.

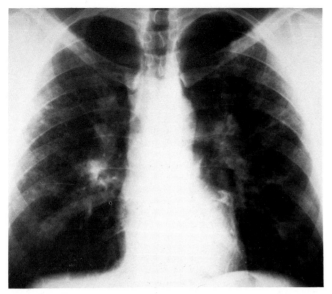

Fig. 3-54. Patient with sarcoidosis characterized by enlarged although poorly defined hilar lymph nodes and poorly defined interstitial densities throughout both midlung fields.

⊖ Effusion, ⊖ Cavitation

LUNG PARENCHYMAL INVOLVEMENT. No radiographic pattern of lung disease stands up and shouts, "I am sarcoidosis!" It often appears as diffuse, interstitial disease characterized by a reticular pattern and small, poorly defined densities (Fig. 3-54). This sort of "dirty lung" is a pattern that can be seen with many disease processes that are primarily interstitial. Occasionally the disease presents with a miliary pattern and is easily confused with tuberculosis. In about 10 percent of patients lung involvement appears alveolar, with large, fluffy, confluent areas of consolidation. Segmental or lobar atelectasis is uncommon but not rare. The atelectasis may result from either bronchial compression caused by adenopathy or an endobronchial sarcoid granuloma obstructing a bronchus. More commonly than not, hilar adenopathy coexists in patients who have parenchymal lung involvement (Fig. 3-55). Pleural effusions and cavitating masses are rare with sarcoidosis. If either feature is present on the chest film, a new diagnosis should be considered.

In some institutions radionuclide scintigraphy utilizing ^{67}Ga-citrate has been used to evaluate the activity of the lung disease. The more active the disease, the greater the gallium uptake in the lungs. Progressive parenchymal activity may indicate the need for treatment, specifically with long-term steroids.

In most patients the pulmonary effects of sarcoid clear with few sequelae. For others progression to chronic fibrocystic disease is relentless with extensive scarring, blebs, and bullae. Complications include fungus balls and pneumothoraces. The result is end-stage pulmonary disease radiographically indistinguishable from the end-stage of many other chronic lung disease. Mortality in sarcoidosis usually results from progressive lung involvement and superimposed cor pulmonale.

Reactions to Specific Agents

Certain agents have direct toxic effects on the lungs and present with radiographic findings that may assist in mak-

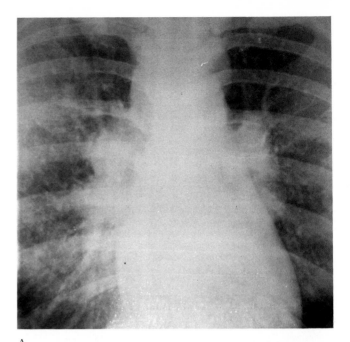

Fig. 3-55. Other manifestations of sarcoidosis. A. Extensive reticular nodular interstitial disease associated with "potato" nodes. B. Predominantly alveolar sarcoidosis characterized by a granular pattern particularly prominent on the right side, with associated bilateral hilar adenopathy.

ing the diagnosis. In general most of these agents are capable of both acute and chronic effects, and the radiographic picture reflects these differences.

DRUG-INDUCED LUNG DISEASE. Most drugs that cause lung changes as undesirable side effects are chemotherapeutic agents. Of these, the most common are methotrexate, bleomycin, busulfan, and BCNU. Other agents include the antimicrobial nitrofurantoin, and a new agent for refractory arrhythmias known as amiodarone. All these agents produce nonspecific interstitial pneumonitis and some alveolar damage.

The early findings on x-ray include a generalized increase in reticular, nodular markings and some fluffy con-

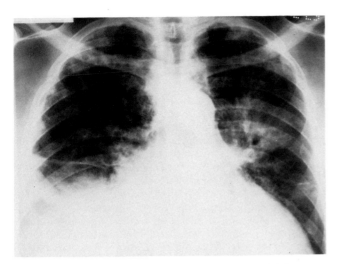

Fig. 3-56. Drug toxicity. Patchy increase in interstitial markings in both lungs particularly prominent in the perihilar regions as a result of amiodarone. Associated right-sided pleural effusion is an uncommon finding in drug toxicity.

fluence if the acute phase is fulminant. In general, the diffuse, streaky densities are indistinguishable from patterns encountered in most of the pneumoconioses and hypersensitivity pneumonitides (Fig. 3-56). Pleural effusions are uncommon. Since many of these patients have cancer, the differential diagnosis of this pattern also includes lymphangitic spread of tumor and atypical pneumonia in a compromised host.

Withdrawal of the offending medication leaves several possible results. Many patients recover essentially all pulmonary function, and abnormal x-ray findings disappear. Others have mild residual deficit and persistence of increased interstitial markings. A few progress to debilitating changes and a pattern of honeycombing and scarring on x-ray.

RADIATION INJURIES. Radiation effects on the lungs are much the same as those described earlier in this section. The acute phase usually starts during or shortly after significant radiation treatment to the chest, while chronic scarring and fibrosis may develop months later. There is one radiographic feature that allows for fairly easy recognition of radiation pneumonitis, either acute or chronic. The x-ray findings are confined precisely to the radiation treatment field. Thus, the x-ray abnormalities are bounded by the sharp lines of the portals and not by any reasonable anatomic boundaries (Fig. 3-57).

OXYGEN TOXICITY. Prolonged exposure to high concentrations and/or pressures of oxygen result in lung changes similar to those described previously. Acutely, the changes are those of alveolar damage and hyaline deposition, causing a fluffy confluent pattern of edema; these findings appear in a matter of days. To a large degree such oxygen toxicity is unavoidable, because the oxygen is necessary to treat an underlying pulmonary catastrophe, shock lung (adult respiratory distress syndrome or ARDS). Radiographically, the changes of shock lung cannot be separated from those of superimposed oxygen toxicity.

The chronic effects of oxygen toxicity resemble the chronic changes of all of the offending agents named in this section. The x-ray pattern of scarring and fibrosis extends from minimal to extensive and debilitating.

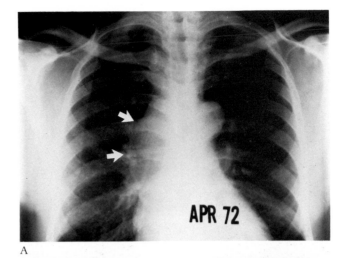

A

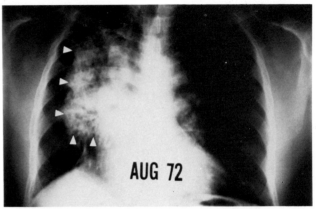

B

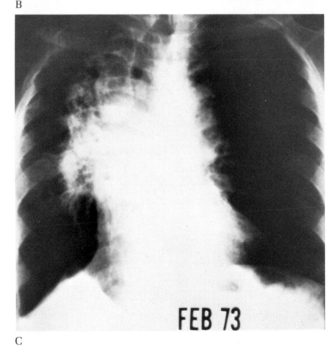

C

Fig. 3-57. Radiation injury. A. Bronchogenic carcinoma with superimposed right hilar adenopathy (arrows) in patient about to receive radiation therapy. B. Extensive radiation pneumonitis 60 days after the completion of radiation therapy, conforming to the sharp edges of the radiation fields (arrowheads). There is already the start of volume loss on the right, with tracheal shift to the right and right diaphragmatic elevation. C. Six months later there is residual radiation fibrosis with more pronounced volume loss on the right.

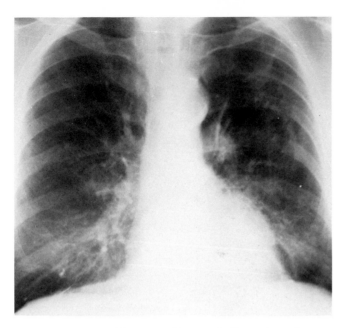

Fig. 3-58. Patient with 25-year history of silo work on the Mississippi River. The nonspecific reticular changes throughout both lungs are presumed to be the result of chronic oxygen toxicity.

SILO FILLER'S DISEASE. Nitrogen dioxide is an uncommon but potent agent for damaging lungs. The fermentation of ripe silage in silos generates oxides of nitrogen and consequently is the source of the disease name. Exposure acutely causes pulmonary edema, and chronic low-grade exposure results in fibrosis (Fig. 3-58). The oxides function as oxidants, and so the disease resembles oxygen toxicity. Since various industrial processes generate nitrogen dioxide, workers in jobs other than silo filler are also at risk for exposure.

Liquid-fueled rockets in another type of silo also have the potential for causing nitrogen dioxide exposure. The rockets use nitrogen tetroxide, a dioxide dimer, as the oxidant for the fuel. One fueling accident caused several deaths from acute toxicity and chronic lung changes in other exposed workers.

Other Interstitial Lung Diseases

There are a large number of diseases, primarily noninfectious inflammatory processes, that have only a limited way of expressing themselves when they involve the lungs. These diseases fall primarily into three categories: (1) collagen vascular disease, (2) interstitial pneumonitis, and (3) granulomatous angiitis. The radiographic pattern of lung disease runs from barely discernible reticular markings through diffuse nodularity to crippling involvement characterized by honeycombing. Some of the diseases tend to have more pulmonary involvement than others, but for any given patient the radiographic appearance alone is inadequate to make the diagnosis.

COLLAGEN VASCULAR DISEASES. The most common chest findings of lupus are effusions, both pleural and pericar-dial. During active phases of the disease, some patients demonstrate small, patchy densities, but significant nodularity or fibrosis is rare.

Of all the collagen diseases, scleroderma consistently demonstrates the most extensive lung findings. Prominent, reticular, nodular markings are seen in the lower half of the lungs and progress to scarring and fibrosis (Fig. 3-59).

Findings in patients with rheumatoid disease tend to fall between lupus and scleroderma in terms of lung involvement. Some patients with rheumatoid disease develop extensive restrictive lung disease, but this is uncommon. On the other hand, pleural effusions are common but often asymptomatic. Rheumatoid disease is also known for its necrobiotic nodules, and patients with such subcutaneous nodules tend to also have them in the lungs. On x-ray they appear as soft-tissue masses 1 to 5 cm in diameter that are usually near pleural surfaces and often cavitate (Fig. 3-60). Patients with any of the other collagen diseases may fit anywhere in the spectrum of no lung involvement to severe lung involvement.

INTERSTITIAL PNEUMONIA. Diseases in this category include desquamative interstitial pneumonia (DIP), lymphoid interstitial pneumonia (LIP), grant cell interstitial pneumonia (GIP), and usual interstitial pneumonia (UIP). Distinctions among the diseases are basically histologic. Radiographically the pattern runs from reticular and nodular changes in the early stages to coarse stranding and honeycombing as a result of chronic fibrosis in the later stages. About 10 percent of patients have no lung findings on x-ray. If there are observed abnormalities, there is a predilection for the lower lobes.

The term *Hammon-Rich syndrome* periodically resurfaces. Originally it was synonymous with interstitial pneumonia until that entity was better explained histologically. Now the eponym seems to be associated with any idiopathic interstitial fibrosis. Its use as a substitute for admitting ignorance is decried.

GRANULOMATOUS ANGIITIS. Two diseases, Wegener's granulomatosis and lymphomatoid granulomatosis, are the primary occupants of this category. Patients with Wegener's have the well-known triad of pulmonary nodules, sinusitis, and glomerulonephritis. The nodules tend to be 1-3 cm in diameter with no predictable distribution (Fig. 3-61), and often cavitate. The disease usually responds to cyclophosphamide. Lymphomatoid granulomatosis tends to have more confluent nodules that congregate at the bases, and there is often an underlying reticular pattern, even when the nodules clear. At least 10 percent of these patients develop lymphoma. The radiographic pattern of granulomatous angiitis most closely resembles that of rheumatoid disease with necrobiotic nodules.

NEUROFIBROMATOSIS. At least 10 percent of patients with von Recklinghausen's neurofibromatosis develop interstitial lung disease. A reticular, nodular pattern develops predominantly at the bases and continues on to extensive fibrosis. There is nothing diagnostic about the pattern nor about the blebs or bullae that may develop near the apices.

Other stigmata of neurofibromatosis should be readily identifiable on the chest film. Cutaneous neurofibromas are superimposed on the lungs as indistinct soft-tissue masses and more should be evident in profile along the lateral chest walls. Posterior mediastinal masses occur commonly and result from either nerve root neurofibromas

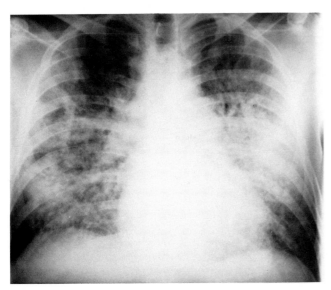

Fig. 3-64. Goodpasture's syndrome, with fluffy, alveolar densities primarily in the midlung fields, sparing the apices and the bases.

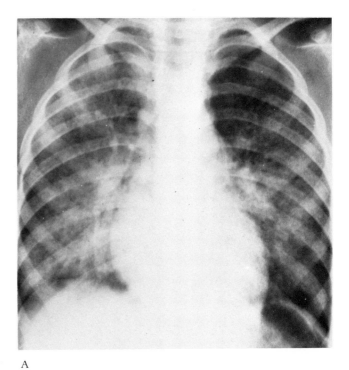

A

...tral stenosis may also cause pulmonary hemosiderosis and end-stage fibrotic lung disease.

OTHER CAUSES OF HEMORRHAGE. Warfarin (Coumadin) toxicity carries the risk of uncontrolled bleeding in the lungs. As with the diseases described earlier, such pulmonary hemorrhage tends to be symmetrical. Several other entities are likely to produce asymmetric hemorrhage. Trauma to the chest often creates a lung contusion that is a focal area of edema and hemorrhage (Fig. 3-66). Parenchymal destruction, as occurs in lung cavitation, can rupture vessels and induce hemorrhage. This is a recognized risk in the cavitating nodules of Wegener's granulomatosis, and such hemorrhage may obscure the underlying characteristic nodules. Vessels crossing tuberculous cavities (Rasmussen's aneurysms) are at risk for the same sort of rupture. A classic x-ray appearance of apical cavitary tuberculosis would be suddenly altered by superimposed fluffy densities while the patient experiences hemoptysis.

Rasmussen's Aneurysm

Atypical Infectious Pneumonias

The classic pneumonia caused by pyogenic bacteria results in a chest x-ray with segmental or lobar consolidation and prominent, branching air bronchograms (see the section on basic principles). The patient is appropriately symptomatic, and the correct antibiotic relieves both symptoms and x-ray abnormalities. But many pneumonias do not fit this pattern, and physicians often have difficulty making them fit into any radiographic pattern.

MYCOPLASMA AND VIRAL PNEUMONIAS. In the past, *mycoplasma* pneumonia has also been known as Eaton agent, pleuropneumonia-like organisms (PPLO), and primary atypical pneumonia. It is a disease commonly encountered in healthy young adults housed in close quarters, such as

B

Fig. 3-65. Five-year-old child with idiopathic pulmonary hemosiderosis. A. Acute phase with fluffy, alveolar consolidation. B. Six days later with essentially complete clearing. Early chronic changes are evident in the donuts (peribronchial thickening) seen in the right hilar region (*arrows*).

Lupus
Uremia
Goodpasture's   Pulmonary
Mitral Stenosis   Renal
Idiopathic   Syndromes

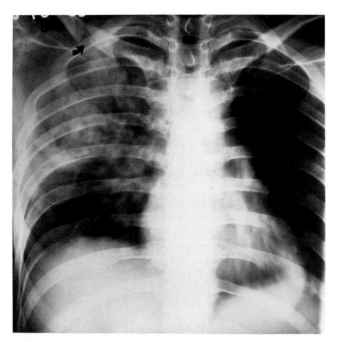

Fig. 3-66. Pulmonary contusion secondary to trauma with patchy, right upper lobe consolidation. Associated right clavicular fracture (*arrow*) is readily evident, but fractures of ribs 2, 3, 4, and 5 are not apparent in this projection.

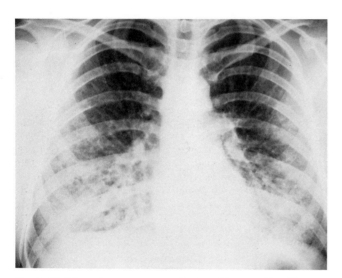

Fig. 3-67. *Mycoplasma* pneumonia in a 21-year-old college senior. Extensive patchy densities were essentially limited to the lower lobes at a time when the patient complained of cough and occasional, low-grade fevers over the previous week. Clearing followed one week of erythromycin.

barracks or college dorms. The radiographic course often begins with increased interstitial markings occurring in a fine to coarse reticular pattern that is often confined to a single lower lobe but is sometimes quite diffuse. After several days superimposed patchy consolidation often develops, quite commonly at both bases (Fig. 3-67). Effusions are rare.

The radiographic appearance is frequently more impressive than the patient's mild symptoms, and radiographic resolution lags behind clinical resolution. Viral pneumonias present essentially the same sequence of increased reticular markings progressing to patchy, nondescript densities. A rare exception is chickenpox pneumonia, said to resemble miliary tuberculosis and leaving in its wake a large number of 2 to 4 mm calcified nodules.

CHLAMYDIA. This group of quasi-viruses, quasi-bacteria may produce pulmonary involvement through either trachoma or psittacosis. Trachoma occurs in adults as well as children, and psittacosis is carried by poultry as well as parrots. There is no dependable radiographic pattern of chlamydial pneumonia. The x-ray findings run the gamut from streaky reticular markings and plate-like atelectasis to patchy, nonlobar consolidation.

LEGIONNAIRES' DISEASE. This disease was originally identified in local outbreaks associated with contaminated central air-conditioning systems. Since then the bacteria have also been implicated in disease in nonepidemic settings, including individual patients with chronic lung disease, alcoholism, renal failure, and immunosuppression from any cause. Unfortunately, the pneumonia associated with Legionnaires' disease has no consistent pattern. Densities may be segmental, perihilar, peripheral, or diffuse. Atelectasis and pleural effusions are common. In short, the radiographic pattern of pneumonia caused by *Legionella* can duplicate the pattern of most any other infectious pneumonia.

Acquired Immune Deficiency Syndrome (AIDS)

An immune-compromised patient used to mean one on high-dose steroids or chemotherapy or someone grossly debilitated by disease. Now the model is the AIDS patient, as well it should be with a doubling of new cases each year and an 80 percent two-year mortality rate.

The pattern on chest x-ray depends upon what combination of one or more of three factors is present. These factors are *Pneumocystis carinii* pneumonia (seen in nearly all patients with AIDS), other opportunistic organisms, and Kaposi's sarcoma. Pneumocystis presents initially with increased reticular markings, radiating mainly from the hilar regions. With the development of a fulminant clinical picture the radiographic pattern progresses to fluffy, confluent alveolar densities, sparing the apices and bases (Fig. 3-68). At this stage the radiographic image closely resembles the appearance and distribution of adult respiratory distress syndrome (ARDS). Resolution with appropriate treatment may take weeks to months and often leaves residual increased interstitial markings.

Other opportunistic invaders include cytomegalovirus, *Mycobacterium avium, M. intracellulare, Cryptococcus, Candida* and other fungi, *Legionella*, and even pyogenic

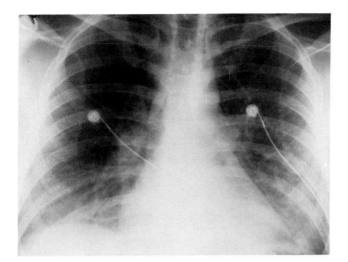

A

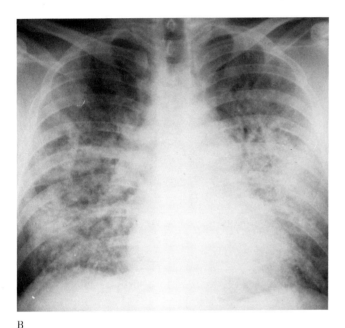

B

Fig. 3-68. *Pneumocystic carinii* pneumonia in a 30-year-old homosexual with AIDS. A. Mild to moderate involvement resulting in general haziness in the mid- and lower lungs. B. Twelve days later the patient is moribund, with fulminant, disseminated disease and a radiographic pattern of shock lung.

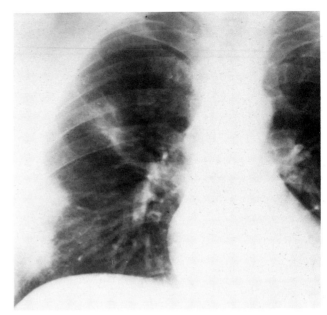

Fig. 3-69. Patchy densities in an asymptomatic AIDS patient, which proved on biopsy to be caused by *Cryptococcus*.

repeated lung biopsies for significant progression of radiographic findings, since the x-ray features are so nonspecific.

Noncardiogenic Pulmonary Edema

The vast majority of patients with pulmonary edema suffer from chronic cardiac disease and congestive heart failure, but many other causes of pulmonary edema exist; these include inhalation of smoke or other noxious fumes, intravenous drug abuse, head trauma, altitude sickness, near drowning, sepsis, anaphylactic reaction, fluid overload, and uremia. The final common pathway for most of these causes is probably increased capillary permeability, but much remains unknown. Direct chemical toxicity certainly plays a role in situations like silo filler's disease and aspiration of gastric contents, but neural reflexes and ischemia may also be significant in many instances.

THE BAT WING PATTERN. The bat wing succinctly describes the basic radiographic pattern of noncardiogenic pulmonary edema. There is fluffy alveolar consolidation radiating from the hilar regions that tends to spare the apices, bases, and periphery of the lungs. Others call it the butterfly pattern (see Fig. 3-2). A delay of up to 24 hours often occurs in the development of the full-blown radiographic features following the initial insult. Kerley A and B lines may also be evident, indicating interstitial as well as alveolar edema (see Fig. 3-8).

The question often arises in the clinical setting whether pulmonary edema is cardiac or noncardiac in origin. Several features on the radiograph may help to answer that question, but no absolute criteria exist. If pulmonary edema exists in conjunction with a normal-sized heart, it is unlikely to be cardiac in origin. In most instances of pulmonary edema secondary to congestive heart failure, car-

bacteria (Fig. 3-69). These invaders have no redeeming radiographic virtues. They usually demonstrate nonhomogeneous patchy densities similar to those in the atypical pneumonias. Even common pyogenic bacteria present with atypical pneumonia because of the host's limited inflammatory response. Kaposi's sarcoma may demonstrate a more nodular appearance, often with associated adenopathy.

The radiographic appearance of AIDS in the chest is made more complex because the three factors described above often complicate each other. Opportunistic invaders are often superimposed on the ever present pneumocystis, and any pneumonia may complicate Kaposi's sarcoma. Consequently the chest x-ray may include any combination of fluffy alveolar edema, reticular markings, patchy densities, and malignant nodules. Some investigators urge

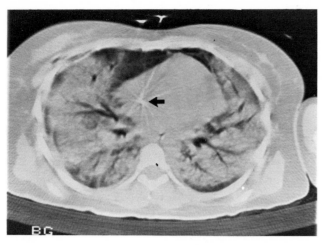

Fig. 3-70. CT image in a patient with shock lung, characterized by dense alveolar filling involving the entire chest and prominent air bronchograms. The stellate shadow (*arrow*) is the CT image of a pacemaker wire going through the right atrium.

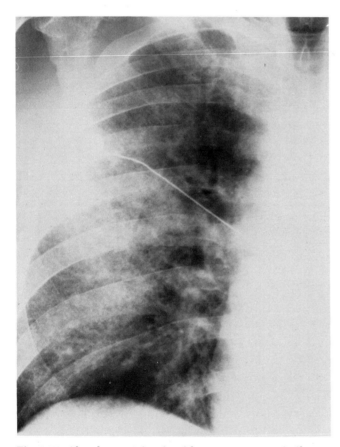

Fig. 3-71. Alveolar proteinosis with an appearance similar to that of pulmonary edema, sparing the apices and the bases.

alveolar proteinosis

vs

alveolar sarcoidosis

diomegaly has been a much earlier feature than pulmonary edema. Of course, exceptions exist. Acute cardiac failure, as in myocardial infarction or papillary muscle rupture, may precipitate pulmonary edema without the cardiac enlargement of chronic heart disease.

Pulmonary edema of chronic heart disease often lacks the bat wing distribution. It frequently involves the lower lobes, so that the edema appears to cascade from the hilar regions to the diaphragms. Other anomalies occur that may confuse the picture of pulmonary edema. Emphysema distorts lung architecture and changes both ventilatory and circulatory patterns. Noncardiogenic pulmonary edema in such patients may be both irregular and asymmetric. In other patients pulmonary edema is unilateral, despite the systemic nature of the insult.

SHOCK LUNG (ADULT RESPIRATORY DISTRESS SYNDROME). Radiographically the pattern of shock lung closely resembles the bat wing pattern of noncardiogenic pulmonary edema, but temporally these entities differ. Uncomplicated pulmonary edema usually clears in hours to days, whereas shock lung persists from days to weeks. Shock lung normally follows significant tissue destruction, such as massive thermal or muscle injuries or septic shock. The lungs need not be directly affected for the radiographic pattern and respiratory distress to develop. The bat wing pattern in shock lung changes with alterations in the pulmonary status of the patient. With improvement, the perihilar densities gradually fade away. With increasing respiratory embarassment and the development of hyaline casts, the radiographic shadows become more dense and granular as they coalesce and progressively fill both lungs (Fig. 3-70). The terminal patient has a diffuse "white-out."

ALVEOLAR PROTEINOSIS. Alveolar proteinosis is an unusual disease that also creates a bat wing, perihilar pattern of pulmonary alveolar filling, secondary to deposition of a proteinaceous material (Fig. 3-71). Alveolar proteinosis may wax and wane over a prolonged course, and this prolonged course, in association with a normal cardiac silhouette, should rule out both congestive heart failure and causes of acute noncardiogenic pulmonary edema. Alveolar proteinosis is most commonly mistaken for the alveolar phase of sarcoidosis on chest films. Many patients with sarcoidosis, however, have been correctly diagnosed by the time the alveolar phase on chest x-ray is reached. Alveolar proteinosis may be complicated by *Nocardia* or other opportunistic infection. Lately it has also been identified in association with immune deficiency syndromes, lymphoma, and leukemia.

Pulmonary Embolism

Pulmonary emboli are elusive. Hunting for them resembles tracking down quarks in cloud chambers, since there is often only circumstantial evidence for the existence of emboli. Statistics confirm the problem. One study showed that two-thirds of proved pulmonary emboli were asymptomatic. Another showed that 17 percent of autopsies on patients who died in hospital revealed a significant pulmonary embolus. Emboli are easier to identify if they result in pulmonary infarcts, but only 10 to 15 percent of emboli go on to infarct lung.

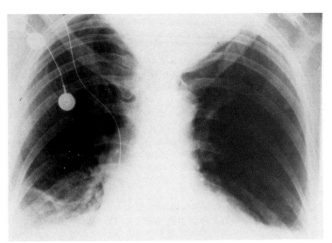

Fig. 3-72. Westermark's sign of pulmonary embolism, with virtually no pulmonary vascular markings evident on the left beyond the hilum when compared to the relatively normal vascular markings on the right.

EMBOLUS WITHOUT INFARCTION. Plain film diagnosis is exceedingly difficult since radiographic findings are not specific. The majority of radiographs following an embolus show no abnormality, but there are several signs that are sometimes useful. An embolus often causes peripheral oligemia, making the area of lung distal to the embolus appear relatively more lucent. This is Westermark's sign, but problems exist in identifying the sign (Fig. 3-72). The oligemia is ephemeral, usually lasting no more than 24 to 48 hours, and good reproducible film quality is essential for observation. Patients at risk often require portable, supine films, where quality control is less than ideal.

The hilar section of the pulmonary artery, proximal to the embolus, often bulges. This bulge may be the result of short-lived increased pulmonary arterial pressure or a large clot within the major pulmonary vessel. Occasionally an embolus causes local edema or hemorrhage, which appear as a radiodensity in the region of the embolus. With such a paucity of reliable radiographic features it is no wonder that many emboli are missed.

Lung Scanning. Radionuclide perfusion and ventilation scintigraphy have become an important part of diagnosing pulmonary emboli. In general, the ventilation scan serves a purpose similar to that of the chest x-ray; that is, it establishes the pattern of aeration. Ventilation should remain unimpaired in the presence of an embolus, and inhalation of a radioactive gas such as xenon-133 should result in a uniform distribution of radioactivity throughout the lungs. Conversely, the perfusion lung scan utilizing intravenous injection of an agent such as ^{99m}Tc macroaggregated albumin demonstrates a "cold spot," or area of diminished radioactivity, peripheral to the embolus. Thus the classic combination for a pulmonary embolus on lung scan is the ventilation-perfusion mismatch (i.e., a segmental or lobar perfusion defect in the presence of a normal ventilation pattern) (Fig. 3-73).

Unfortunately, most radionuclide lung scans provide somewhat less than certain results in the diagnosis of pulmonary embolus. Even the ideal ventilation-perfusion mismatch is only interpreted as being highly probable for embolus. Lung scans are customarily reported in degrees that range from low to intermediate to indeterminate to high probability of embolus. Only a normal finding is absolute (relatively). Lung scans are probably less accurate

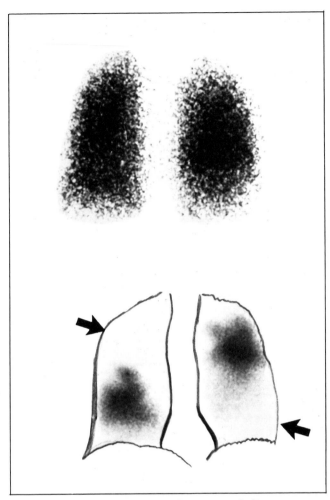

Fig. 3-73. High probability for pulmonary embolism. Ventilation and perfusion lung scans: At the top is the ventilation scan demonstrating essentially normal ventilation consistent with the normal chest x-ray; below is the perfusion scan in the anterior projection, demonstrating cold areas in the right upper lung field (*arrow*) and the left lower lung field (*arrow*). (Lung margins drawn in to demonstrate the anticipated distribution of the radioactivity if no emboli were present.)

than pulmonary arteriograms. In one recent comparative study an embolus was found on arteriography in 15 percent of patients with low probability scans, 32 percent with intermediate scans, 39 percent with indeterminate scans, and 66 percent with high probability scans. Yet other studies have shown better correlation between radionuclide studies and arteriograms.

Many times situations exist where it is vital to know if a patient has suffered a pulmonary embolus. Under those sets of circumstances the probabilities associated with interpretation of chest films and lung scans are not good enough. The pulmonary arteriogram is the definitive study. A filling defect in a vessel that either partially or completely obstructs it constitutes inequivocal evidence of an embolus. A vessel cut-off constitutes a finding only slightly less absolute on the arteriogram (Fig. 3-74).

EMBOLUS WITH INFARCTION. Infarcted lung is radiodense, indistinguishable in density from atelectasis or consolidation on x-ray. Infarctions have several features that help to distinguish them from other lung densities. Infarc-

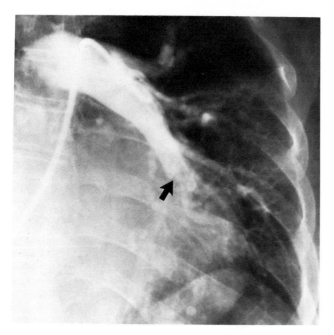

Fig. 3-74. Pulmonary arteriogram demonstrating a vessel cut-off (*arrow*) characteristic of a pulmonary embolus.

tions often appear triangular, with the apex directed to the hilum and the base contiguous with the pleura (Fig. 3-75). The apex is often called Hampton's hump, and this sign reflects the bulge of infarcted lung as opposed to an area of atelectasis, which would more likely be flat or concave as a result of volume loss. Pleural effusions commonly accompany infarcts.

Resolution of the radiodense infarct occurs in one to three weeks, whereas hemorrhage or edema of an uncomplicated embolus clears in several days. The pattern of resolution differs from that of consolidated lung, in that the latter resolves by gradually reaerating the affected volume and fading away. Infarcts resolve by decreasing in volume in the same manner that ice cubes melt.

In a sense, lung infarction complicates the interpretation of a ventilation-perfusion lung scan. The lung infarct creates matching perfusion and ventilation defects, as does pneumonia or atelectasis. However, the perfusion defect associated with an infarct is often larger than the corresponding density seen on x-ray. Additional areas of mismatched defects, suggesting other emboli without infarction, are also helpful in diagnosing pulmonary embolus in the presence of infarction.

Mediastinal Masses

The mediastinum is that space in the chest that includes all organs except the lungs and their pleurae. Although it is one continuous space, it is usually divided into front, middle, and back. The divisions are functional, with certain pathologies being characteristic of certain spaces. Whether the anterior mediastinum extends to the posterior edge of the heart in one definition, or only two-thirds that distance in another definition, is not important; the significance of division lies in the fact that a different set of diagnostic possibilities exists for a mass in one compartment than for a mass in another.

In this discussion, the mediastinum is divided into anterior, middle, and posterior portions. The anterior mediastinum extends from the sternum to just anterior to the trachea and includes the heart. The middle mediastinum extends to the anterior margin of the vertebrae and includes the trachea and esophagus. The posterior mediastinum extends back from the anterior lip of the vertebrae and includes the spinal cord and nerve roots. Even as a functional division, this system is less than perfect, as there are significant entities that appear in more than one compartment. In general, CT is the diagnostic study of choice to evaluate all three areas.

ANTERIOR MEDIASTINUM. Thymoma. The thymus appears as a prominent, twin-lobed, soft-tissue mass on pediatric chest films. It rests on the heart and fills most of the space behind the sternum on a young child's lateral chest radiograph. After early childhood the thymus is seen again on a chest radiograph only if it abnormally increases in size.

Radiographically, thymomas appear bumpy or smooth as they extend beyond one or both sides of the mediastinal shadow on the PA chest film, usually just above the heart. Some may even have calcifications. A significant association exists between the thymus and myasthenia gravis. Up to 15 percent of patients with myasthenia have thymomas, and many patients with myasthenia improve after thymectomy, even if no thymoma is present. Computed tomogra-

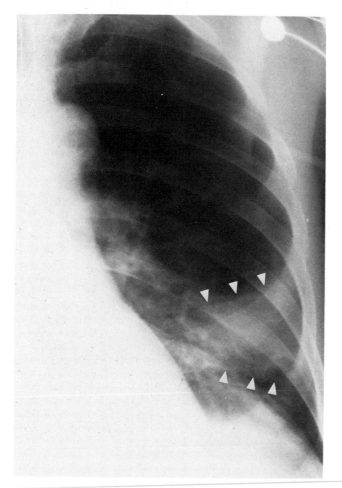

Fig. 3-75. Pulmonary infarction characterized by a triangular soft-tissue density (*arrowheads*) with its base along the chest wall pointing toward the hilum.

phy is ideal for delineating the extent of thymic enlargement. If an obvious mass is present on chest films of a patient with myasthenia, CT examination is important to clarify its size and proximity to sensitive structures preoperatively. If no obvious mass is present in a patient with myasthenia, thymectomy can be reasonably performed without a CT scan.

Teratoma. Teratomas are tumors that occur in the same region as thymomas. Most teratomas appear during young adulthood, whereas most thymomas occur in middle age. Both tumors tend to be benign, but each has potential for malignancy. Computed tomography may demonstrate cystic parts from the ectodermal component of teratomas, but other tumors in the same region may demonstrate cystic degeneration.

Substernal Thyroid. It is frequently unclear if a substernal thyroid is an extension of the normal thyroid gland or a distinct, aberrant tissue mass. Computed tomography clearly identifies the former, with radiographic evidence of tracheal deviation and contiguity of the thyroid and its substernal continuation. The latter situation, an aberrant tissue mass, presents more diagnostic problems. Radionuclide scintigraphy utilizing ^{131}I is positive in over half of patients with mediastinal thyroids. The remainder, however, have nonfunctional thyroidal tissue and fall into the same diagnostic dilemma as patients with other anterior mediastinal masses (Fig. 3-76).

Adenopathy. Enlarged lymph nodes may appear bumpy or smooth, as may any of the masses mentioned earlier in this section. They contain no distinguishing radiographic features. Hodgkin's disease frequently has its first nodal enlargement in this region (Fig. 3-77). The substernal lymph nodes include the internal mammary chain, which is made up of regional draining nodes from the breasts, and consequently adenopathy secondary to breast malignancy may also appear in this region. The affected nodes in adenopathy are usually not as prominent as in Hodgkin's disease, but often appear as discrete shadows behind the sternum on the lateral radiograph.

The anterior mediastinum is also a frequent site for a small number of more esoteric masses. These include germ cell tumors, hygromas, parathyroid tumors, and lipomas. Excess steroids, either endogenous or exogenous, cause proliferation of fat tissue and widen the entire mediastinal shadow. Ascending aortic aneurysms also exist in the anterior mediastinum, as do pericardial cysts. Both should be easily identified on CT examination.

Radiologic evaluation of an anterior mediastinal mass should be very limited. After ^{131}I scintigraphy has ruled out a functioning thyroid mass, CT of the thorax should be performed. Computed tomography usually separates an aneurysm from other masses. Once an aneurysm has been excluded, mediastinoscopy and biopsy are necessary since there are no radiographically distinguishing features among the more common masses cited previously.

MIDDLE MEDIASTINUM. Lymph Nodes. Enlarged lymph nodes account for most of the masses in the middle mediastinum. Most of the nodes are paratracheal and carinal, although bronchopulmonary nodes may also be enlarged if there is primary lung disease. The causes of nodal enlargement include lymphoma, leukemia, pulmonary and esophageal carcinoma, and infection—especially granulomatous disease (see Fig. 3-53). In general, middle mediastinal adenopathy appears smaller and lumpier than

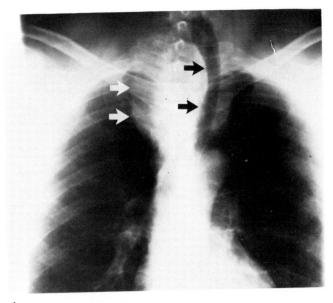

A

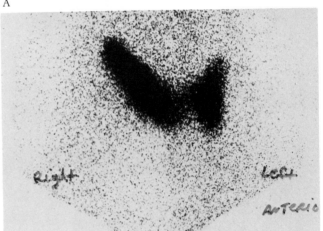

B

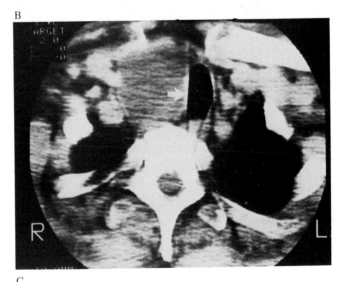

C

Fig. 3-76. Substernal mass. A. Chest film demonstrates a mass at the top of the chest (*white arrows*), displacing the trachea to the left (*black arrows*). B. Radionuclide study utilizing ^{131}I demonstrates no functioning thyroid tissue below the normal thyroid gland. C. CT section near the lung apices demonstrates that the mass is less radiodense than soft tissue and therefore cystic. Note how the trachea is flattened and pushed across the midline (*arrow*).

106

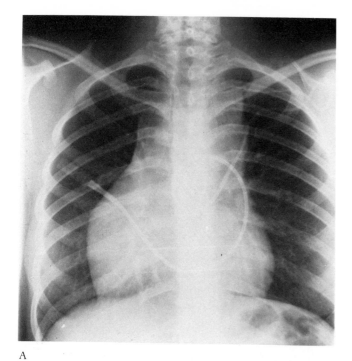

A

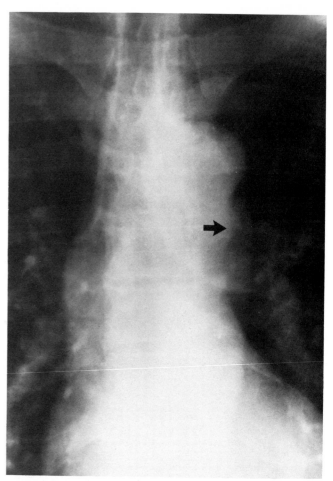

Fig. 3-78. Middle mediastinal lymph node enlargement. Soft tissue bulge (*arrow*) representing adenopathy in the aorticopulmonary window is secondary to oatcell carcinoma. The patient six months earlier demonstrated no bulge.

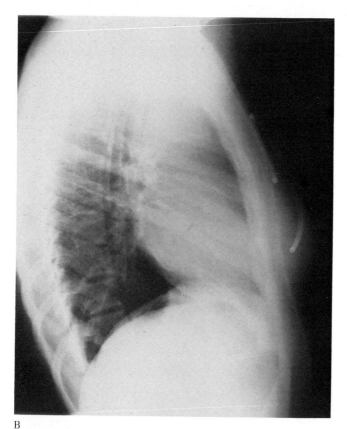

B

Fig. 3-77. Hodgkin's disease in a 20-year-old woman. A. PA chest film demonstrating soft-tissue mass superimposed on the heart and extending up to the clavicles. Superimposed on the chest is a chemotherapy catheter. B. Lateral projection demonstrating that the heart is not enlarged and that the entire anterior mediastinum above the heart is filled in with adenopathy.

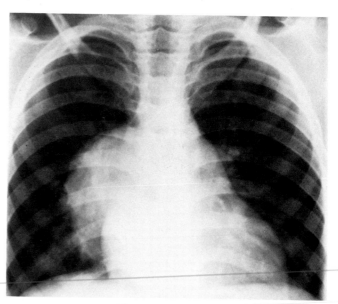

Fig. 3-79. Large bronchogenic cyst originating below the carina.

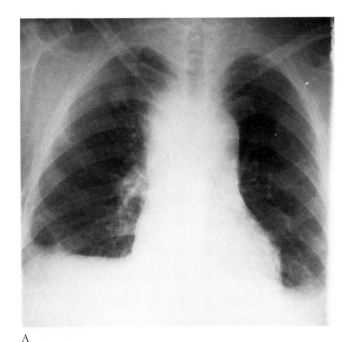

A

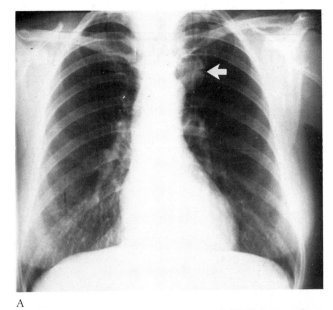

A

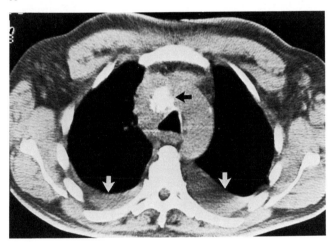

B

Fig. 3-80. Superior vena cava obstruction. A. PA chest film demonstrating a large mass obscuring the aortic arch as well as bilateral pleural effusions. B. CT section demonstrating the mass contiguous with the aortic arch and completely surrounding the trachea. The dilated, obstructed vena cava is demonstrated by the pooled contrast material (*black arrow*) that had been injected through the arm. Note the pleural effusions layering out posteriorly (*white arrows*) during this supine study.

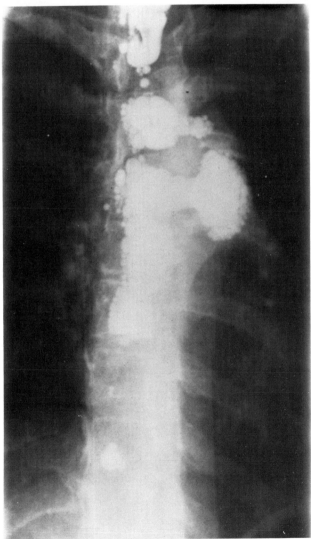

B

Fig. 3-81. Posterior mediastinal mass in a patient with von Recklinghausen's neurofibromatosis. A. Small soft tissue mass (*arrow*) on the PA chest film. B. Myelogram demonstrates contrast material filling this mass, proving that it is an intrathoracic meningocele.

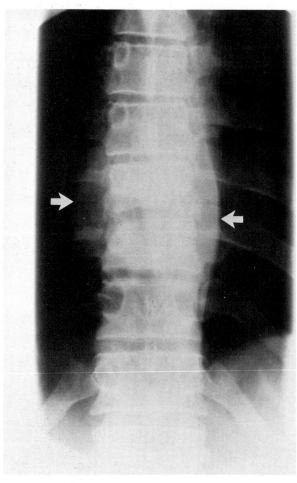

A

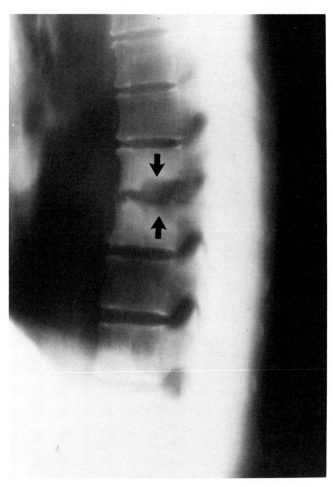

B

Fig. 3-82. Posterior mediastinal mass associated with vertebral infection. A. AP spine film demonstrating posterior mediastinal bulge bilaterally (*arrows*). B. Tomographic section in the lateral projection demonstrating destructive changes involving two adjacent vertebral bodies (*arrows*) characteristic of osteomyelitis originating in disk space.

the large anterior mediastinal shadows, and in the lateral projection most of the masses tend to be perihilar (Fig. 3-78).

Cystic Masses. Several cystic structures also appear in this compartment. Bronchogenic cysts most commonly present as rounded, asymptomatic, soft-tissue masses, usually below the carina (Fig. 3-79). Computed tomography confirms their cystic, noninfiltrating nature and excludes enlarged nodes. Esophageal duplications and neurenteric cysts are usually found just posterior to the esophagus, and the latter occasionally display connections to the spine and associated spinal anomalies. Hiatal hernias sometimes present as middle mediastinal masses resting on the diaphragm directly behind the heart. Changes in the size of the mass and a characteristic air-fluid level on the chest radiograph make the diagnosis straightforward.

Vascular Structures. Abnormal vascular structures may also present as middle mediastinal masses. An aortic arch aneurysm appears as a bulge along the upper portion of the mediastinal shadow and is often inseparable from the aortic knob on the PA chest film. Abnormally dilated main pulmonary arteries may resemble lung masses on conventional chest radiographs, and right paratracheal adenopathy may be simulated by an unusually distended azygous vein coursing over the right main bronchus to empty into the superior vena cava. Computed tomography confirms the vascular nature of all these masses.

Superior vena cava obstruction often creates significant

diagnostic as well as therapeutic problems. Caval obstruction most commonly results from lung cancer and consequent mediastinal adenopathy. If obstruction is acute, the patient may develop sudden neck and facial edema or upper extremity edema or both, depending on the site of obstruction. Venography is usually satisfactory for identifying the site of the block, but venography in combination with CT is superior since it identifies both the site and extent of block (Fig. 3-80). Posttreatment studies are often carried out using radionuclide venography, since visualizing anatomy is less significant in this situation than evaluating flow through previously obstructed vessels.

The greater diagnostic dilemma arises months later when the patient develops recurrent vascular obstruction that is more chronic and less obtrusive than the original obstruction. Diagnostic studies are now far less fruitful than they were originally. Treatment, whether by surgery or radiation therapy, has destroyed normal tissue planes and stimulated scarring. It is often unclear after both CT and venography if recurrent caval obstruction is due to recurrent tumor or posttreatment fibrosis.

POSTERIOR MEDIASTINUM. Most posterior mediastinal masses develop along the paravertebral gutters. Most are

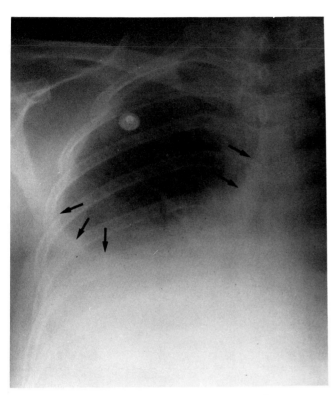

Fig. 3-83. A large pleural effusion demonstrating the meniscus (*arrows*).

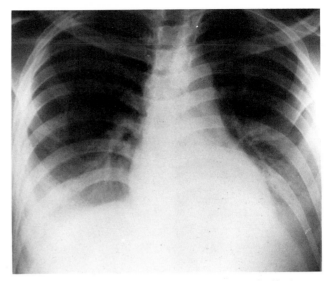

Fig. 3-84. Semierect patient with bilateral pleural effusions shows gradual decrease in density away from the diaphragms. Diaphragms are obliterated by the extensive pleural fluid inferiorly.

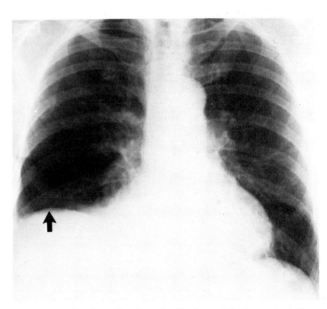

Fig. 3-85. Subpulmonic pleural effusion with characteristic lateral displacement of the apex of the right hemidiaphragm (*arrow*).

neural in origin and are often asymptomatic, appearing as unexpected findings on chest films made for other purposes. Cell types include neurofibromas, neurilemmomas, ganglioneuromas, and neuroblastomas. When large enough, these often invade adjacent structures, and some are malignant. If the tumor arises in a nerve root within the canal, it frequently widens the intervertebral foramen as it grows out. Computed tomography is excellent for evaluating such a mass, both in terms of size and local invasiveness. There are, however, no clues to propensity for metastasis without biopsy.

Paraspinal bulging also results from other vertebral problems. Meningeal herniations, or meningoceles, are a frequent finding in von Recklinghausen's disease, independent of the neurofibromas (Fig. 3-81). Vertebral infection or hemorrhage often result in a paravertebral mass, as does extramedullary hematopoesis, a complication of severe hereditary anemias (Fig. 3-82). All these entities should be readily identifiable on CT once the bulge has been noted on plain films.

Descending aortic aneurysms also appear as mediastinal bulges. Much of the normal aorta is anterior to the spine, but aneurysmal dilatation appears adjacent to the spine on the left and may even erode vertebrae. Computed tomography confirms the diagnosis, but an arteriogram is usually necessary to determine the degree of clot versus the degree of functional lumen in the diseased aorta.

Pleural Disease

The two layers of lung covering that comprise the pleura provide a site for fluid accumulation, tumor growth, and bacterial proliferation. The presence of adjacent lung gives

the necessary radiographic contrast to evaluate pleural disease with reasonable accuracy. Computed tomography has done much to raise this level of accuracy over the accuracy achievable with conventional films.

PLEURAL EFFUSIONS. The most common problem affecting the pleural space is the accumulation of unwanted fluid. Pleural effusions have many causes but are most commonly the result of either decompensated congestive heart failure or pulmonary infection. Radiographic appearance of pleural fluid depends primarily on three factors, (1) the amount of fluid, (2) the position of the patient, and (3) any restrictions on the movement of the fluid.

A pleural effusion in an erect patient can be imagined as having the shape of a tea cup, the lung being the tea. Thus, the lower portion of the lung is surrounded uniformly by

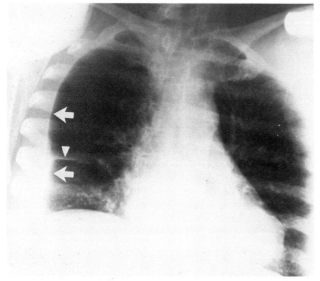

Fig. 3-86. Right side down decubitus view demonstrating layering out of the pleural effusion along the right chest wall (*arrows*) and into the horizontal fissure (*arrowhead*). The patient shown is the same as in Fig. 3-85 with subpulmonic effusion.

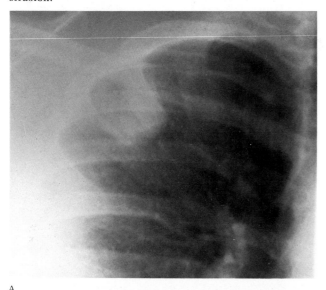

A

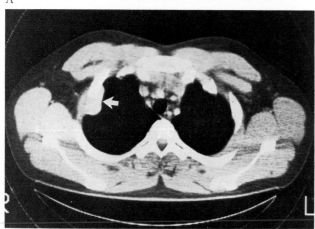

B

Fig. 3-87. Pleural-based mass. A. PA chest film demonstrating characteristic lack of complete margination. B. CT section demonstrating more clearly the outline of this pleural based neurofibroma (*arrow*).

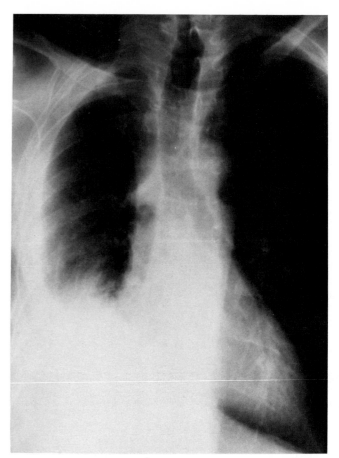

Fig. 3-88. Malignant mesothelioma constricting and encasing the entire right lung.

the effusion, which presses upon the lung all around its circumference. Radiographically this results in a soft-tissue density at the lung base, from the surrounding fluid, with a meniscus-like shape at the edges (Fig. 3-83). A point is reached when the amount of pleural fluid becomes great enough that its pressure upon the lung exceeds the pressure keeping the lung expanded, and atelectasis results at the lung base. Clearly the tea cup analogy falls apart at this point, because tea cups never crush tea. It is conceivable that a pleural effusion may become so extensive that it opacifies the entire hemithorax. At the other extreme, a very small pleural effusion may result only in the blunting of a normally sharp costophrenic angle.

Patients with pleural effusions are often radiographed in bed in a semierect position; thus the pleural fluid layers out posteriorly and inferiorly, and on the portable chest film gives the appearance of added density over the lung base that gradually fades away higher in the chest (Fig. 3-84). This appearance may be confused with pneumonia.

Occasionally a pleural effusion may not develop a meniscus in the costophrenic angle in the upright position; instead, fluid may be caught between the lung and diaphragm. The only clue to this "subpulmonic" effusion is lateral displacement of the apex of the diaphragm (Fig. 3-85). When the features of an effusion are not obvious on conventional chest films, a cross-table lateral projection, with the patient lying with the affected side down (decubitus position), should demonstrate the fluid layering along the dependent chest wall (Fig. 3-86). If the pleural fluid is purulent, fibrinous, or full of clot, its motility is reduced. Adhesions from previous pleuritis have the same

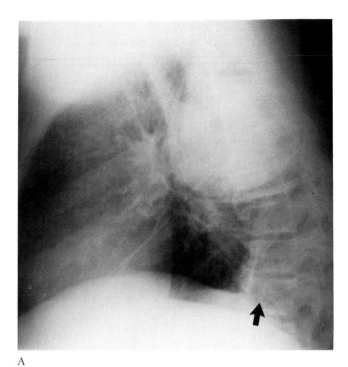

A

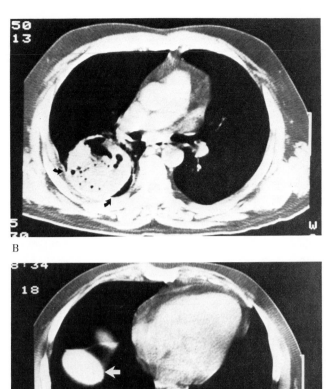

B

C

Fig. 3-89. Lung abscess and empyema in the same patient. A. Lateral chest film demonstrating a large mass posteriorly and superiorly and a less evident mass at the base posteriorly obliterating the right hemidiaphragm posteriorly (*arrow*). B. Tomographic section near the level of the carina showing the large, rounded mass posteriorly, with multiple pockets of air representing an abscess. Note the acute angles (*arrows*) that the mass makes with the adjacent pleura. C. Tomographic section at the level of the dome of the right diaphragm (*arrow*) demonstrating the posterior empyema characterized by its lenticular shape (*arrowheads*) and lack of acute angles.

effect. In such situations, the fluid neither conforms to the standard configurations nor layers out appropriately in the decubitus position. The fluid may resemble a pleural mass, in which case ultrasound or CT scan may help determine its real nature.

Pleuritis and pleural fluid may leave permanent scars in the form of pleural thickening or blunting of a costophrenic angle that does not change over time. This appearance is quite common following interpersonal conflicts (e.g., stabbings, shootings) involving the chest.

PLEURAL MASSES. Most discrete pleural masses appear on x-ray as soft-tissue shadows outlined by lung. If the lesion happens to be radiographed *en face*, it appears round with margins made sharp by surrounding aerated lung. In this circumstance the pleural mass is indistinguishable from a lung mass. If the discrete pleural lesion is x-rayed so that it is not *en face*, it has an appearance characterized by a clear margin only on its lung side and no margin on its pleural side. This lack of complete margination is the hallmark of the discrete pleural mass (Fig. 3-87). Pleura-based tumors include fibromas, lipomas, metastases, and localized benign mesotheliomas.

Asbestos-related malignant mesothelioma significantly differs in appearance from a discrete pleural mass. Malignant mesothelioma develops as a diffusely thickened, lumpy pleura frequently extending around much of the lung before diagnosis. There are often associated pleural effusions that are quite frequently bloody. Mesothelial in-

volvement can be so extensive that it dramatically restricts underlying pulmonary function (Fig. 3-88). Computed tomography is very useful for evaluating the initial extent of mesothelial involvement, as well as results of treatment.

EMPYEMA VERSUS ABSCESS. A pulmonary abscess is a loculate accumulation of pus in the lung parenchyma, whereas empyema is an accumulation of pus in the pleural space. The difference between empyema and abscess is more than semantic, because treatment differs dramatically for the two. Abscesses require prolonged antibiotics, postural drainage, and in some situations repeated bronchoscopy. Empyemas require external tube drainage. If, for instance, an abscess were mistakenly diagnosed as an empyema and treated via a chest tube, the abscess would be compounded by an empyema as the pleural space became contaminated; a bronchopleural fistula would result. Thus, it is vitally important to distinguish radiographically between abscess and empyema.

An abscess tends to appear round on chest films, and where it is contiguous with the pleura and chest wall an acute angle should be evident. As opposed to the appearance of an abscess, an empyema displaces lung from the chest wall, resulting in a lenticular shape and obtuse angles with the chest wall. Ultrasound may be helpful in confirming fluid in the pleural space, but CT is the best diagnostic tool. Computed tomography is better than conventional films for demonstrating the significant shapes, angles, and fluid accumulations (Fig. 3-89). In addition, CT often demonstrates the thickened, split pleura that envelops an empyema and is characteristic of it.

Bibliography

Basic principles of pulmonary disease
Felson, B. *Chest Roentgenology.* Philadelphia: Saunders, 1973. Chaps. 2 and 3.
Heitzman, E. R. *The Lung: Radiologic-Pathologic Correlations* (2nd ed.). St. Louis: Mosby, 1984. Chaps. 5 and 12.
Tuddenham, W. J. Editorial. *Radiographics* 4:865, 1984.

Lung neoplasms
Hill, C. A. Bronchioloalveolar carcinoma: A review. *Radiology* 150:15, 1984.
Janower, M. L., and Blennerhassett, J. B. Lymphangitic spread of metastatic cancer to the lung: A radiologic-pathologic classification. *Radiology* 101:267, 1971.
Libschitz, H. I. CT of mediastinal lymph nodes in lung cancer: Is there a "state of the art"? (editorial). *A.J.R.* 141:1081, 1983.
Muhm, J. R., et al. Lung cancer detected during a screening program using four-month chest radiographs. *Radiology* 148:609, 1983.
Steckel, R. J., and Kagan, A. R. Diagnostic persistence in working up metastatic cancer with an unknown primary site. *Radiology* 134:367, 1980.
Stewart, J. F., et al. Unknown primary adenocarcinoma: Incidence of overinvestigation and natural history. *Br. Med. J.* 1:1530, 1979.
Webb, W. R. The pleural tail sign. *Radiology* 127:309, 1978.
Woodring, J. H., Fried, A. M., and Chuang, V. P. Solitary cavities of the lung: Diagnostic implications of cavity wall thickness. *A.J.R.* 135:1269, 1980.

The solitary pulmonary nodule
Godwin, J. D., et al. Distinguishing benign from malignant pulmonary nodules by computed tomography. *Radiology* 144:349, 1982.
Siegelman, S. S., et al. Computed tomography of the solitary pulmonary nodule. *Semin. Roentgenol.* 19:165, 1984.

Upper airway disease
Bass, E. Widened superior mediastinum with acute and chronic pulmonary symptoms. *J.A.M.A.* 239:753, 1978.
Fraser, R. G., and Paré, J. A. P. *Diagnosis of Diseases of the Chest* (2nd ed.). Philadelphia: Saunders, 1977. Vol. 3, Chap. 11.

Chronic obstructive pulmonary disease
Clinicopathological exercises (alpha₁ antitrypsin deficiency). *N. Engl. J. Med.* 287:763, 1972.
Clinicopathological exercises (COPD). *N. Engl. J. Med.* 289:1132, 1973.
Heitzman, E. R. *The Lung: Radiologic-Pathologic Correlations* (2nd ed.). St. Louis: Mosby, 1984. Chap. 11.

Pneumoconioses
Bouhuys, A., and Peters, J. M. Medical progress: Control of environmental lung disease. *N. Engl. J. Med.* 283(11):573, 1970.
Rabinowitz, J. G., et al. A comparative study of mesothelioma and asbestosis using computed tomography and conventional chest radiography. *Radiology* 144:453, 1982.
Ziskind, M. M. Occupational pulmonary disease. *Clin. Symp.* 30(4), 1978.

Tuberculosis and fungal diseases
Choyke, P. L., et al. Adult-onset pulmonary tuberculosis. *Radiology* 148:357, 1983.
Connell Jr., J. V., and Muhm, J. R. Radiographic manifestations of pulmonary histoplasmosis: A 10-year review. *Radiology* 121:281, 1976.
Klein, D. L., and Gamsu, G. Review: Thoracic manifestations of aspergillosis. *A.J.R.* 134:543, 1980.
Palmer, P. E. S. Pulmonary tuberculosis: Usual and unusual radiographic presentations. *Semin. Roentgenol.* 14:204, 1979.
Rabinowitz, J. G., Busch, J., and Buttram, W. R. Pulmonary manifestations of blastomycosis. *Radiology* 120:25, 1976.
Tuddenham, W. J. *Chest Disease Syllabus* (2nd series), Set 8. Chicago: American College of Radiology, 1975.

Weider, S., et al. Pulmonary artery occlusion due to histoplasmosis. *A.J.R.* 138:243, 1982.

Bronchiectasis
Nadel, H. R., et al. The immotile cilia syndrome: Radiological manifestations. *Radiology* 154:651, 1985.

Aspiration pneumonia
Ginai, A. Z., et al. Experimental evaluation of various available contrast agents for use in the upper gastrointestinal tract in case of suspected leakage: Effects on lungs. *Br. J. Radiol.* 57:895, 1984.
Heitzman, E. R. *The Lung: Radiologic Pathologic Correlations* (2nd ed.). St. Louis: Mosby, 1984. Chap. 7.

Pulmonary eosinophilia
Castleman, B., Scully, R. E., and McNeely, B. U. Presentation of case 22-1972: Case records of Massachusetts General Hospital. *N. Engl. J. Med.* 286(22):1205, 1972.

Sarcoidosis
Fajman, W. A., et al. Assessing the activity of sarcoidosis: Quantitative ⁶⁷Ga-citrate imaging. *A.J.R.* 142:683, 1984.
Rabinowitz, J. G., Ulreich, S., and Soriano, C. The usual unusual manifestations of sarcoidosis and the "hilar-haze": A new diagnostic aid. *Am. J. Roentgenol.* 120:821, 1974.
Rockoff, S. D., and Rohatgi, P. K. Unusual manifestations of thoracic sarcoidosis. *A.J.R.* 144:513, 1985.

Reactions to specific agents
Roswit, B., and White, D. C. Severe radiation injuries of the lung. *Am. J. Roentgenol.* 129:127, 1977.
Sostman, H. D., Putman, C. E., and Gamsu. G. Diagnosis of chemotherapy lung. *A.J.R.* 136:33, 1981.
Yockey, C. C., Eden, B. M., and Byrd, R. B. The McConnell missile accident: Clinical spectrum of nitrogen dioxide exposure. *J.A.M.A.* 244(11):1221, 1980.

Other interstitial lung diseases
Genereaux, G. P. The end-stage lung. *Radiology* 116:279, 1975.
Martin, E. Leiomyomatous lung lesions: A proposed classification. *A.J.R.* 141:269, 1983.
Wechsler, R. J., et al. Chest radiograph in lymphomatoid granulomatosis: Comparison with Wegener granulomatosis. *A.J.R.* 142:79, 1984.

Pulmonary hemorrhage
Herman, P. G., et al. The pulmonary-renal syndrome. *Am. J. Roentgenol.* 130:1141, 1978.
Schwartz, E. E., et al. Pulmonary hemorrhage in renal disease: Goodpasture's syndrome and other causes. *Radiology* 122:39, 1977.

Atypical infectious pneumonias
Fairbank, J. T., et al. The chest radiograph in Legionnaires' disease. *Radiology* 147:33, 1983.

Acquired immune deficiency syndrome (AIDS)
Cohen, B. A., et al. Pulmonary complications of AIDS: Radiologic features. *A.J.R.* 143:115, 1984.
McCauley, D. I., et al. Radiographic patterns of opportunistic lung infections and Kaposi sarcoma in homosexual men. *A.J.R.* 139:653, 1982.

Noncardiogenic pulmonary edema
Joffe, N. The adult respiratory distress syndrome. *Am. J. Roentgenol.* 122:719, 1984.
Putman, C. E., et al. Radiographic manifestations of acute smoke inhalation. *Am. J. Roentgenol.* 129:865, 1977.
Reed, J. C. *Chest Radiology: Patterns and Differential Diagnosis.* Chicago: Year Book, 1981. Chap. 14.
Scully, R. E., Mark, E. J., and McNeely, B. U. (eds.). Case records of the Massachusetts General Hospital: Weekly clinicopathological exercises. Case 14-1984. *N. Engl. J. Med.* 310(14): 915, 1984.

Pulmonary embolism

Braun, S. D., et al. Ventilation-perfusion scanning and pulmonary angiography: Correlation in clinical high-probability
pulmonary embolism. *A.J.R.* 143:977, 1984.

Figley, M. M., Gerdes, A. J., and Ricketts, H. J. Radiographic aspects of pulmonary embolism. *Semin. Roentgenol.* 2(4):389,
1967.

Fraser, R. G., and Paré, J. A. P. *Diagnosis of Diseases of the Chest*
(2nd ed.). Philadelphia: Saunders, 1977. Vol. 2, Chap. 9.

Hull, R. D., et al. Pulmonary angiography, ventilation lung scanning, and venography for clinically suspected pulmonary embolism with abnormal perfusion lung scan. *Ann. Intern. Med.*
98(6):891, 1983.

Mediastinal masses

Fon, G. T., et al. Computed tomography of the anterior mediastinum in myasthenia gravis. *Radiology* 142:135, 1982.

Fraser, R. G., and Paré, J. A. P. *Diagnosis of Diseases of the Chest*
(2nd ed.). Philadelphia: Saunders, 1977. Vol. 3, Chap. 16.

Glazer, G. M., Axel, L., and Moss, A. A. CT diagnosis of mediastinal thyroid. *A.J.R.* 138:495, 1982.

Pleural disease

Dedrick, C. G., et al. Computed tomography of localized pleural
mesothelioma. *A.J.R.* 144:275, 1985.

Mirvis, S., et al. CT of malignant pleural mesothelioma. *A.J.R.*
140:665, 1983.

Stark, D. D., et al. Differentiating lung abscess and empyema: Radiography and computed tomography. *A.J.R.* 141:163,
1983.

4. Genitourinary Disease

Jack G. Rabinowitz

Congenital Abnormalities

DUPLICATION. Duplication of the collecting system is a well-known cause of enlarged kidneys. It can involve either one or both kidneys and is easily demonstrated on excretory urography. Two or more renal collecting systems associated with an equal number of ureters establishes the diagnosis. When two complete ureters join a single kidney, the ureter draining the upper pole terminates in an ectopic location inferior to the insertion of the lower pole ureter. The ectopic ureter in females is inserted easily into either the vagina or the perineum, whereas in males it may be inserted into the posterior urethra, the seminal vesicle, or even the vas deferens. Ectopic ureters are frequently associated with ureteroceles and obstruction of the corresponding ureter; this anomaly has a higher incidence in females.

As a result of ureteroceles, the upper pole of the kidney is dilated and displaces the inferior collecting system of the kidney. Once the ureter is obstructed, the upper pole calyces are either difficult or impossible to visualize during intravenous urography. The upper pole appears as a radiolucent mass during the total opacification phase at radiography and as a sonolucent structure at ultrasonography. The existence of an obstructing calyx is suggested by the configuration of the lower calyceal group. This group is depressed, rotated downward and outward, and its appearance has been likened to a drooping lily (Fig. 4-1). An excessive amount of renal tissue appears above the depressed collecting system; the obstructed calyces may eventually opacify if residual functioning renal tissue remains within the duplicated area.

The ureterocele is recognized at radiography as a smooth, mucosal mass located within the region of the trigone. In the early phases of contrast filling of the bladder, the ureterocele appears as a well-defined, lucent, space-occupying mass (Fig. 4-2), which varies in size and may be large enough to fill the entire bladder lumen. Ureteroceles may eventually fill with contrast material if the parenchyma associated with the affected calyx is viable. The presence of the lesion near the trigone is often responsible for producing ipsilateral reflux into the lower pole, and it is also not unusual for a large ureterocele to obliterate the entire trigone and obstruct the opposite ureter.

Ultrasonography is also useful in evaluating ureteroceles. A spherical or linear echogenic density is seen within the sonolucent bladder, and dilatated ureters complete the picture. Presently, surgery for ureteroceles consists of removal of the upper pole of the kidney and its corresponding ureter to within a few centimeters of the bladder. The ureteroceles are drained and left in situ.

HORSESHOE KIDNEY. The metanephric blastema lies in the most caudal portion in the 5 mm embryo. Growth of this part of the embryo carries the kidney cephalad higher into the posterior portion of the developing abdominal cavity. In the early stages, the renal pelvis is directed anteriorly and the lower poles are more closely proximated than the upper poles. Only a slight medial shift of the

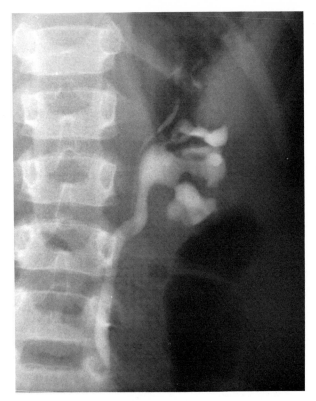

A

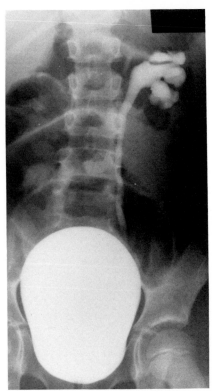

B

Fig. 4-1. Duplication. A. A double collecting system is seen on the left. The inferior system is dilatated. B. On a retrograde examination, contrast refluxes into the lower system. The downward and outward orientation of the calyces (drooping lily appearance) is easily recognized.

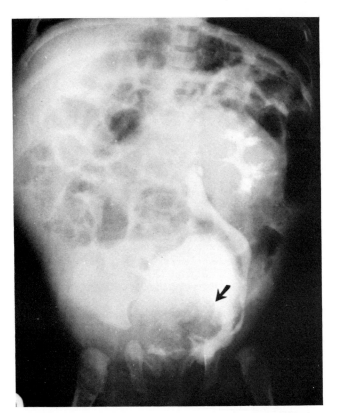

Fig. 4-2. Ureterocele. A large filling defect (*arrow*) is located on the right side of the bladder. The ureter and collecting systems on the ipsilateral side are completely obstructed. Note also the degree obstruction on the opposite side.

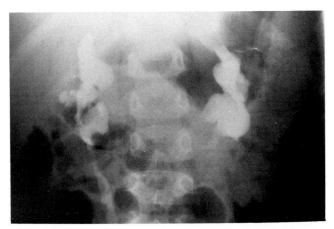

Fig. 4-3. Horseshoe kidney. Both kidneys lie close to the vertebral bodies. The lower poles are directed medially. The calyces are distorted and dilatated bilaterally.

lower poles is necessary to bring them into approximation and produce a horseshoe kidney. The frequency of fusion of the upper poles is unknown, but the degree of fusion varies from near contact of the external surfaces to complete integration of the parenchyma. Horseshoe kidney may present some clinical confusion, since the kidney is easily palpated and the axis of the kidney abnormally rotated. Radiographically, both kidneys are positioned close to the vertebral column, with the inferior parts of the kidneys rotated medially (Fig. 4-3). The connecting soft tissue is frequently seen superimposed across the midline of the abdomen, and the calyces appear deformed because of the faulty rotation; this distorted appearance is often mistaken for obstruction or a space-occupying mass.

CROSSED RENAL ECTOPIA. Crossed renal ectopia is another positional anomaly that may be misinterpreted as an abnormal renal mass on palpation. Embryologically, one kidney shifts to the center and ascends on the contralateral side. Fusion with the other kidney may be incomplete (crossed renal ectopia) or so complete as to form a single renal mass (crossed renal fused ectopia). The findings are basically the same, regardless of what imaging modality is used. One kidney is noticeably absent on one side and two renal structures, each complete with a normal complement of calyces, pelvis, and ureters, are present on the opposite side. The ureters, however, terminate in their proper location within the bladder trigone, and therefore the ureter draining the ectopic kidney must cross the midline to reach its respective kidney.

Pelvic kidney is another form of ectopia that is often mistaken for tumor. This form of ectopia results from failure of the embryonic kidney to ascend from its original location within the pelvis. Fusion of both renal blastema has also been known to occur in this location.

CONGENITAL HYPOPLASIA. The hypoplastic kidney is defined as a congenitally small kidney resulting from a quantitative deficiency in the metanephric primordia. As a result, there is an overall decrease in the number of renal lobes as well as in the number of nephrons contained in each lobe. Generally, in unilateral renal hypoplasia normal function is maintained, although the opposite kidney appears enlarged. Bilateral hypoplasia leads to renal failure and to other complications. The most salient radiographic feature of congenital hypoplasia is basically a small kidney with fewer calyces than the corresponding enlarged contralateral kidney. The hypoplastic kidney usually contains an adequate amount of functioning nephrons. The Ask-Upmark kidney, a form of segmental renal hypoplasia, was believed at one time to represent a form of congenital hypoplasia. However, the more recent literature has demonstrated this disease state to be the end result of recurrent infections, with resulting scar formation.

Reflux Uropathy

Vesicoureteral reflux is defined as the abnormal backflow of urine from the bladder into the ureter. Reflux is of major concern because it ultimately destroys a clearly defined population of nephrons and is associated with chronic pyelonephritis, renal scarring, and potential renal failure.

Intrarenal reflux of infected urine into susceptible compound papillae is considered the mechanism most responsible for renal scarring. Abnormal embryologic development of the ureteral bud and long-standing sterile reflux are other mechanisms that have been proposed to account for the development of renal scars. In general, the prevention of reflux depends on the existence of certain normal anatomic relationships between the ureter and bladder. These include (1) oblique entry of the ureter into a fixed posterolateral portion in the floor of the bladder, (2) adequate length of the ureter transversing the bladder wall and especially under the bladder mucosa, (3) adequate detrusor, or muscle support, of the intramural and submucosal ureter, and (4) a 4 : 1 or 5 : 1 ratio of submucosal tunnel length to ureteral diameter. Primary reflux occurs when any of these conditions are altered, that is, the ureteral orifice is displaced laterally, the submucosal ureter is foreshortened, or the diameter ratio is decreased.

In 1981, an international classification of vesicoureteral reflux was established, based mainly on findings on voiding cystourethrogram. Five grades of vesicoureteral reflux were described: Grade 1 is reflux into the ureter alone; grade 2 is reflux into ureter, pelvis, and calyces, with no dilatation and normal calyceal fornices; grade 3 is mild dilatation and moderate tortuosity of ureter and mild to moderate dilatation of the renal pelvis, with slight blunting of the fornices; grade 4 is moderate dilatation and tortuosity of ureter and moderate dilatation of renal pelvis and calyces; grade 5 is gross dilatation of renal pelvis, and calyces and tortuosity of ureter.

Vesicoureteral reflux occurs in about 0.5 to 1.0 percent of asymptomatic children. This is in strong contrast to the 25 to 50 percent incidence noted in children being investigated for recurrent urinary tract infection. The presence of renal scarring in children with no documented evidence of previous urinary tract infection has been attributed to the result of an early single infection, the so-called big bang theory.

Pyelonephritis

ACUTE. Acute pyelonephritis is defined as an acute inflammatory disease of the kidney, caused by bacteria. Based on clinical and radiographic findings, two forms of pyelonephritis, uncomplicated and complicated, seem to exist. The acute uncomplicated form is a relatively common lesion, involving approximately 30 percent of women under the age of 40. In general, in many individuals it occurs as a single episode that causes little or no damage to the kidney, although some physicians believe that a single infection may be sufficient to produce scarring in children (the big bang theory). Pathogenic organisms can reach the kidney through a variety of routes, but ascending infection is the most common in general and results from ureteral and subsequent intrarenal reflux. Hematogenous infection is also common. However, involvement through the lymphatics is probably nonexistent. The majority of bacteria causing ascending pyelonephritis originate from gut flora that abnormally colonize the vaginal introitus. These bacteria possess an ability to adhere that allows them to attach either to uromucous or epithelial cells, thus preventing them from being washed out. In addition, the endotoxins produced by these bacteria impede ureteral motility, causing dilatation that results in ureteral reflux.

Radiographic Features. Radiographic changes associated with acute pyelonephritis are encountered infrequently,

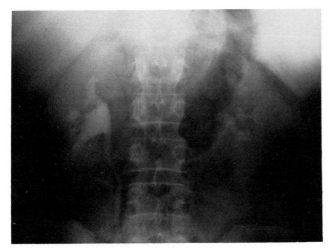

Fig. 4-4. Acute pyelonephritis. Conventional urography reveals an enlarged left kidney with poor opacification of the collecting systems.

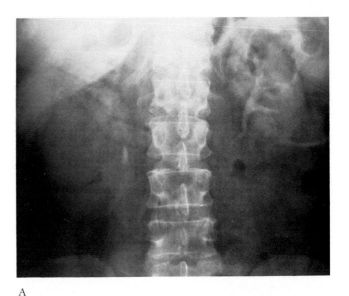

A

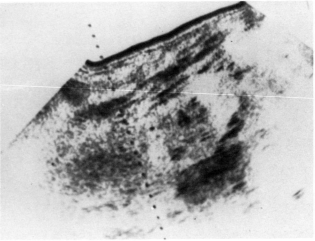

B

Fig. 4-5. Acute bacterial nephritis. A. The right kidney is enlarged, with a suggested space-occupying mass displacing the calyces. B. Sonographic features: Enlarged kidney containing a poorly echogenic mass with ill-defined borders.

with only 25 percent of patients demonstrating abnormal radiographic features. These consist of enlargement of the kidney or kidneys, decreased density of contrast, delayed opacification, and dilatation of the collecting system (Fig. 4-4). In general the manifestations suggesting the more complicated form are enlargement of the kidneys, dilatation of the collecting system, and delayed opacification. The latter may be manifested by decreased or absent function on urographic examination (Fig. 4-5A). The underlying process is an interstitial bacterial pyelonephritis consisting of multiple collections of microabscesses localized to part or all of the kidney. The disease is seen predominantly in females and diabetics, is basically caused by gram-negative organisms, and may present either as a focal or diffuse lesion. The term *acute bacterial nephritis* best describes it. The majority of such infections are hematogenous in origin, with microabscesses mainly localized to the cortex, where they excite an intense inflammatory reaction that spreads rapidly into the perirenal tissues through the intrarenal lymphatics. If untreated, the lesions subsequently coalesce to form one large abscess. The basic radiographic findings consist of an enlarged kidney with a surrounding perinephric process. Swelling is either localized or diffuse. Since the infection is mainly localized to the interstitium, it spreads to the internal structures evenly. The initial radiographic features are associated with perinephric disease, loss of renal outline and motility, increased localized density within the surrounding tissues, and displacement of the kidney. In those cases presenting with absent renal function it is often necessary to exclude pyonephrosis. At one time this distinction was accomplished by retrograde pyelography; however, this procedure has a certain degree of morbidity and is no longer required. Ultrasound and CT best demonstrate pyonephrosis and unquestionably should be the initial diagnostic modalities. The sonographic features of pyonephrosis are obvious and demonstrate large, dilated collecting systems with internal echoes of varying sorts. The findings of acute bacterial nephritis in both CT and ultrasound consist of an increase in overall size of the kidney, which contains within it a poorly echogenic mass with ill-defined borders (Fig. 4-5).

Focal pyelonephritis on occasion simulates renal abscess or tumor on CT and ultrasound, and arteriography may then be used to exclude this possibility. Arteriograms do not reveal true masses. Vessels are not displaced but are separated, attenuated, and elongated, and show decreased perfusion in the area of involvement. Moreover, the corticomedullary junction, which is normally sharp and well-defined, is also absent.

The lesion may resolve without liquification and necrosis if early and appropriate antibiotics are administered. If untreated, it will develop into an abscess.

CHRONIC. In all probability most cases of chronic pyelonephritis begin in childhood as a result of vesicoureteral reflux and renal infection. However, it is not unusual for severe and recurrent infections in adults to produce renal changes that are associated with chronic pyelonephritis.

The polar regions of the kidney or kidneys are primarily affected when reflux is present. The end result is parenchymal atrophy and ballooning of the corresponding calyx. In general, these findings can be patchy or generalized, and the overall impression is a small, scarred kidney with clubbed calyces (Fig. 4-6).

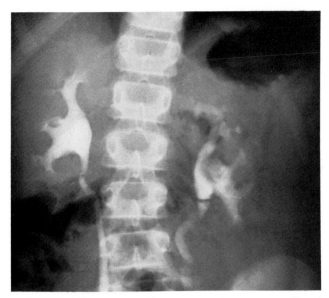

Fig. 4-6. Chronic pyelonephritis. The left kidney is small and irregular. All the calyces are rounded and clubbed.

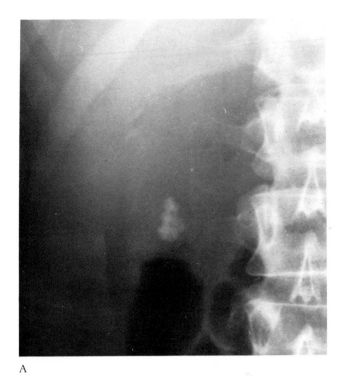

A

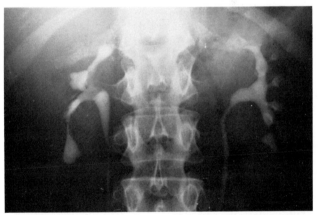

B

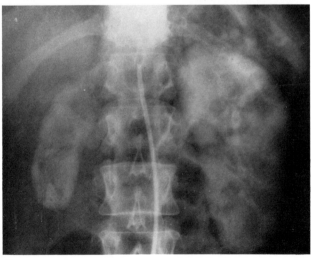

C

Fig. 4-7. Chronic pyelonephritis: Tuberculosis. A. A mottled calcification is present within the lower pole of the right kidney. B. The calyces are distorted and blunted. C. The nephrogram reveals a small irregular scarred kidney.

XANTHOGRANULOMATOUS. Xanthogranulomatous pyelonephritis (XP) is a chronic inflammatory reaction within the kidney that is characterized by the formation of lipoid-laden cells. Lesions may either diffusely involve the entire kidney or present as focal lesions simulating tumor replacement of the renal parenchyma. Histologically, the center of the process is frequently necrotic and is surrounded by a cellular reaction that is filled with the lipoid-laden cells characterizing the lesion. Granulomas and associated fibrosis become more evident within the periphery of the lesion. Long-standing kidney infections and staghorn calculi are the two major predisposing clinical features usually associated with this form of pyelonephritis. Other associated features are female predominance and an overwhelming involvement of *Proteus* organisms and *Escherichia coli*.

Radiographic Features. Radiographic features of XP vary depending on the distribution of the process within the kidney. Focal lesions present as a space-occupying mass within a kidney that in most cases functions well. The calyceal structures are distorted and displaced, as with any space-occupying mass. Although diffuse XP generally replaces the entire kidney, a minimal amount of functioning parenchyma remain in a small percentage of cases. Xanthogranulomatous pyelonephritis is best documented and diagnosed by either sonography or CT (Fig. 4-8). Sonography shows the mass with scattered anechoic and hypoechoic areas that correspond to the enlarged irregular calyces, with granulomatous tissue within the surrounding inflammatory reaction. The parenchyma in general appear thickened, since the inflammatory tissue produces low-level echoes similar to the normal renal parenchyma. The presence of abundant lipoid-laden cells and inflammatory tissue produces central areas of low attenuation on CT. Despite the accuracy of these modalities, it is occasionally difficult to differentiate a focal lesion from a tumor. Angiography may be helpful in this respect, since lesions are hypovascular and none of the features consistent with tumor vascularity are present. A hypovascular hypernephroma may demonstrate similar angiographic features.

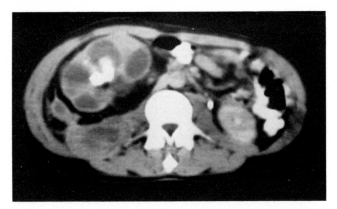

Fig. 4-8. Xanthogranulomatous pyelonephritis: Computed tomography shows the right kidney markedly enlarged and displaced. A large **staghorn calculus** is located within the pelvis causing obstruction. The surrounding parenchyma is nevertheless thickened and irregular.

GENITOURINARY TUBERCULOSIS. Genitourinary tuberculosis results from hematogenous spread of tuberculous bacilli from a primary pulmonary focus. The genitourinary tract is the second most common site of tuberculosis. Bacilli settle within the periglomerular capillaries, forming granuloma. These lesions are usually bilateral, stable, and asymptomatic, and in most patients they remain latent. Alteration in the patient's defense mechanisms causes reactivation of these foci, with further necrosis and enlargement resulting in ulcerocavernous lesions that may spread to eventually involve the calyces, renal pelvis, ureter, and bladder. Such multiplicity of involvement is characteristic of genitourinary tuberculosis. Pathologic features of genitourinary tuberculosis are ulceration, wall thickening, and fibrosis that often results in stricture formation. Calcification within areas of caseation is common. The term *autonephrectomy* has been applied to total destruction of the kidney by the tuberculous process and its replacement by calcification.

In general, establishment of the diagnosis is often difficult. However, the presence of sterile pyuria should alert the clinician to the possibility of underlying tuberculosis. Radiographic evidence of pulmonary tuberculosis (active or inactive) is absent in more than 50 percent of cases.

Radiographic Features. The radiographic features of renal tuberculosis correspond to the pathologic changes. Parenchymal calcification, which occurs in areas of caseation, is quite distinct and diagnostic (Fig. 4-7A). Its outline is irregular and varies in size from small areas of involvement to the entire kidney in cases where autonephrectomy has occurred.

Urographic findings of tuberculosis become apparent when the lesion has ulcerated into the calyx, producing a small or large cavity that fills with contrast (Fig. 4-7B). Before this becomes obvious, dilatation of the calyces as well as irregularity of the lesion's contour suggest the presence of necrosis within the pyramids. When contrast is visualized outside the calyx, its features strongly resemble those of papillary necrosis. However, tuberculosis is the primary consideration if and when the infundibulum or other parts of the urinary tract are involved. When scarring transpires, parts of the calyx become pinched off and appear amputated. Coalescence of multiple adjacent calyces results in a larger cavitary lesion.

Cicatrization occurs in other portions of the urinary tract (e.g., the ureter). Multiple strictures of the ureter are a typ-

ical finding. Although cicatrization and end-stage scarring generally produce a small kidney (Fig. 4-7C), ureteral involvement may be associated with obstruction and resultant hydronephrosis. In summary, the findings of what appear to be changes of papillary necrosis, scarring, and calcification represent the hallmarks of tuberculosis.

Computed tomography contributes significantly to establishing a diagnosis, determining the extent of the disease, and following its course with treatment. Many of the features on conventional studies described earlier are apparent on CT. However, small, early, ulcerating lesions are best detected by urography. Thickening of the wall of a calyx, the pelvis, or a ureter are best seen by CT and are extremely suggestive of the diagnosis.

Obstructive Disease

Hydronephrosis is the most common renal mass discovered in the newborn period. Obstruction at the ureteropelvic junction is the most frequent cause of this lesion. On occasion, and especially in males in the first year of life, ureteropelvic obstruction may be bilateral. In the older child, however, ureteropelvic obstruction for some reason more commonly affects the left side. Ureteropelvic obstruction is predominantly a congenital lesion, although acquired stenosis following chronic inflammatory disease also occurs. One or more strictures comprise the main pathologic findings. Bands, polyps, adynamic segments, vascular ischemia, ureteral kinking, anomalous vessels, and abnormal muscle development within the ureteral wall are unusual causes of obstruction. Vessels passing over the ureteropelvic junction have also been incriminated. These apparently are not the primary cause of obstruction, but on the basis of their location may aggravate the underlying lesion. The replacement of spiral muscle by an excessive collection of longitudinal muscle in the ureteral wall has been observed in a number of cases. This developmental anomaly may prove to be an important factor, since it does result in poor distensibility.

Obstruction of the ureter beyond the ureteropelvic junction is also caused by a variety of lesions. These include ureteral valve obstruction, congenital as well as traumatic stenosis, urethral polyps, urethral stones, blood clots, and lesions producing extrinsic compression, such as retrocaval ureter, enlarged lymph nodes, and retroperitoneal neoplasms that compress or invade the ureter. Ureteral valves are unusual congenital lesions that rarely produce obstruction and frequently disappear within the first six months of life. Intraureteral tumors in infants and children are extremely rare. Fibrous polyps are typically found in the upper third of the ureter and produce intermittent renal obstruction.

DIAGNOSTIC EXAMINATIONS. Intravenous urography and ultrasonography are the main diagnostic examinations needed to evaluate urinary tract obstruction. Supine radiographs of the abdomen often demonstrate a mass at the site of the enlarged kidney in cases with a high degree of obstruction, and a portion of the mass may extend across the midline. In the neonatal period this finding usually distinguishes ureteropelvic junction obstruction from a small multicystic kidney. Renal function in general depends on the amount of residual renal parenchyma and is therefore quite variable (Fig. 4-9). In advanced cases, hours may be

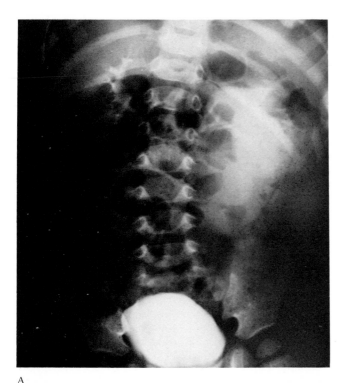

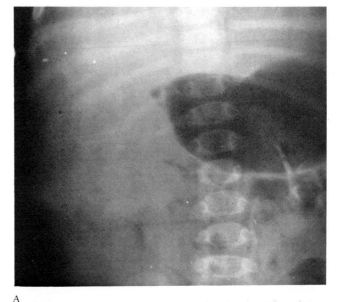

A

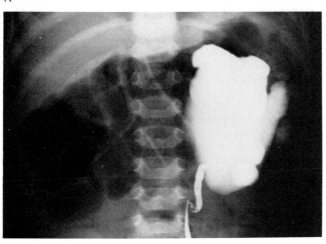

B

Fig. 4-9. Ureteropelvic junction obstruction. A. Delayed film taken during intravenous pyelogram reveals a slightly opacified but markedly dilatated renal pelvis on the left. The ureter is not visualized. B. Retrograde study demonstrates a collapsed and small ureter associated with a markedly dilatated pelvis and calyces.

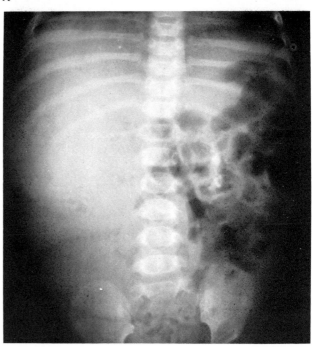

B

Fig. 4-10. Ureteropelvic obstruction. A. A 10-minute film reveals a large mass on the right displacing adjacent viscera. At this time no opacification is seen although multiple lucent areas are noted within. B. A film taken one hour later shows a markedly dilated pelvis filled with diluted contrast that extends across the midline.

required for sufficient contrast material to collect within the calyceal system (Fig. 4-10). Efforts to identify the normal and collapsed ureter should be made by altering the position of the patient. In a supine patient distal ureteral obstruction may mimic proximal obstruction, since retained urine in the ureter may act as a hydrostatic blockade. Antegrade pyelography by direct subcutaneous injection into the renal pelvis is presently being used more frequently in cases where renal function is inadequate for diagnosis. This study easily distinguishes obstruction at the ureteropelvic junction from more distal lesions. However, ultrasound is a more benign technique and in most instances locates the site of the obstruction. Sonography moreover does not rely on renal function and therefore provides instantaneous results and determines the amount of residual cortical tissue.

RADIOGRAPHIC FINDINGS. Basically, radiographic findings of ureteral obstruction are recognized by the changes that occur in the ureter at the site of obstruction. Certain characteristic changes help to distinguish the underlying cause. For example, a ureteral valve is a sharply defined lucent band that projects into the middle of the ureter. Congenital stenosis and stricture can be indistinguishable.

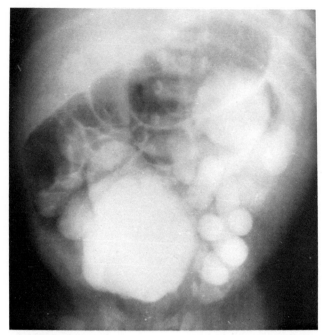

A

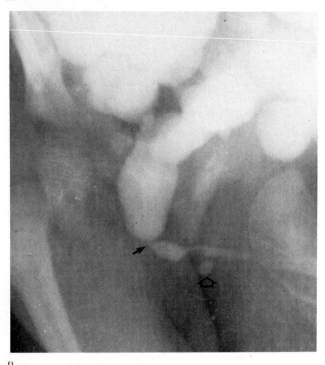

B

Fig. 4-11. Posterior urethral valves. A. The urographic study reveals massive bilateral obstruction. Both ureters are dilatated and tortuous and the bladder is moderately trabeculated. B. The voiding cystourethrogram reveals marked dilatation of the posterior urethra, with obstruction at the external sphincter (*arrow*). There is an incidental finding of a dilatated urethral gland (*open arrow*).

However, congenital stenosis is more likely to occur in the distal ureter above the ureterovesical junction, whereas stricture is more typically found in the middle third of the ureter. A fibrous polyp presents as a filling defect that is indistinguishable from a blood clot or nonopaque calculus. The ureter in lesser degrees of obstruction is only slightly dilated. With progressive degrees of obstruction, increasing dilatation and widening become apparent.

The majority of causes of bilateral and unilateral obstruction are similar (Fig. 4-11A). Posterior urethral valves are the most common cause of bilateral obstruction in infants and children. The diagnosis of posterior urethral valves is best established during voiding cystourethrogram (Fig. 4-11B). The posterior urethra is markedly dilated and the valves can be seen as linear lucencies extending from the verumontanum distally toward the external sphincter. Occasionally, valves have been noted to extend proximally; a membranous form has also been described. In the adult, prostatic hypertrophy and carcinoma are the most common causes in men and carcinoma of the cervix is the most common cause in women.

Other forms of obstructive disease are caused by lesions outside the ureter, such as retroperitoneal fibrosis, radiation fibrosis, and retroperitoneal masses (e.g., tumors). Retroperitoneal fibrosis is a fibrotic process that principally involves the retroperitoneal structures. It can be idiopathic and associated with systemic connective tissue disorders (e.g., fibrous mesenteritis, thyroiditis, cholangitis) or can be provoked by neoplasms, leaking aortic abdominal aortic aneurysm, or in some instances by long-standing ingestion of methysergide. The diagnosis of retroperitoneal fibrosis is made predominantly utilizing imaging techniques that demonstrate the classic findings of medial deviation and narrowing of the ureters near the lower lumbar spine (Fig. 4-12). Mild proximal hydronephrosis and hydroureter are usually present. This alteration is the end result of a fibrotic retraction that envelops the ureter, interfering more with peristalsis than mechanically obstructing the ureter. It must be emphasized that a degree of medial deviation is found in a small percentage of normal individuals. Deviation of the right ureter must be distinguished from a retrocaval ureter, which assumes an S-shaped medial curvature at approximately L_3. An important feature of retroperitoneal fibrosis, aside from the ureteral deviation noted on ultrasonography and CT, is the presence of a soft-tissue fibrotic mass located anterior to the lumbar spine, adjacent to the great vessels and surrounding the ureters. Enlarged lymph nodes associated with lymphoma or metastatic disease also cause deviation of the ureters, but generally in a direction opposite to that noted in retroperitoneal fibrosis. Lymph nodes in this location lie medial to the ureters, and subsequent enlargement projects the ureters laterally (Fig. 4-13). However, within the osseous pelvis the lymph nodes are anatomically located more laterally in relation to the ureter, and as a result the ureters are then displaced medially. This inverse relationship allows for easy recognition of enlarged lymph nodes in the retroperitoneum.

Papillary Necrosis

Many factors contribute to the development of papillary necrosis; among these are diabetes mellitus, urinary tract infection, renal vein thrombosis, hypertension, obstruction, sickle cell disease, and analgesic nephropathy. The pathologic changes of papillary necrosis have been well

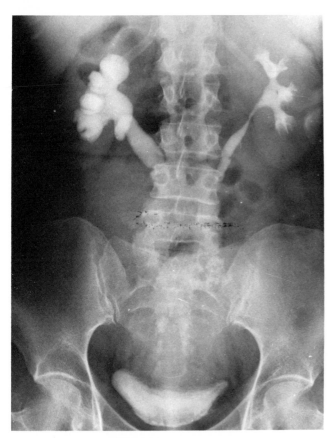

Fig. 4-12. Retroperitoneal fibrosis. Both kidneys are obstructed. The ureters are deviated medially and obstructed at the level of L4. At this level, the fibrotic process is seen as an increased amount of mass density.

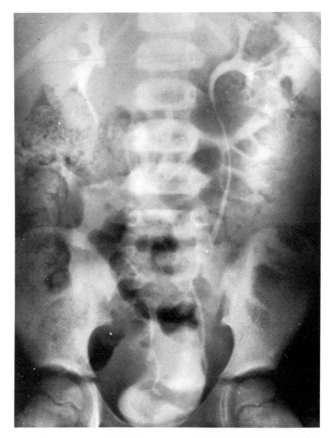

Fig. 4-13. Retroperitoneal lymph node enlargement. Urogram in patient with Hodgkin's disease demonstrates deviation of middle third of ureter and medial deviation of distal ureter. Note indentation on right side of bladder by enlarged lymph nodes.

studied in analgesic nephropathy. The severity of these changes varies according to the amount of drugs ingested. Analgesic nephropathy occurs most often in middle-aged and elderly women with a long history of ingesting large amounts of analgesics. The incidence of nephropathy is particularly high in hot climates, suggesting the possibility that dehydration may potentiate the effect. Another unusual complication associated with long-standing analgesic ingestion is the formation of transitional cell carcinoma, which is found more often in patients who consume large amounts of drugs.

The major cause of papillary necrosis is medullary ischemia. The initial damage occurs at the level of the loop of Henle and the vasa recta. As the disease progresses, there is subsequent loss of these loops along with destruction of the epithelium of the vasa recta. In advanced cases, diffuse fibrosis and chronic inflammatory cell infiltration associated with tubular atrophy and glomerular hyalinization occur within the interstitium.

RADIOGRAPHIC FINDINGS. Two major configurations, medullary and papillary, comprise the radiographic findings of papillary necrosis on conventional urographic studies. In the early and acute phases, diminished secretion of contrast material in the affected area occurs, with subsequent necrosis of the papillae. Central cavitation with subsequent sloughing results in a configuration that is termed the medullary form, whereas the term papillary is associated with necrosis and sloughing of an entire papilla (Fig. 4-14). As a result the radiographic features in the medullary form are recognized as tracts that extend from

the fornix of the calyx into the lateral apsect of the medulla. A central round or oval collection of contrast is generally associated with the papillary form. In some situations, the necrotic tissue fails to slough and the diagnosis can be suggested only after calcium has precipitated within the necrotic tissue. Necrotic tissue passing down the pelvocalyceal system and ureter can cause ureteral obstruction. The obstructing defect is obviously nonopaque and is radiographically indistinguishable from blood clots. Late stages of papillary necrosis are manifested by calyces that are round or saccular in appearance and represent communication of the necrotic areas with the calyx. The overall size of the kidney remains normal in most cases involving analgesic abuse, although with severe and chronic involvement kidneys eventually decrease in size. In this stage, kidney contour is generally irregular due to atrophy and fibrosis.

Calculous Disease of the Genitourinary Tract

Nephrolithiasis and nephrocalcinosis describe the two major types of stone formation that occur within the kidney. *Nephrolithiasis* is categorized as the presence of renal stones within the collecting system, located either within a calyx of the kidney or the pelvis, while *nephrocalcinosis* refers to the precipitation of calcification within the renal

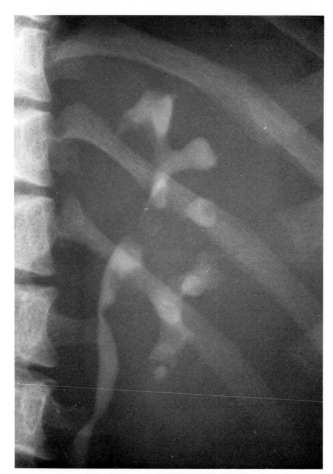

Fig. 4-14. Papillary necrosis: Sickle cell disease. The calyces are all blunted. There is a circular collection of contrast located within the lower pole papilla.

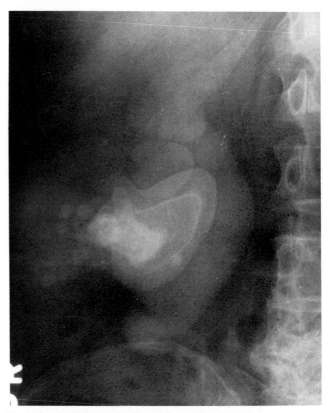

Fig. 4-15. Staghorn calculus. A large, lamellated calculus occupies the renal pelvis as well as some of the adjacent calyces. Multiple calculi are also present. The collecting system is dilatated and poorly opacified.

parenchyma. Calculi occupying either all or a large part of the renal collecting system are referred to as *staghorn calculi.*

NEPHROLITHIASIS. A variety of calculi form within the urogenital tract, some of which occur as the result of recognized or unknown urinary tract abnormalities, while others develop following infestation by crystalline complexes in association with obstruction or a chronically infected urinary tract. Basically, stones are classified as either opaque or nonopaque. Only densely opaque stones, consisting mainly of calcium oxalate and calcium phosphate, are well visualized on conventional abdominal studies. These stones develop idiopathically, although oxalate stones are not found frequently in patients with Crohn's disease. Slightly opaque calculi, such as cysteine and struvite calculi, are poorly and infrequently noted on routine studies. Struvite stones are both common and important since they are associated with chronic urinary tract infections, especially those due to urea-splitting organisms. Struvite stones are composed of magnesium ammonium phosphate and are often laminated. These calculi, along with cysteine stones, have a strong tendency to form staghorn calculi (Fig. 4-15). Apparently, calcium oxalate and calcium phosphate calculi are also prone to forming staghorn calculi. Uric acid stones are generally small and radiolucent, unless they contain calcium. Twenty-five percent of patients with uric acid stones have associated gout and twenty-five percent of patients with gout also develop uric acid stones.

The common presenting symptoms of urinary tract calculi are gross hematuria, renal colic, urosepsis, and abdominal flank pain. This presentation is usually sufficient for diagnosis. The main urologic feature is dilatation of the collecting system proximal to the obstructing calculus, which appears as a meniscus-shaped defect at the point of obstruction. In a certain percentage of cases in which the calculus is opaque, the stone may be visualized projecting along the anatomic pathway of the ureter on the conventional abdominal film (Fig. 4-16A). The overall urologic findings in general depend greatly upon the size of the obstructing calculus. Occasionally, with the presence of small stones, the entire intravenous pyelogram may appear completely normal. Localized spasm and minimal ureteral dilatation may be sufficient evidence to suggest the diagnosis. Larger calculi produce complete obstruction impeding progress of contrast beyond the level of the stone. With resulting loss of peristalsis the ureter appears tube-like, and the term *columnization* is used to describe this appearance (Fig. 4-16B). The renal pelvis and calyces are also dilated. Because of the obstruction, tubular secretion is impaired and overall opacification of the kidney is delayed. This can be demonstrated by performance of a nephrogram early in the study. During the nephrographic stage, the entire kidney becomes dense. Distinction between cortex and medulla, and eventually between the collecting systems, becomes apparent as the contrast slowly perfuses throughout the kidney. Delayed studies are therefore necessary to demonstrate the dilatation, as well as the site of the obstruction. Bear in mind that these stones frequently lie within the osseous pelvis, and as a result are often difficult to see (Fig. 4-16A). Oblique studies are frequently required to demonstrate the distal portion of the ureter. Patients with severe renal colic due to

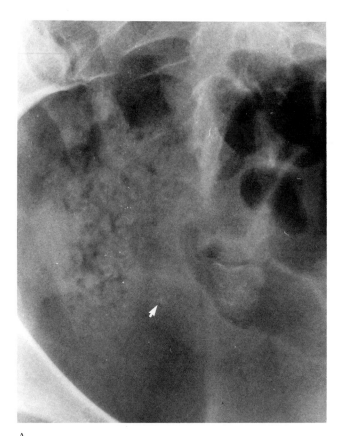

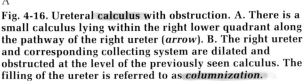

A

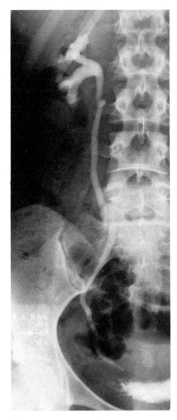

B

Fig. 4-16. Ureteral calculus with obstruction. A. There is a small calculus lying within the right lower quadrant along the pathway of the right ureter (*arrow*). B. The right ureter and corresponding collecting system are dilated and obstructed at the level of the previously seen calculus. The filling of the ureter is referred to as *columnization*.

acute obstruction occasionally manifest peripelvic and perirenal extravasation of contrast during excretory urography. Increased ureteral pressure as well as increased peristaltic activity result in detachment of the capsule at the forniceal junction, allowing for urine extravasation.

NEPHROCALCINOSIS. The patterns of nephrocalcinosis are often suggestive of underlying disease. For example, when patterns are localized to an area in the kidney, lymphoma, infection, or old infarct must be considered. Widespread calcification loculated within the renal medulla is associated with the various hypercalcemic states, medullary sponge kidney, sarcoidosis, and renal tubular necrosis (Fig. 4-17). It is often difficult to be specific about the diagnosis, but the associated clinical and radiographic findings, and at times even the character of the calcifications, often narrow the possibilities. The type of calcifications seen in renal tubular acidosis, for example, are dense, typically uniform, and bilateral.

Renal Cysts

A variety of classifications corresponding to specific disease states has been presented thus far. However, as many different forms of cystic lesions arise in the kidney alone, classification is relatively confusing and no specific clas-

sifications are attempted in this chapter. Renal cysts are discussed instead as simple cysts, polycystic disease, multicystic kidney, and medullary cystic disease.

SIMPLE CYSTS. Simple cysts are relatively common renal lesions and appear in a variety of sizes and numbers. When multiple, they mimic adult polycystic disease; when single, they may resemble tumors. The pathogenesis of simple cysts is unknown. Tubular obstruction, vascular block, and ischemia all have been proposed as causes for its development. Cysts appear most often within the cortex, but are also found within the medullary portion of the renal parenchyma. The gross pathologic examination of the renal cortex demonstrates rounded, thin-walled translucent masses that are filled with clear, thin, straw-colored fluid. Occasionally hemorrhage or infection thickens the cyst wall to produce a brownish or blackish appearance. Most cysts are asymptomatic, but in some cases pressure on the renal parenchyma may cause hematuria, pain, or discomfort. Rarely an emergent cyst may enlarge within the hilum of the kidney, causing obstruction of one or more calyces.

Radiographic Features. The abdominal film is of little value in diagnosing the renal cyst. The lesion is recognizable as a nonspecific mass. In about 1 to 2 percent of cases layers of calcium deposit on the wall of the cyst and appear as a thin, curvilinear, peripheral, radiopaque line that resembles an egg shell. This appearance is unfortunately not pathognomonic, since the actual incidence of this type of calcification is higher in renal tumors. Irregular collections of calcification located within the mass, however, are far more characteristic for neoplasm. The urographic manifestations of a cyst are best seen during the nephrogram. The

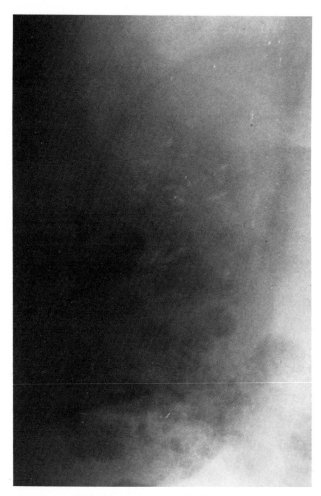

Fig. 4-17. Nephrocalcinosis. Multiple small calculi are scattered throughout the renal cortex.

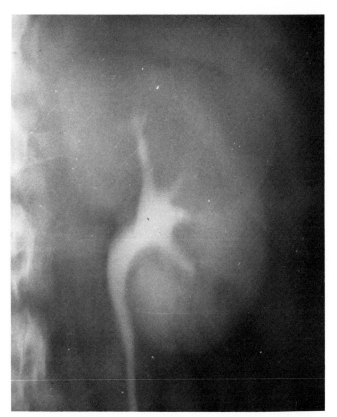

Fig. 4-18. Renal cyst: Nephrogram: A lucent mass arising from the lateral upper pole of the left kidney is seen on the nephrogram. The wall is fine and pencil-thin. Note the beak-like parenchymal defect as the cyst emerges from the kidney.

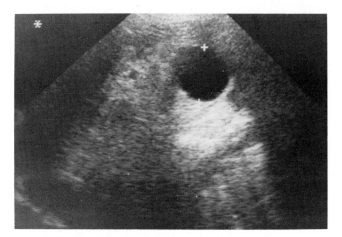

Fig. 4-19. Cyst: Ultrasonography. Echo-free mass is seen, with posterior acoustic enhancement.

cyst appears lucent, and if it bulges outside the confines of the kidney the outline of the wall may be visualized as a sharply defined, curvilinear structure (Fig. 4-18). A beak-like defect in the parenchyma appears at the point where the cyst wall emerges from the surface of the kidney. Cysts embedded well within the kidney cause considerable distortion of the calyces and pelvis. These findings appear similar to any expanding mass and are not absolute. The calyces, however, remain intact, a finding not always made in patients with renal tumor. Other conventional techniques, such as nephrotomography, help differentiate cysts from tumors.

The arteriographic features of cysts and tumors are similar in many ways. The cyst is a nonvascular mass; as a result the intrarenal vessels are usually stretched and displaced around the lesion, and changes of neovascularity are not encountered. During the nephrographic phase the characteristic feature of hypolucency within the cyst is well demonstrated.

Ultrasonography. Sonographic evaluation of a renal mass is of vital diagnostic importance. Three major sonographic features are associated with cystic lesions: (1) they are echo-free, even in high-gain settings; (2) they have smooth, well-defined walls; and (3) they demonstrate posterior acoustic enhancement (Fig. 4-19).

Computed Tomography. The characteristic features of a renal cyst seen on computed tomography resemble a com-

bination of those found on nephrotomography and ultrasound, and consist of the presence of a mass that basically demonstrates a very low attenuation, equivalent to that of water density (Fig. 4-20). Any variation in these criteria may indicate the presence of an underlying neoplasm.

Needle Aspiration. This procedure is done in situations where the above studies are not conclusive. The technique is essentially simple and carries little morbidity to the patient. To be extremely accurate, rigid diagnostic criteria must be adhered to. Essentially, clear cystic fluid having a low fat, protein, and lactic acid dehydrogenates content

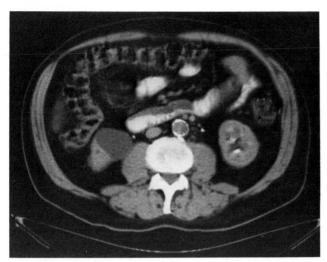

Fig. 4-20. Cyst: Large, low-density, well-marginated mass extending outside confines of kidney. Density of the lesion is equivalent to that of water and slightly below that of surrounding soft-tissue.

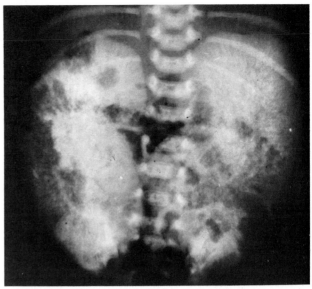

Fig. 4-21. Infantile polycystic kidneys: neonatal form. Nephrogram shows kidneys occupying almost the entire abdomen and demonstrating a striated appearance.

must be obtained. For additional confirmation, a double contrast study can be done by replacing all the aspirated fluid with contrast medium and making multiple exposures in various projections to ensure that the cyst wall is completely smooth and regular throughout.

The usual prognosis of a simple cyst is excellent. The incidence of an associated neoplasm developing within a nonresected cyst is highly uncommon. The coexistence of nonrelated cysts and tumors developing in different locations within the kidney is only 1 percent. This incidence is much higher in patients with underlying congenital lesions (e.g., von Hippel-Lindau disease).

POLYCYSTIC DISEASE. Polycystic disease of the kidney is a spectrum of inherited diseases that may be broadly divided into childhood and adult varieties. The childhood form is autosomal recessive, with variable cystic involvement of the renal and liver parenchyma. The adult form is autosomal dominant and affects mainly the kidneys.

Infantile Polycystic Disease. The infantile form is an uncommon disease that demonstrates a spectrum of renal and liver abnormalities. As a result, three clinicoradiologic forms emerge: (1) neonatal, (2) intermediate or infantile, noted in the first decade of life, and (3) juvenile, manifested at the end of the first decade or later. The most severe renal abnormalities predominate in the neonatal form and account for the poor prognosis. Only minimal renal changes are present in the juvenile form. However, the pathologic changes of periportal fibrosis and bile duct hyperplasia in the liver assume a greater degree of importance, and patients present with clinical findings of portal hypertension. In the neonatal and infantile form the kidneys are markedly enlarged, occupying almost the entire abdomen but still maintaining a reniform configuration (Figs. 4-21, 4-22). The outer surface is studded with small cysts, and on cross-section demonstrates enlarged, cystic, elongated tubules that radiate through the entire kidney. The urographic appearance is characteristic. Renal function is poor and during the nephrographic phase a striated appearance due to the dilated tubules is observed (see Figs. 4-21, 4-22). The kidneys in the juvenile form are not remarkably enlarged, function well, and in some patients

Juvenile: Portal Hypertension

may be almost completely normal (Fig. 4-23A). However, ectatic ducts are often opacified in the renal pyramids. Enlarged spleen, esophageal varices, and so forth are some of the radiographic features of portal hypertension that may be encountered (Fig. 4-23B).

Adult Polycystic Disease. Adult polycystic disease is the most common form of polycystic disease encountered in clinical practice. The lesion is transmitted as an autosomal dominant trait and is almost always bilateral. In about one-third of the cases, cysts are also found in the liver, pancreas, and lung (Fig. 4-24). In a recent study done with CT, the incidence of associated cysts in the liver was found to be as high as 74 percent. This finding is of significance, considering the increased longevity of these patients. In addition, approximately 15 percent of the patients with adult polycystic disease have one or more cerebral aneurysms, and rupture of these is responsible for the early mortality noted in these patients.

Liver
Pancreas
Lung
Aneurys.

The pathologic features of this form of cystic disease are characterized by an abnormal, irregular intermixture of normal and abnormal tubules and nephrons. The cysts can arise from any part of the nephron. Although the lesion may be present at birth, in most instances a certain length of time is required for cysts to enlarge in order to produce clinical symptoms. As a result, the diagnosis is usually not made until the fourth or fifth decade of life, although the disease has been described in infants and children. The kidneys are enlarged and are almost completely replaced by a multitude of cysts of varying sizes. Only occasionally are flecks of calcium noted in the walls of the cysts. In the early stages of the disease renal function is not impaired and the calyceal structures are easily demonstrated. The latter are frequently deformed and displaced by the adjacent cystic masses (Fig. 4-24A). Calyceal structures may appear irregular and elongated but are almost never eroded or destroyed. The remaining interstitial parenchyma is thickened and irregular, and during the nephrographic phase demonstrates a distinctive swiss-cheese appearance due to the presence of radiolucent cysts (Fig. 4-24B). This latter appearance is also present on both ultrasound and computed tomography. These modalities are very helpful

Infantile
Kidney
Liver

Adult: most common
Bilateral
Auto Dom

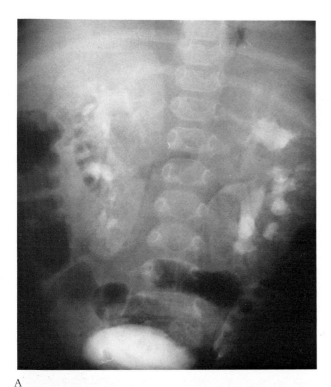

A

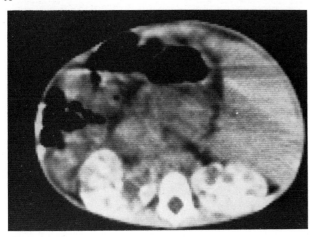

B

Fig. 4-22. Infantile polycystic kidneys: Intermediate or infantile form. A. The kidneys are markedly enlarged with corresponding elongation and distortion of the collecting systems. Contrast is also retained within dilatated tubules that radiate toward the periphery of the kidney. B. In same patient, CT shows multiple cystic spaces to be more apparent within the renal structures (probably a conformation of the dilated tubules).

in establishing the presence or absence of tumors and have replaced angiography in this regard.

Polycystic disease should not be mistaken for the multiple simple cysts that are not infrequently encountered in the elderly. The kidneys in these patients are usually not enlarged, and the cysts are fewer in number. However, the kidneys found in tuberous sclerosis may also contain multiple cysts that resemble polycystic disease. Multiple cystic abnormalities have also been described in the Laurence-Moon-Biedl syndrome (Fig. 4-25).

MULTICYSTIC KIDNEY. Multicystic kidney usually presents in neonates as an asymptomatic unilateral flank

not enlarged

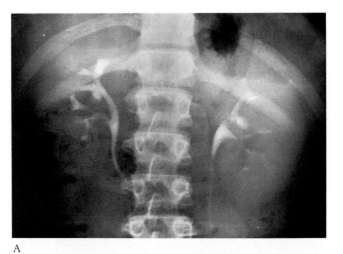

A

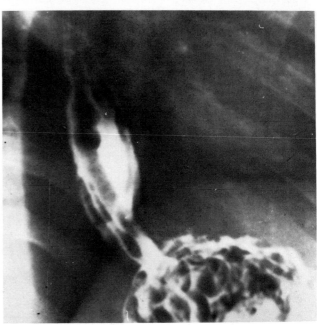

B

Fig. 4-23. Infantile polycystic disease: Juvenile form. A. Both kidneys are only moderately enlarged and aside from minimal distortion of the calyces, appear almost normal. B. Esophagram reveals esophageal varices with the lower end of the esophagus and fundus of the stomach.

mass. It is the most common abdominal mass discovered within the first twenty-four hours of life and is overall the second most common abdominal mass occurring in the neonatal period. Contralateral renal anomalies, such as multicystic dysplastic kidney and congenital ureteropelvic obstruction, are found in approximately one-third of the cases. When bilateral multicystic disease occurs, it is accompanied by Potter's syndrome, which is fatal. The multicystic kidney probably represents one part in the spectrum of abnormalities that evolve from ureteropelvic junction obstruction, in which atresia is most often noted as the basic defect. This concept is supported by the occasional finding of well-developed, functioning renal tissue in the multicystic kidney and by the high association of contralateral renal abnormalities. The ureter on the involved side almost always ends blindly, and ipsilateral hemitrigonal atrophy is found when the entire ureter is absent. Pathogenesis of the multicystic kidney is unknown

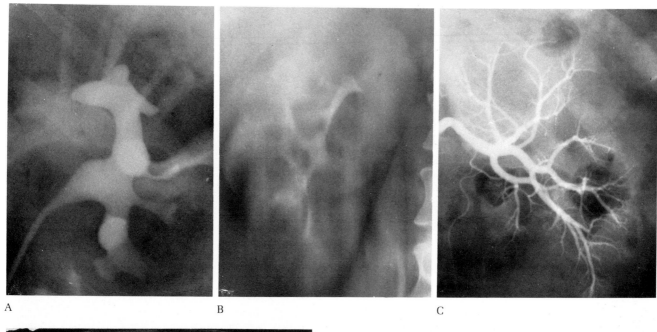

A   B   C

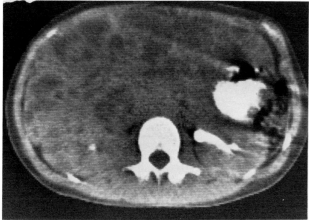

D

**Fig. 4-24. Polycystic disease: Autosomal dominant. A.
Intravenous urogram. The calyces are stretched and distorted
by adjacent cystic masses. B. Nephrogram. Collecting system
distortion caused by multiple lucent masses are well
visualized. C. Arteriogram. Similar distortion of vessels is
produced by the cystic lesions. D. Computed tomography.
Lucent, well-defined cysts occupy most of the liver. Left
kidney is also diffusely replaced by low density cystic spaces.**

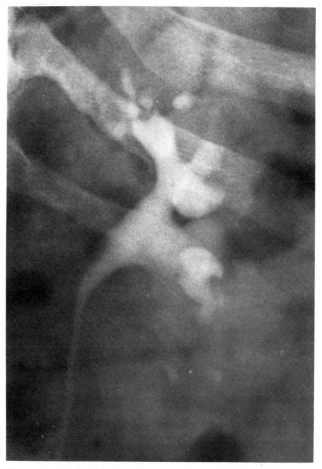

**Fig. 4-25. Cystic changes: Laurence-Moon-Biedl syndrome.
Contrast is present within multiple small cyst spaces within
the upper pole of the kidney. Other dysplastic and cystic
changes are noted in the lower pole.**

but is believed to be sustained from an injury or vascular
incident, which results in atresia and absent development
of the proximal ureter, pelvis, and calyceal structures because of deranged growth and branching of the ureteral
bud. The arteries supplying such kidneys are often either
atretic or hypoplastic.

Multicystic kidney is generally a harmless, asymptomatic mass consisting of dysplastic renal tissue with multiple grape-like cysts of varying size. The need for surgical
removal is questionable, but surgery is often still under-
taken because of the remote possibility of neoplasm developing in the dysplastic tissue.

Diagnostic Findings. Ultrasonography in most instances is
the diagnostic method of choice. Findings consist of semi-
lucent cystic structures containing multiple septi (Fig. 4-

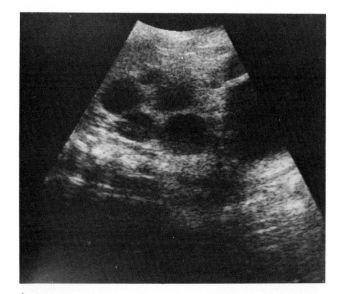

A

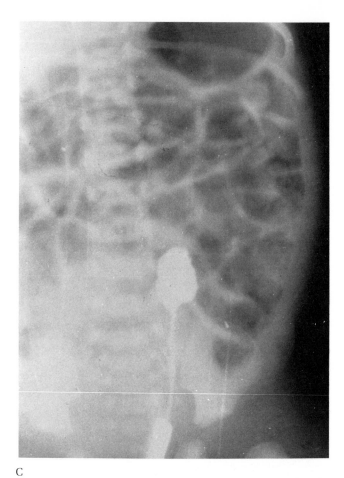

C

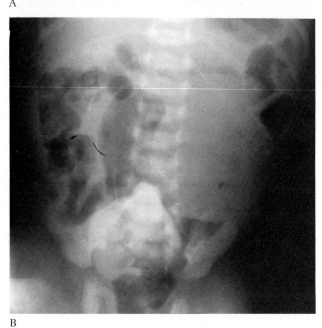

B

Fig. 4-26. Multicystic kidney. A. Ultrasound. Multiple, lucent cystic structures of varying sizes are associated with a single large cystic structure in the left kidney. B. Intravenous pyelogram, delayed 25-minute film, reveals a nonfunctioning mass within the left portion of the abdomen. The right kidney is visible. C. Retrograde study reveals an atretic ureter with extravasation of contrast.

26A), which differs from findings in hydronephrotic kidney caused by ureteropelvic obstruction. In this disorder, residual parenchymal tissue and dilated renal calyces that communicate with the pelvis are demonstrated. A nonfunctioning renal mass that may displace intestinal gas is the main urographic feature (Fig. 4-26B), which is more evident in the cross-table lateral view. In a few cases, however, the walls of the cyst have been shown to contain remnants of cortical tissue that opacify during the total body opacification phase. Reflux into a blindly ending ureter can occur during voiding cystourethrography (Fig. 4-26C). In the adult, an undiagnosed multicystic dysplastic kidney is occasionally discovered as a calcified, rounded, cystic mass.

MEDULLARY SPONGE KIDNEY. Medullary sponge kidney is a developmental defect characterized by either cylindrical or sacular cystic dilatation of the collecting tubules in one or more renal papillae. Renal function in general is not impaired and cysts in other organ structures are not encountered. Pathologically, the medulla and renal pyramids are enlarged because of the dilated tubules. Calcium deposition occurs in 32 percent of cases within the dilated tubules. Symptoms related to these calculi often call attention to the condition. The exact cause of this lesion is not known, but in all probability it is a developmental defect affecting the formation of the collecting tubules. The diagnosis is usually made by excretory urography. In the early stage of the lesion, contrast stagnates in the collecting tubules and produces a characteristic streak-like appearance within the papillae. With increasing severity of the lesion, the streaks become more linear and obvious and eventually progress to form tiny cysts (Fig. 4-27). The term *bouquet of flowers* was originally used to describe the appearance of these cysts when associated with contrast in the adjacent calyx.

The ultrasonographic appearance of the medullary sponge kidney is not defined too clearly, since the abundant sinus fat and overlying muscle may obscure the medulla. In children the dilated tubules strikingly enhance pyramidal demonstration.

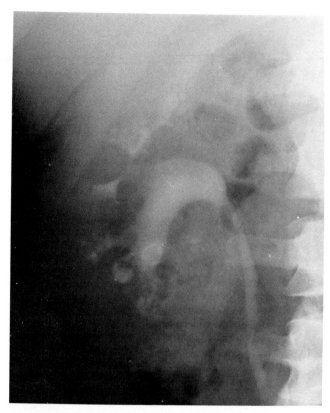

Fig. 4-27. Medullary sponge kidney. Multiple cystic collections of varying sizes are located within all the renal papillae.

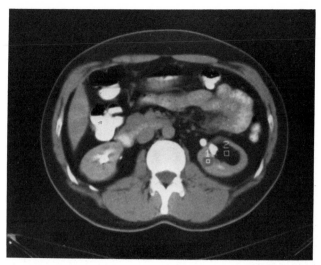

Fig. 4-28. Angiomyolipoma: Computed tomography. A large, cyst-like lesion within the center of the kidney. The density of the lesion is equal to that of fat tissue surrounding the kidney.

Benign Tumors

ADENOMAS. Adenomas are common benign tumors that occur as single or multiple yellowish-gray nodules within the renal cortex immediately below the renal capsule. The overall incidence of these lesions noted at necropsy varies from 0.8 to 3.0 percent. The smaller lesions are most often incidental findings, although tumors of large size can cause a localized bulge of the renal surface and project sufficiently into the parenchyma to disturb the collecting system. Histologically, three cell types have been described; these are papillary, tubular, and alveolar. Each type may be solid or cystic in nature, although the vascular supply in each is quite modest in most instances.

The majority of adenomas are asymptomatic and are usually discovered accidentally. The neoplastic nature of these lesions is problematic, since they show little or no tendency to grow during a five-year interval. Despite their benign histologic appearance, many pathologists consider these tumors malignant if they measure more than 5 cm in diameter.

Urographic Features. The majority of adrenal adenomas are too small to reveal any abnormality on routine urographic studies. The early change is usually an alteration in the renal contour, which may easily pass unnoticed. Larger, more centrally growing lesions produce displacement and pressure changes of the adjacent calyces. This distortion is smooth and regular and no areas of erosion or destruction are encountered, regardless of the size of the lesion. During

the nephrographic phase, the lesion in 80 percent of cases is lucent because of the hypovascular nature of the lesion. However, a mass-like density is present both on CT and ultrasound (e.g., a well-defined echogenic mass on ultrasound and a soft-tissue mass on CT).

ANGIOMYOLIPOMA (HAMARTOMA). Angiomyolipomas are benign mesenchymal lesions commonly found in patients with tuberous sclerosis. In these patients, the tumors are frequently multiple and involve both kidneys. Angiomyolipomas are also known to occur sporadically as solitary lesions and in this situation are found almost exclusively in women approximately 40 years of age. The tumor is composed, as the name implies, of multiple tissue elements (e.g., blood vessel, smooth muscle, and adipose tissue). These elements vary in consistency from one tumor to another. Grossly, the mass appears yellow and lobulated, and is firm and more friable than fatty tissue, which it can resemble. Distant metastasis has never been reported, although local infiltration by tumor does occur. The presenting symptoms are pain, mass, and hematuria due to hemorrhage because of tumor necrosis. The conventional urographic studies are nonspecific, since a large, single, space-occupying mass that may be indistinguishable from hypernephroma is seen. However, CT and ultrasound are capable of detecting the presence of fat within the tumor and a correct diagnosis can be often made (Fig. 4-28). The angiographic findings are relatively characteristic, but unfortunately are not always distinguishable from hypernephromas. For example, early shunting with venous filling as seen in hypernephroma is not noted in angiomyolipomas.

Malignant Tumors

WILMS' TUMOR. Wilms' tumor is the most common renal neoplasm encountered in children and accounts for approximately 30 percent of all neoplasms in this age group. It is presently the most curable of childhood malignancies, with survival rates of more than 80 percent currently being

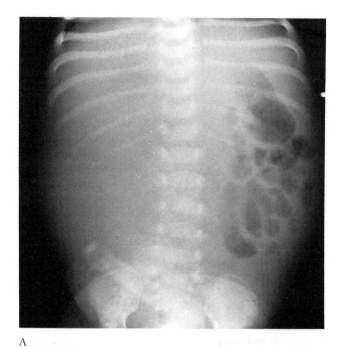

A

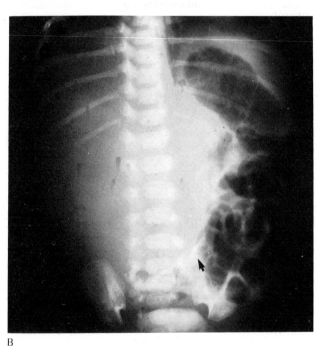

B

Fig. 4-29. Mesoblastic nephroma. A. Abdominal film. A large mass occupies the major part of the patient's abdomen. B. Intravenous urogram. The mass displaces the collecting system over the sacrum and left iliac bone (*arrow*).

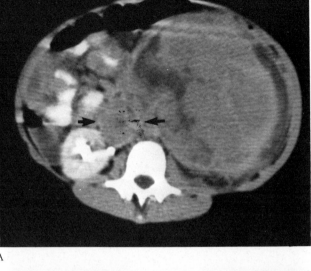

A

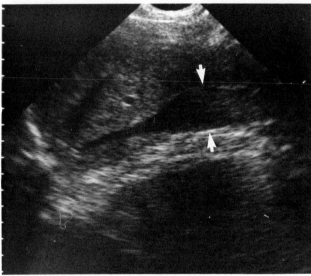

B

Fig. 4-30. Wilms' tumor: Ultrasound and computed tomography. A. Computed tomography confirms the presence of this mass in the kidney. Tumor thrombosis is also present in I.V.C. (*arrows*). B. Ultrasound. The inferior vena cava (I.V.C.) is widened and contains a tumor thrombus (*arrows*). The intrahepatic portion of the I.V.C. is normal.

achieved. The tumor is most frequently seen in children below age 5, with peak incidence at around 3 years of age. It is rarely noted in infants below age 6 months. What was once defined as neonatal Wilms' tumor is now recognized as a benign hamartoma (mesoblastic nephroma). Almost all solid tumors in the neonate are of this origin and carry an excellent prognosis (Fig. 4-29). Benign hamartoma manifests many of the radiographic features of Wilms' tumor, but in contrast to Wilms' tumor is derived from a single cell line consisting of bundles of fibroblasts.

The symptoms of Wilms' tumor are minimal and the lesion is usually detected as an abdominal swelling or mass.

Good Px

Hematuria is not a frequent symptom, in contrast to renal tumors found in the adult. Wilms' tumor may be associated with other abnormalities, such as aniridia, hemihypertrophy, and Beckwith-Wiedemann syndrome. Bilateral tumors present in younger children on the average and are more common in males.

Wilms' tumors are rapidly growing, solid tumors composed of cells derived from multiple blastemas. At the time of discovery they are fairly large, bulky masses but are frequently contained for the most part within the renal capsule, a feature important in determining the ultimate outcome for the patient. The radiographic features of Wilms' tumor consist predominantly of a large soft-tissue mass that may displace adjacent viscera. The tumor rarely extends across the midline of the body, since it is contained within the renal capsule. Calcification occurs infre-

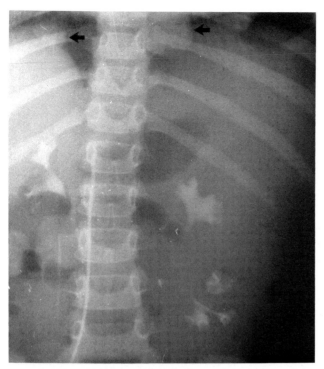

Fig. 4-31. Wilms' tumor with metastases. The left upper and middle calyceal group are displaced by a mass. Pulmonary metastases are already noted within both lower lung fields (*arrows*).

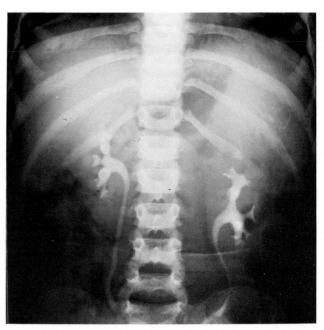

Fig. 4-32. Neuroblastoma. There is a large mass within the left upper quadrant, displacing the kidney symmetrically and uniformly downward. Linear and spotty areas of calcification are noted within the mass.

No Ca++   4-10% Bilateral

quently and is seen in only approximately 5 percent of masses. During the total body opacification phase of the urogram, a combination of solid and lucent components due to necrosis and hemorrhage are encountered. Ultrasonography is presently considered the initial modality when evaluating abdominal masses; it demonstrates a mass with a mixture of echogenic and nonechogenic changes. Findings of a similar type are made on CT (Fig. 4-30). The excretory urogram is typical for an intrarenal mass, with main features consisting of considerable distortion, elongation, and compression of the adjacent pelvocalyceal structures located in the immediate vicinity of the tumor (Fig. 4-31). Hydronephrosis and decreased renal function are observed when the tumor compresses the renal pelvis or the remaining renal parenchyma. A nonopacifying kidney may occur without obstruction when the tumor infiltrates the kidney or occludes the renal vein. Arteriography is no longer essential in the diagnostic evaluation of Wilms' tumor. It can be useful in excluding neoplasm in the opposite kidney, involvement of the liver, and other associated conditions. These considerations are presently better determined through the use of ultrasound or CT (Fig. 4-30B). Wilms' tumor is bilateral in 4 to 10 percent of cases. Although 65 percent of cases may be diagnosed at the initial study, the remaining cases may require 3 to 10 years before the lesion is detected in the opposite kidney. Wilms' tumor can metastasize to the lungs, a finding made in 8 to 15 percent of cases at the initial examination (Fig. 4-31). *Wilms: meta → lung*

NEUROBLASTOMA. The overall incidence of neuroblastoma is almost equivalent to that of Wilms' tumor. However, in contrast to Wilms' tumor, this lesion can be encountered in younger infants. Neuroblastomas can occur anywhere along the sympathetic chain, although the ma-

younger kids

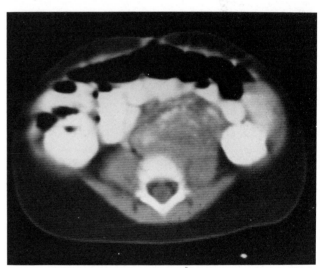

Fig. 4-33. Neuroblastoma: Computed tomography. A large mass is present within the lower lumbar region, with mottled and irregular areas of calcification and necrosis.

jority are suprarenal in origin (Fig. 4-32). Extraadrenal renal neuroblastomas have been observed in the organ of Zuckerkandl within the lower abdomen, pelvis, and upper thoracic area (Fig. 4-33). Tumors that occur in the upper thoracic region in the posterior mediastinum may produce erosions in the adjacent verterbral bodies, vertebra, and ribs and carry a much better prognosis than tumors located below the diaphragm.   *→ Bone*

Neuroblastomas disseminate rapidly to liver, bone marrow, orbit, and skin. Spread into neighboring lymph nodes produces widening of the paravertebral soft tissues, a feature that may be seen in the lower thorax and is occasionally the earliest radiographic manifestation of the disease. Calcification is fairly typical in this lesion, and is encountered in 50 percent of cases (Figs. 4-32, 4-33). The tumor is not encapsulated and often extends across the midline. The extrarenal location of the tumor easily differentiates it

Crosses midline
(+) Calcification (50%)
younger

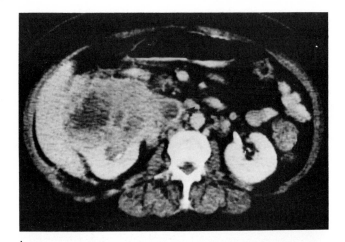

A

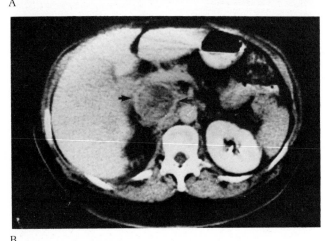

B

Fig. 4-34. Hypernephroma: Computed tomography. A. A large mass arises anteriorly from the kidney with multiple areas of necrosis. The inferior vena cava is dilated and filled with tumor thrombus. B. A more cephalic tomographic cut at the level of the liver better demonstrates the tumor thrombus within the I.V.C. (arrows).

Entire kidney displaced from Wilms' tumor. The entire kidney along with its calyceal structures is displaced uniformly (Fig. 4-32). Metastatic distribution is also different. Neuroblastoma spreads commonly to the bones, whereas Wilms' tumor affects the lungs. Associated clinical symptoms referable to the excess secretion of catecholamines have also been seen in neuroblastoma patients; these symptoms are occasionally the first indication of the presence of neuroblastoma and consist of fever, hypertension, and diarrhea. Bizarre myoclonic seizure and cerebellar symptoms have also been reported.

HYPERNEPHROMA OR ADENOCARCINOMA. Renal cell carcinoma or hypernephroma is a common renal tumor of tubular origin. Approximately 20,000 new cases of this carcinoma occur each year in the United States. These tumors have a peak incidence in relatively young individuals (the mean age is 55 years) and demonstrate strong male dominance. The lesion is unfortunately not often diagnosed early because of the absence of symptoms. The classic triad of hematuria, palpable mass, and weight loss are generally late manifestations occuring in less than 15 percent of patients. The ultimate prognosis depends on the histo-

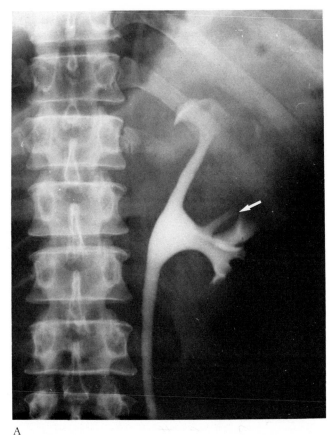

A

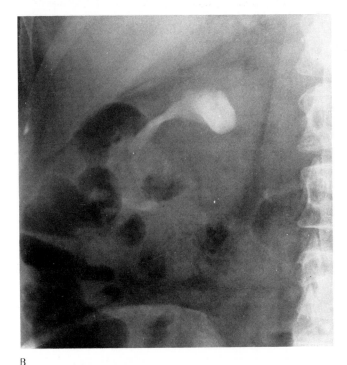

B

Fig. 4-35. Hypernephroma. A. Retrograde study reveals a large, space-occupying mass involving the mid- and upper pole of the left kidney. The upper pole calyces are elongated and associated with downward displacement of the middle pole calyces. One middle pole calyx is amputated (arrow). B. A large, space-occupying mass is present within the major portion of the kidney. The visualized calyces are deformed and dilatated due to partial obstruction by the mass.

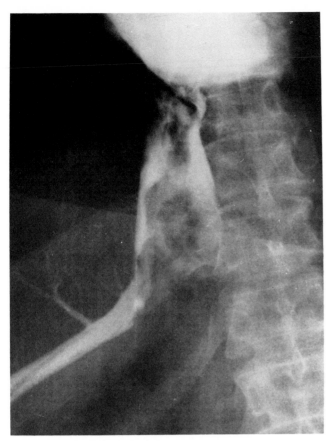

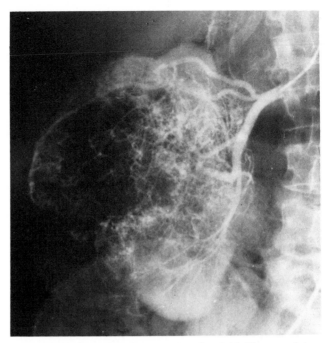

Fig. 4-37. Hypernephroma: Angiography. A highly vascular tumor occupies most of the kidney. Part of the mass extends outside the medial and lateral kidney borders.

Fig. 4-36. I.V.C.: Tumor thrombus. The lumen of the inferior vena cava is filled by an irregular soft-tissue mass that extends into the right atrium.

logic character, as well as the staging, of the lesion. The various stages are:

1. The tumor is confined to the kidney.
2. The tumor extends outside the kidney into the perirenal fat, but is confined within Gerota's fascia.
3. The tumor involves the renal veins, the renal lymph nodes, and the vena cava.
4. The tumor involves distant as well as adjacent organs.

The lesion is frequently diagnosed or at minimum is suspected by either ultrasound, CT, or conventional radiology. Basically, the findings consist of a mass arising within the kidney. As a result, the overall kidney is enlarged, lobular, and irregular. Ultrasonography demonstrates a mass containing multiple echoes, and a correspondingly high-density lesion is encountered on CT (Fig. 4-34). The calyceal structures on conventional urographic studies are generally distorted and demonstrate elongation and irregularity. Encroachment upon the collecting system by the mass causes flattening and elongation and occasionally filling defects (Fig. 4-35A). Large tumors are known to completely obliterate the pelvis, causing obstruction with impairment of renal function (Fig. 4-35B). Invasion of the renal vein is a well-known complication (Figs. 4-34B, 4-36), as is usual involvement of the surrounding nodes. Invasion of the renal vein not only accounts for complete loss of function of the kidney, but also worsens the general outlook of the lesion.

Although angiography has received little attention recently because of the advantages of CT and ultrasonography, there are many who still use this procedure in order

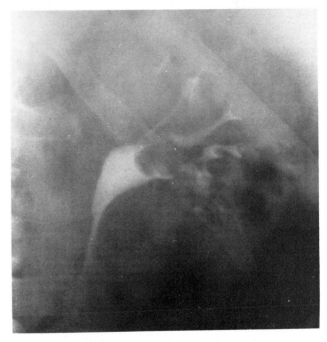

Fig. 4-38. Transitional cell tumor. A small, irregular mass occupies the proximal portion of the renal pelvis. A portion of pelvis and an associated infundibulum are obliterated.

to trace the entire vascular supply and to determine the vascular nature of the lesion in cases of doubt (Fig. 4-37, 4-38). The lesion's vascular nature is not always specific, since lesions with a minimal vascular supply, severe necrosis, or hemorrhage may be difficult to distinguish from cysts. Ultrasonography and CT are excellent modalities for distinguishing solid neoplasms from cysts, but despite the excellence of these procedures, there are some lesions in which the diagnosis may still remain unclear. Calcification is occasionally visualized within the tumor and is quite

Cortical Ca⁺⁺

significant when nonperipheral in location. Tumors are echogenic on ultrasound, but can also present as basically echo-free masses with low-level internal echoes.

UROEPITHELIAL CARCINOMAS. Uroepithelial tumors occur most commonly late in middle age and affect men more frequently than women, at a ratio approximately of 2 : 1. Transitional cell carcinoma and the less common squamous cell carcinoma are the two main histologic types encountered. Transitional cell tumors vary in their morphologic presentation and also correspondingly in their degrees of malignancy. The less invasive and aggressive lesions are grossly papillary, whereas nonpapillary transitional tumors are invasive and more aggressive. Squamous cell carcinoma is almost entirely infiltrative and therefore highly malignant. Papillary cell carcinomas are commonly multicentric. However, when the lesion presents as a solitary tumor it is most frequently located in the renal pelvis. A second tumor discovered is almost always on the same side.

In most cases, patients present with the triad of hematuria, pain, and a palpable mass. The latter is usually the result of an obstructing hydronephrosis or is due to the extension of tumor outside the renal area. The radiographic findings are usually diagnostic and typically present as a filling defect associated with destructive changes within the renal pelvis or calyx (Fig. 4-38). Small lesions may be subtle and are often mistaken for a blood clot or vessel. The more aggressive lesions also infiltrate the surrounding renal parenchyma; this behavior is most often noted with squamous carcinomas. Chronic infections and calculi are predisposing conditions associated with squamous carcinomas of kidney.

Transitional cell tumors arising within the ureter or bladder demonstrate similar radiographic features (e.g., an intraluminal mass or constriction) despite the different locations. Frequently, tumors arising within the bladder present as large, fungating papillary masses that extend through the bladder wall into the surrounding tissue. Papillary tumors in the ureter enlarge within the lumen, causing the ureter to subsequently widen. This presentation is characteristic and differentiates papillary tumors from most other obstructing ureteral lesions.

Decreased Renal Function

Decreased renal function generally indicates underlying renal parenchymal disease. The radiographic assessment of the kidney allows the physician to analyze renal size and contour as well as the configuration of the calyces and the adjacent papillae. Renal size is estimated by measuring renal length, which is generally approximately 10 to 12 cm. The left kidney is always larger than the right. Ultrasonography and tomography are the two principal means of determining renal size. The measurements obtained on ultrasound are always smaller because of the magnification factor associated with tomography. Ultrasound also affords the opportunity to study the internal architecture of the kidney in order to exclude obstruction as the primary or contributing factor.

Excretory urography is of little value, particularly if the serum creatinine level is above 5 mg/dl. However, the size and contour of the kidney can be evaluated during the nephrographic phase. The addition of tomography at this time potentiates the detail. Small kidneys with irregular

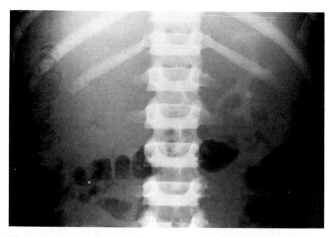

Fig. 4-39. Acute glomerulonephritis: Decreased Renal Function. Both kidneys are enlarged, with only minimal contrast noted within the left kidney. The collecting system in this kidney is due to the intraparenchymal inflammatory changes and edema.

scarred contours often represent significant renal disease, particularly when associated with decreased renal function. Bear in mind that in the early stages of chronic renal disease the kidney may be of normal size. In chronic atrophic pyelonephritis, the kidney is generally small, the contour irregularly scarred, and the calyces underlying the scars abnormal. These findings differ from the changes associated with renal infarction, since the calyces underlying the cortical abnormalities are basically normal.

Angiography is of no diagnostic significance, although specific alterations in the intrarenal vessels are apparent. The branches are pruned, narrowed, and irregular and are associated with decreased flow in many of the conditions causing parenchymal disease.

Acute renal failure can be described as a clinical syndrome with abrupt and frequently reversible transient decrease in renal function. Many terms, such as acute tubular necrosis, crush syndrome, and lower nephron nephrosis have been used to describe the condition. Basically, acute renal failure results from injury or poisoning of the renal tubules (e.g., mercury or lead poisoning or the use of anesthetic drugs). Intravenous contrast studies may also precipitate an acute decrease in function in patients with underlying renal disease. The actual pathogenesis of acute renal failure is not completely understood. Factors such as possible blocked effusion of filtrate, tubular blockade, and tubular cell edema have been considered responsible for the radiographic process. The radiographic findings of the urinary tract in patients with acute renal failure simply demonstrate a prolonged or absent nephrogram (Fig. 4-39). The study does allow for assessment of anatomic appearance, renal size, and contour. Angiography in acute renal failure is of no significance.

Intrarenal Arterial Aneurysms

The diagnosis of renal arterial aneurysm is basically established via angiography. Occasionally, it may be suggested on abdominal films by the presence of curvilinear calcifications that lie adjacent to or cause displacement or pressure defects of the collecting systems during the urographic study. Periarteritis is the most widely diagnosed

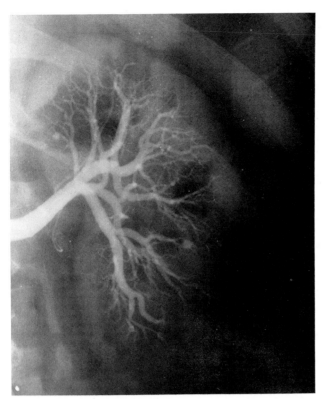

Fig. 4-40. Polyarteritis. Arteriographic study reveals multiple small aneurysms within the kidney.

systemic angiitis associated with intrarenal arterial aneurysms (Fig. 4-40). Multiple studies seem to indicate that some of these aneurysms are reversible following therapy. Similar abnormalities involving the vessels and associated aneurysms have been seen with mycotic aneurysms following drug abuse.

Renal Infarction

Acute renal infarction occurs following arterial or venous occlusion. The majority of these lesions involve a branch vessel; only rarely is an entire kidney, or even a major segment of a kidney, affected. Emboli as a cause of arterial occlusion are found more frequently than thrombosis. The former often arise from a heart damaged by such conditions as rheumatic heart disease, bacterial endocarditis, or myocardial infarction. Another important clinical factor that results in renal ischemia is abdominal trauma, which may take the form of severe contusion, rupture of the vascular pedicle, or thrombosis of the renal artery. The overall symptoms of acute renal infarction vary from minimal changes encountered with small lesions to abrupt onset of severe abdominal pain, nausea, vomiting, hematuria, and shock in cases where a major vessel is involved. In early phases of large vessel occlusion, overall size and configuration of the kidney are not altered although excretion of contrast material is impeded on excretory urography. The presence of a normal collecting system noted on retrograde pyelography is diagnostic. The radiographic findings of venous occlusion as the cause of renal infarction varies slightly, since interstitial hemorrhage is the main pathologic feature. As a result, the kidney may be enlarged, and varying degrees of contrast secretion are encountered (Fig.

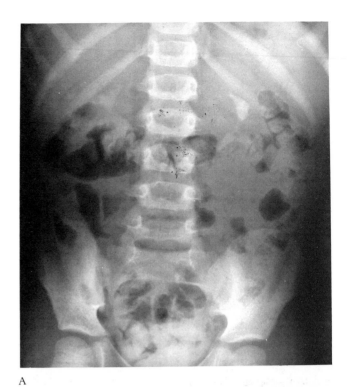

A

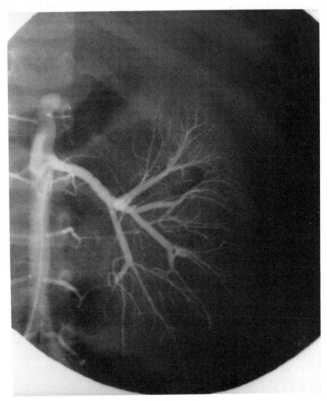

B

Fig. 4-41. Renal infarction. A. Both kidneys are poorly visualized. The inferior pole on the left is swollen and not opacified. B. Arteriographic study shows poor perfusion of the lower pole. The vessels are elongated and appear pruned, particularly when compared to corresponding vessels within the upper pole. These findings are compatible with ischemic changes.

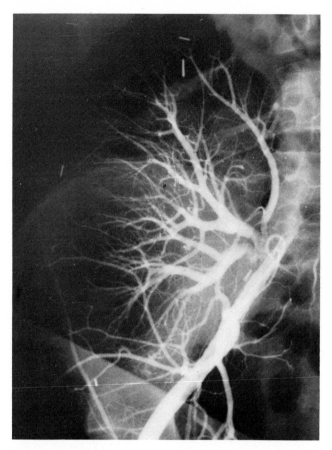

Fig. 4-42. Renal transplant, rejection: Arteriographic study. The kidney is enlarged and the arteries are stretched and pruned.

4-41A). The urographic findings of small renal infarcts vary according to the age of the lesion. In the early stages, a defect corresponding to the absence of perfusion in the involved area may be detected in the nephrogram. The base of the defect is juxtaposed to the outer margin of the kidney. Selective renal angiography often provides important information in the early phase. The embolus may be seen as a filling defect within, or as an abrupt termination of, a branch vessel. The involved vessel may not opacify or may retain contrast material longer than unoccluded vessels of similar size. The infarcted area eventually contracts, causing depression of the renal contour at the site of the infarction in approximately 4 weeks. However, the underlying collecting system usually remains normal. Renal angiogram performed at this time may demonstrate an irregular vessel, prolonged retention of contrast material, or no opacification of the affected vessel. However, the embolus is no longer visualized as a filling defect at this time. Bear in mind that renal arteriography is always required to exclude occlusion of the renal pedicle or thrombosis of the renal artery in those patients who present in a shock state following an episode of abdominal trauma.

Renal Transplantation

Radiology assumes a very important role in evaluating the pre- and posttransplant kidney. Urologic complications following renal transplantation occur in about 10 percent of patients. The most important complications noted in the posttransplant period include extravasation, obstruction, hemorrhage, rejection, and tubular necrosis. These can be well-documented by a variety of imaging techniques.

Extravasation on the basis of leakage arises either from the ureter or at the site of the ureterocystotomy. The clinical features are usually pain and fever. Excretory urograms often demonstrate extravasation of the urine but rarely the actual site of the leak. Radioisotope scanning and sonograms are also helpful in demonstrating this phenomenon.

Obstruction commonly occurs at the ureterovesicular junction as a result of an inadequate opening or calculus occlusion, most often by a uric acid stone. The conventional urogram is generally adequate to suggest this diagnosis.

More complicated problems, such as rejection or tubular necrosis, are best diagnosed by nuclear scintigraphy and ultrasound. It is important to distinguish these entities since therapy is different for each. The kidneys are enlarged, and use of excretory urography is limited, since it only shows an enlarged kidney with poor function, if any. The value of arteriography has also decreased in the past few years, although the changes that occur within arteries can be diagnostic. In the more severe forms of rejection, the intralobar and other peripheral vessels are stretched, irregular, and occluded in some branches (Fig. 4-42). The nephrogram is nonhomogeneous due to presence of microinfarcts. Although the vessels in acute tubular necrosis may show similar changes, they are often not quite as dramatically altered.

The nuclear renogram is probably the most important diagnostic test in distinguishing between acute rejection and acute tubular necrosis. In general, both renal perfusion and excretion are diminished in rejection, whereas in acute tubular necrosis the perfusion remains normal, while secretion is diminished.

Sonography has also proved worthwhile in suggesting the diagnosis of rejection. The finding is considered positive if the renal size increases 20 percent in overall length and demonstrates parenchymal foci of diminished or increased echogenecity, reflecting necrosis, hemorrhage, and so forth. No gross abnormalities have been detected in acute tubular necrosis. Ultrasound also helps identify other findings that may be present, such as hemorrhage, blood clots, and perinephric collections.

Bibliography

Haller, J. O., and Schnieder, M. *Pediatric Ultrasound*. Chicago: Year Book, 1980.

Mellins, H. Z. Cystic dilatation of the upper urinary tract: A radiologist's development model. *Radiology* 153:291, 1984.

Potter, E. L. *Normal and Abnormal Development of the Kidney*. Chicago: Year Book, 1972.

Rabinowitz, J. G. *Pediatric Radiology*. Philadelphia: Lippincott, 1978.

Rabinowitz, J. G., and Parvey, L. S. Genitourinary Disorders. In J. G. Teplich and M. E. Haskin, *Roentgenologic Diagnosis*. Philadelphia: Saunders, 1981. Pp. 2269–2303.

5. Oncology

Janet L. Potter

This chapter covers common malignancies with special imaging problems or imaging protocols that are applicable to a wide variety of neoplasms. The initial goal of oncologic imaging is to help make a diagnosis expeditiously and inexpensively. With rare exceptions, imaging does not provide a tissue diagnosis. The x-ray, ultrasound, or MRI appearance and the location of a lesion can only suggest a diagnosis and identify locations where tissue may be obtained with minimal patient morbidity. The second goal of imaging is to accurately determine the clinical stage of the malignancy. The third goal is to identify an inexpensive, low-risk imaging modality to follow remission or progression of a known tumor during treatment. However, when patients are enrolled in oncologic investigational protocols, a more costly follow-up examination may be required to permit accurate measurements. (For example, liver metastases can routinely be followed with radionuclide liver-spleen scan at half the cost of CT, but measurement accuracy is often inadequate to distinguish between response and partial response rates.) The final goal of oncologic imaging is to inexpensively demonstrate recurrences or distant metastases and to accurately define anatomy and tumor extent for planning palliative therapy (e.g., radiation ports or surgical approach) when needed.

The revolution of the last decade in imaging modalities has dramatically changed many staging protocols. In general, for initial diagnosis and work-up, CT has replaced bipedal lymphangiography in abdominal and pelvic malignancies, routine chest tomography in primary lung and metastatic disease, and angiography in vascular, cerebral, and renal cancers. Ultrasound applications continue to expand as technical expertise and equipment improve. In some diseases and patient populations, ultrasound is equivalent to CT in accuracy in staging, although its anatomic definition is usually less accurate than that of CT. The lower cost and lack of radiation may increase acceptance of ultrasound staging as improved cost/benefit ratios are documented. Magnetic resonance imaging use is increasing as the units become more readily available. In MRI there is no ionizing radiation, and the inherently high tissue contrast and ability to image directly in any plane are also important factors when considering MRI. The high cost of MRI (often twice that of CT) is a significant drawback. Magnetic resonance imaging can provide quantitative measurements from tissue, which it is hoped will permit in vivo distinction of benignancy and malignancy, but early results are not promising. There are no large comparative studies yet available to determine whether the increased cost of an MRI scan is justified by an improvement in diagnostic accuracy or patient management.

Breast Cancer

Carcinoma of the breast is the most common malignant tumor of women in the United States. It is estimated that 1 of every 12 women develops breast cancer in her lifetime. Each year more than 100,000 new cases are diagnosed and approximately 36,000 women die of the disease. Risk factors include a family history of breast cancer (especially in a premenopausal mother, sister, or aunt), personal history of breast cancer, nulliparity, late first pregnancy, obesity, and high levels of dietary fat, among others. Male breast cancer is rare, accounting for less than 1 percent of all breast cancer.

Ninety percent of breast carcinomas arise from ductal epithelium and the remaining 10 percent from lobular tissue. The doubling time of breast cancer is highly variable, with ranges extending up to 3 or 4 years. The lobular carcinomas and several of less common ductal carcinomas (e.g., medullary, colloid, and intraductal) are relatively low-grade tumors that carry a significantly better prognosis than the typical infiltrating ductal carcinoma.

The most common presentation is a palpable mass detected by the woman. Under these circumstances the malignancy has usually spread to regional lymph nodes (stage II or III). Ten-year survival when the tumor is limited to the breast (stage I) is greater than 90 percent, but drops precipitously to less than 50 percent with stage III disease (i.e., tumor > 5 cm with involved axillary nodes). Detection of breast cancer in its earliest stages offers the best opportunity for cure. By the time a breast cancer is palpable, the tumor is approximately 1 cm in size. Twenty percent of such cancers have already spread to the axillary lymph nodes. Physical examination alone detects less than half of cancers that are 1 cm or smaller; mammography alone detects 80 percent. Combined mammography and physical examination increase detection accuracy to greater than 90 percent.

Metastatic disease may occur for up to 20 years after diagnosis, although the majority occur in the first 5 to 7 years. The most common distant metastatic sites in declining order of frequency are bone, liver, lung, and brain.

MAMMOGRAPHY. Mammography is performed by two different radiographic methods: (1) film-screen mammography, and (2) xeromammography. Film-screen uses an intensifying screen to decrease the number of x-rays required and a fine-grain, high-resolution film. The result is a conventional black and white radiograph of the breast. Xeromammography is a modification of the xerographic photocopy process and produces a blue and white image on paper. When performed using proper technique, the two methods are equivalent in diagnostic quality. There is, however, a significant difference in radiation exposure; the xeromammogram results in a radiation dose 5 to 10 times greater than the film-screen examination. The initial advantage of xeromammography was that it could be performed on conventional x-ray equipment. However, in the past few years the cost of a dedicated mammography unit has decreased, making film-screen equipment cost competitive with that of a xerographic processor.

Breast cancers usually present mammographically as masses or clustered microcalcifications. The typical cancer has irregular margins with fine spiculations radiating from a mass (Fig. 5-1). Many breast cancers are well-circumscribed, even when quite large, but they almost always reveal at least a small irregularity or "tail" (Fig. 5-2). Perfectly smooth, round masses are usually benign. An ultrasound examination employing a standard small parts transducer (as is used to examine the thyroid gland) distinguishes cystic from solid masses. Cysts can be aspirated for cytologic evaluation (Fig. 5-3). Most solitary solid masses, even when well-circumscribed, require biopsy to rule out malignancy. If the classic coarse calcifications of a degenerating fibroadenoma are identified (Fig. 5-4), or the mass has been present and stable in size for several years, suspicion of malignancy is much reduced.

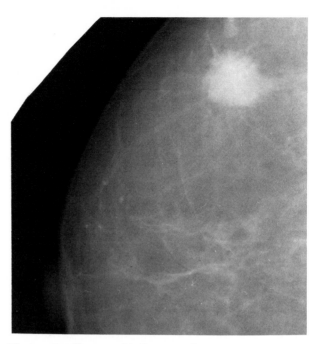

Fig. 5-1. Small mass with fine speculations extending outward into breast parenchyma is a common mammographic appearance of breast carcinoma.

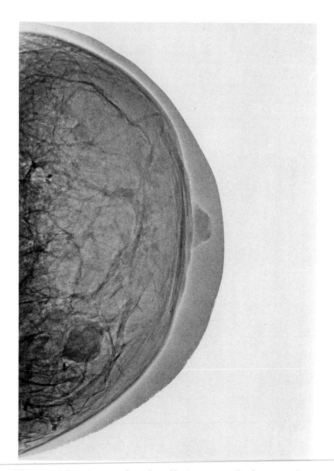

Fig. 5-2. Mass is round and well-circumscribed except for small "tail" (*arrow*) that increases suspicion of malignancy.

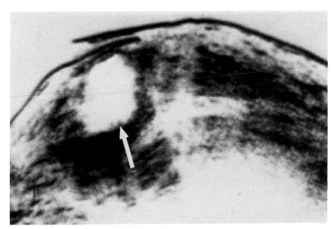

Fig. 5-3. Ultrasound of cyst showing thickening of inner wall (*arrow*) suspicious for malignancy. Biopsy revealed an intracystic adenocarcinoma.

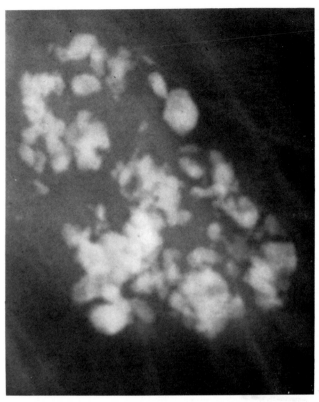

Fig. 5-4. Degenerating fibroadenoma with classic coarse calcifications.

Microcalcification is the second most usual mammographic sign of malignancy (Fig. 5-5). These calcifications are typically very small and are clustered in one region of the breast. Approximately 50 percent of breast cancers calcify, and the calcifications are often evident before a mass is palpable or visible on mammography. Benign calcifications are very common. The typical benign calcification is large, coarse, and rounded or curvilinear (Fig. 5-6).

Other mammographic signs of malignancy include distortion of the normal breast architecture in a localized area, asymmetric density, isolated asymmetric ductal dilatation, and skin thickening (Fig. 5-7).

Nonpalpable lesions must be preoperatively localized under mammographic guidance. The most commonly used technique is the hooked wire method (Fig. 5-8). Once the wire is in place it must be removed surgically. The localization procedure may be performed at one center and the outpatient surgical biopsy at another location.

Ancillary techniques used to improve mammographic distinction of benignancy and malignancy include magnification mammography, galactography, and injection of air. Magnification requires a dedicated mammogram unit with a small focal spot, and allows enlargement of a small mass to better define margins and improve resolution of small or indeterminate calcifications. Galactography involves cannulation of a breast duct and injection of contrast, and is used to demonstrate intraductal papillomas and early intraductal carcinomas. After the x-rays are completed, methylene blue can be injected into the abnormal duct to localize the lesion for the surgeon. The injection of air around masses is not commonly performed but can be used to better outline the margins of a well-circumscribed mass. X-rays then demonstrate marginal irregularities more readily.

Indications for Mammography. Mammography is performed in women with palpable breast masses to evaluate for malignant characteristics of the mass and to survey both breasts for nonpalpable cancer (Fig. 5-9). Except for women under the age of 25, a mammogram should be performed preoperatively in any woman scheduled for breast surgery or biopsy. Other indications for mammography are a history of breast cancer, recent onset nipple retraction, bloody or serous discharge (especially from a single duct), unexplained axillary adenopathy, or focal skin dimpling.

Screening of asymptomatic women is the most important use of mammography. For women age 50 and older, annual screening unequivocally reduces breast cancer morbidity and mortality. For women between the ages of 40 and 49, randomized, controlled studies on modern mammographic technique have not yet been completed. There is, however, substantial indirect evidence from the Breast Cancer Detection Demonstration Projects (BCDDP) that women age 40 to 49 do benefit significantly from screening. The American Cancer Society guidelines for mammographic screening recommend a baseline study between the ages of 35 and 40, screening examinations at one- or two-year intervals between ages 40 and 50 (dependent on risk), and annual screening after age 50. Breast cancer incidence rises rapidly between age 40 and 49 and is the leading cause of death among women age 40 to 45. For these reasons and because of the indirect evidence of mortality reduction through screening, it is anticipated that annual rather than biannual screening should improve survival in the 40- to 49-year age group.

Radiation Exposure. Radiation risk of annual screening is a question of much concern to women and their physicians. The carcinogenic effect of radiation at exposures over 100 rads is well-documented. Long-term follow-up of individuals exposed to radiation in nuclear war, radiation accidents, and x-ray treatments reveals a linear relationship between radiation dose and development of breast cancer. The greatest risk of breast cancer induction is in the peripubertal female when breast tissue is developing. Cancer develops after a 10- to 25-year latency period. No observable increased risk has been identified in women exposed after age 30. There is no equivalent human data to statis-

142

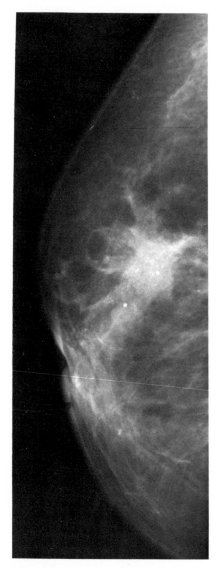

Fig. 5-5. Tiny, clustered calcifications typical of a breast carcinoma.

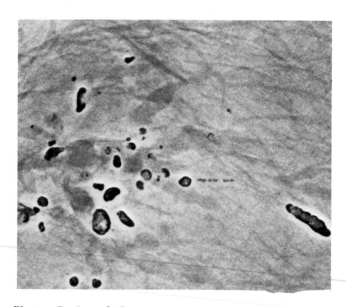

Fig. 5-6. Benign calcifications are large and rounded or curvilinear.

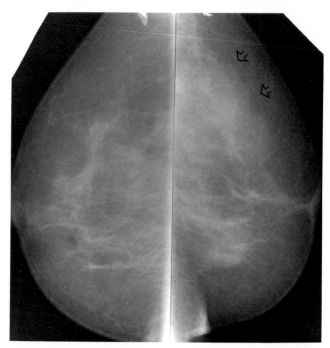

Fig. 5-7. Bilateral mediolateral projections reveal asymmetric architecture (*arrows*). Biopsy revealed infiltrating lobular carcinoma.

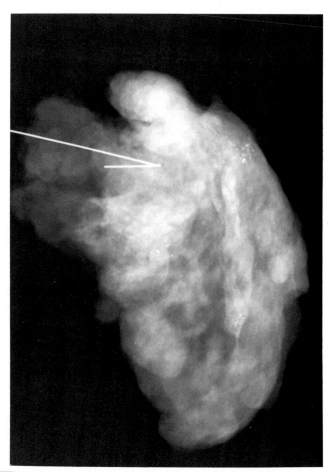

Fig. 5-8. Hooked wire in place localizing nonpalpable clustered microcalcifications. Biopsy specimens are radiographed to ensure that the lesion in question has been surgically removed.

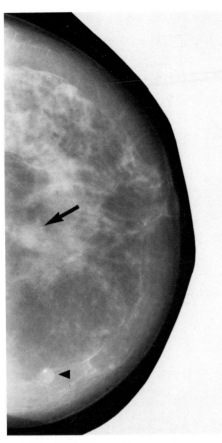

Fig. 5-9. Arrowhead indicates palpable mass that on biopsy was a fibroadenoma. Arrow marks nonpalpable carcinoma identified on prebiopsy screening mammogram.

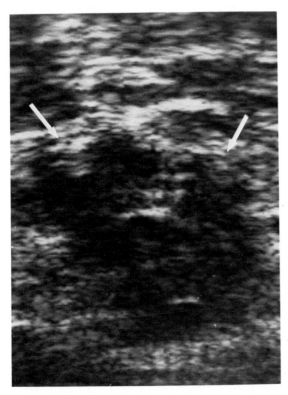

Fig. 5-10. Breast cancer frequently has low-level echoes (*arrows*) in contrast to normally echogenic breast tissue. Study was performed on a dedicated water-bath breast scanner.

tically evaluate breast cancer risk at doses under 100 rads. Animal models indicate that at these low exposure levels the relationship between radiation dose and carcinogenesis is not linear but is even lower than expected. If a woman undergoes annual film-screen mammography (two views per breast) from age 40 to 70, she receives a total accumulated midbreast dose of approximately 21 rads per breast. Risk/benefit analyses have been made by numerous investigators. Even assuming that the rate of carcinogenesis is the same at low-level exposures as it is above 100 rads, the worst case estimate is that screening induces one excess breast cancer per year per million women examined (after a 10- to 25-year latency period). The natural incidence of breast cancer in the United States is 800 cases per million women per year at age 40 and 2,500 cases per million women per year at age 65.

OTHER BREAST IMAGING TECHNIQUES. The superiority of mammography over every other available technique for the detection of early breast cancer has been well-documented. All other breast imaging modalities have unacceptably high false negative rates when subjected to randomized, controlled studies in double-blind comparison with mammography. The other modalities may have roles as adjuncts to mammography in selected clinical situations, but none is scientifically justified as a sole screening tool.

Ultrasound, using standard diagnostic equipment with high frequency transducers, can determine whether a mass is cystic or solid. Dedicated breast ultrasound, using a specially designed water path scanning device, is a useful adjunct to mammography in the dense or glandular breast. The low-level echoes characteristic of malignancy are obvious against the echogenic background of breast tissue (Fig. 5-10). In the patient with multiple cysts or a localized area of fibrocystic disease, ultrasound may identify tumor disguised by adjacent cysts.

Diaphanography, or transillumination, identifies suspicious focal areas of decreased light transmission. The technique is based on the preferential infrared absorption of nitrogen-rich compounds that are increased in malignant cells. The light source has a high proportion of near-infrared wavelengths, and diaphanography uses infrared-sensitive film to enhance detection of the nitrogen spectrum. The potential role of diaphanography is not known. Controlled studies with comparison to mammogrpahy are not yet complete, and even the ability of the technique to supplement mammographic diagnosis is not yet established.

Thermography is a method of measuring body temperature as absolute values or as a thermal map (or image). Temperature differences of as little as 0.1°C can be detected. The technique is based on the demonstration that breast cancer produces hotter thermal signals than normal breast tissue. Numerous techniques and types of equipment are available to make the measurements. Thermography, like ultrasound, has an unacceptably high false-negative rate and therefore is useless as a screening device. There is evidence that patients with abnormal thermograms are more likely to develop breast cancer at some future time. However, normal thermogram does not exclude breast cancer.

Other modalities that have been used in diagnosis are CT and MRI. Computed tomography is accurate, but the radiation dose is unacceptable. Magnetic resonance imaging is new and is still undergoing major technologic developments. It is desirable in breast diagnosis because there is no radiation risk, but the cost of a mammographic

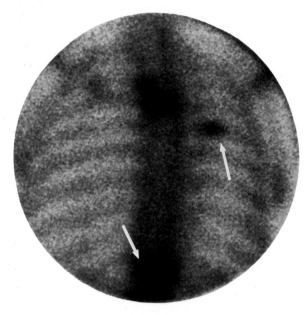

Fig. 5-11. Radionuclide bone scan with several areas of increased uptake (*arrows*) in bony thorax suspicious for metastases in a woman with clinical stage III breast cancer.

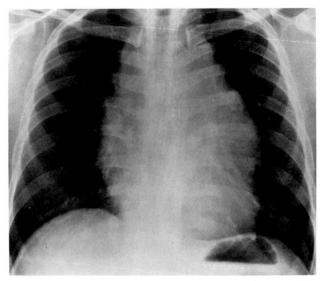

Fig. 5-12. Markedly widened mediastinum secondary to large adenopathy in patient with non-Hodgkin's lymphoma.

examination on a whole-body scanner may be prohibitive for screening purposes. Preliminary studies comparing mammography and MRI are still in the early phases, and the role and sensitivity of MRI in detecting breast cancer will not be known for several years.

Staging and Follow-up. The purpose of imaging is to document distant metastases that would upgrade stage III disease to stage IV. A positive bone scan can be found in up to 25 percent of stage III patients (Fig. 5-11). A standard staging work-up includes routine two-view baseline chest x-ray, radionuclide bone scan, and radionuclide liver-spleen scan. Brain metastases are infrequent at presentation and baseline imaging is not cost effective. When brain metastases are suspected, CT is the procedure of choice for diagnosing brain involvement.

In stage I or stage II disease, the incidence of bone metastases is so low that routine bone scans are not indicated. A two-view chest x-ray is warranted to serve as a baseline.

Lymphoma

Lymphomas are malignant neoplasms arising from lymph nodes or lymphoid tissues of visceral organs. They are subdivided into two histopathologically distinct types, Hodgkin's disease and the non-Hodgkin's lymphomas. The heterogenous non-Hodgkin's lymphomas are further subdivided into lymphocytic, histiocytic, mixed, pleomorphic, and Burkitt's forms. Approximately 7,100 new cases of Hodgkin's and 24,000 new cases of non-Hodgkin's disease are diagnosed each year in the United States. Hodgkin's disease has a bimodal age distribution with one peak incidence between ages 15 and 35 and a second peak incidence after age 50. Non-Hodgkin's lymphomas can oc-

cur at any age, but incidence generally increases with advancing age. Hodgkin's disease arises from the lymph nodes in 90 percent of cases, whereas the non-Hodgkin's lymphomas are of nodal origin in less than 60 percent. The most common clinical presentation in all types of lymphoma is painless enlargement of a peripheral lymph node. Splenomegaly or a palpable abdominal mass are frequent presentations of the non-Hodgkin's lymphomas.

RADIOGRAPHIC MANIFESTATIONS. Mediastinal lymph node enlargement is the most common radiographic finding, occurring in approximately 50 percent of Hodgkin's and 30 percent of the non-Hodgkin's lymphomas. Typically, it is the thoracic anterior and superior mediastinal nodes that are enlarged (Fig. 5-12). Pulmonary parenchymal involvement most often occurs by extension from the mediastinum along the peribronchial lymphatics, which can produce a coarse, reticulonodular pattern, ill-defined patchy densities, or poorly circumscribed nodules (Fig. 5-13). Pulmonary Hodgkin's disease may cavitate in the lung, simulating an infectious process. Primary pulmonary involvement without mediastinal lymphadenopathy is rare.

The gastrointestinal tract is involved in approximately 30 percent of non-Hodgkin's lymphomas but in less than 10 percent of cases of Hodgkin's disease. The most common sites are stomach and small bowel where lymphoma can simulate a variety of benign and malignant conditions, including peptic ulcer disease, scirrhous carcinoma, or malabsorption syndromes (Figs. 5-14 and 5-15). Small bowel involvement is more common in the non-Hodgkin's lymphomas. The diffuse histiocytic subtype may spread submucosally, invade the mesentery, and produce large masses that separate and displace bowel loops (Figs. 5-16 and 5-17).

Colonic lymphoma can assume a variety of radiographic appearances. In contrast to the short segment involvement of colonic adenocarcinoma, lymphoma often produces a large lesion involving a relatively long segment. The most common site is the cecum (Fig. 5-18). Occasionally the

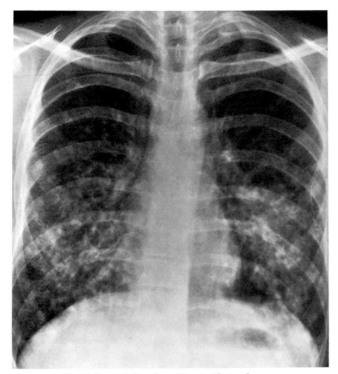

Fig. 5-13. Multiple nodular densities in the pulmonary parenchyma in association with hilar adenopathy in recurrent Hodgkin's disease.

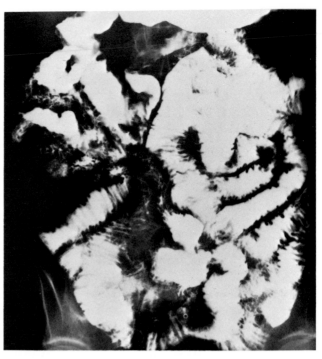

Fig. 5-15. Fold thickening, mild dilatation and separation of multiple small bowel loops caused by a non-Hodgkin's lymphoma.

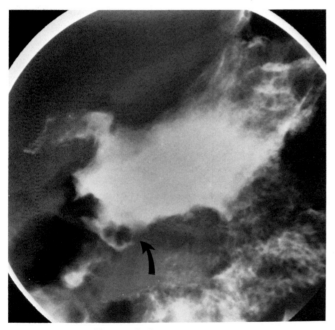

Fig. 5-14. Mass effect and ulceration in gastric antrum (*arrow*) produced by Hodgkin's disease.

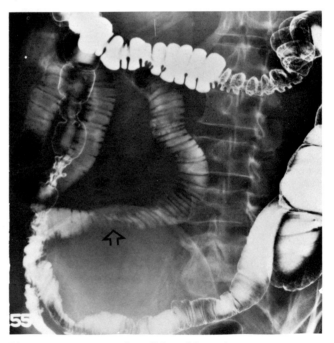

Fig. 5-16. Separation of small bowel loops by mesenteric invasion with only a short segment of submucosal involvement (*arrow*) by diffuse histiocytic lymphoma (DHL).

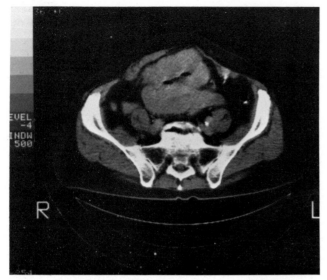

Fig. 5-17. Computed tomography scan of same patient as Fig. 5-16, showing large mesenteric mass with bowel wall involvement in DHL.

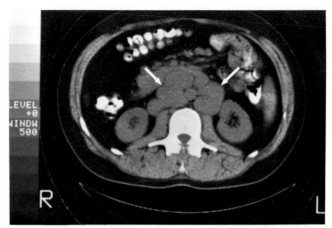

Fig. 5-19. Bulky retroperitoneal adenopathy (*arrows*) in Hodgkin's disease.

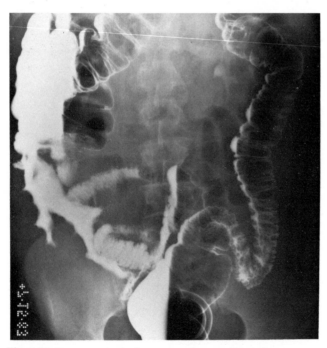

Fig. 5-18. Long segment of cecum and ascending colon involved by a bulky lymphoma.

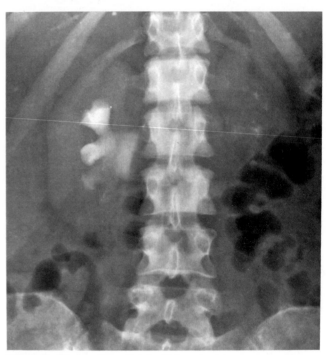

Fig. 5-20. Obstruction of right kidney by large paraaortic adenopathy.

lymphoma presents as a diffuse nodular pattern typical of multiple polyposis syndromes.

Splenic and liver involvement frequently occur, but in many cases the CT appearance is normal, even in the presence of extensive infiltration. The pancreas and less commonly the renal parenchyma may also reveal tumor infiltration.

Retroperitoneal lymphadenopathy is easily visualized by CT (Fig. 5-19). Direct spread from enlarged nodes may produce paravertebral masses, vertebral body erosion, or extradural lesions that result in spinal cord compression.

Hydronephrosis may result from ureteral obstruction by enlarged nodes (Fig. 5-20). The inferior vena cava may be compressed and produce lower extremity edema.

Extranodal sites include bone, thyroid, testis, ovary, and salivary gland. Bone involvement is usually secondary to hematogenous spread, but primary bone lymphomas can occur. Bone lesions are commonly lytic and indistinguishable from other types of metastases but with a predilection for the pelvis, femur, tibia, or humerus. In Hodgkin's disease bone lesions may be both osteoblastic and lytic. Brain involvement is uncommon and is most often seen in the younger patient.

STAGING. Once the diagnosis of lymphoma is established, a thorough staging of disease extent is necessary to select

Table 5-1. Ann Arbor Staging Classification

Stage I	Involvement of a single lymph node region (I) or single extralymphatic site (IE)
Stage II	Involvement of two or more lymph node regions on the same side of diaphragm (II) or a solitary extralymphatic site and one more lymph node areas on the same side of diaphragm (IIE)
Stage III	Involvement of lymph node regions on both sides of diaphragm (III) accompanied by spleen involvement (IIIS) or by solitary involvement of an extralymphatic organ or site (IIIE), or both (IIISE)
Stage IV	Diffuse involvement of extralymphatic sites with or without lymph node enlargement

appropriate therapy and to estimate prognosis. The traditional staging system is the Ann Arbor Staging Classification (Table 5-1). This system is valuable in managing patients with Hodgkin's disease but frequently fails to provide a reliable prognosis for non-Hodgkin's lymphoma. Histopathologic classification of the non-Hodgkin's lymphomas provides a more accurate prognosis. The Ann Arbor system, however, is applied to both types of lymphomas. Patients are assigned a clinical stage based on physical examination, laboratory results, and radiographic studies. Treatment plans are based on the pathologic stage, which is arrived at after appropriate biopsies are evaluated.

Radiographic staging has two purposes: (1) to demonstrate extent of disease, and (2) to document measurable disease that can be noninvasively followed during therapy. Studies include a chest x-ray, CT of abdomen and pelvis, and a bipedal lymphangiogram. Chest CT may also be necessary for more complete staging. The chest x-ray identifies mediastinal or lung involvement. The abdominal and pelvic CT scan demonstrates adenopathy, identifies evidence of visceral organ involvement, and defines the extent of mesenteric masses. If the upper abdominal paraaortic nodes are enlarged, there is a high probability that there is splenic and hepatic involvement. Nodal enlargement is the only criterion by which CT defines lymphomatous infiltration. False positive results by CT using size as an indicator of the presence of lymphoma are rare, but the absence of lymphadenopathy does not exclude lymphoma (Fig. 5-21). Therefore, when CT reveals no evidence of intraabdominal lymphoma, the more invasive bipedal lymphangiogram is necessary. Lymphangiography has an 80 to 90 percent accuracy rate in the lymphomas; false positives are rare. The accuracy rate above the level of L_2 decreases because of incomplete filling of the higher nodes. For this reason, CT and lymphangiography are complementary examinations. Because of patient discomfort associated with cannulating and filling foot lymphatics with contrast, a lymphangiogram is often eliminated if the CT scan is unequivocally positive. Many institutions, however, do routinely require both studies, citing improved staging accuracy and ability to follow treatment response with routine abdominal x-rays as parameters outweighing the one-time discomfort of lymphangiography.

RADIOGRAPHIC FOLLOW-UP. Treatment response is followed by the least invasive, lowest-cost modality that can provide accurate measurement of residual disease. In mediastinal adenopathy a chest x-ray suffices in the majority of cases. The large abdominal masses of diffuse histiocytic lymphoma may be followed by ultrasound examination,

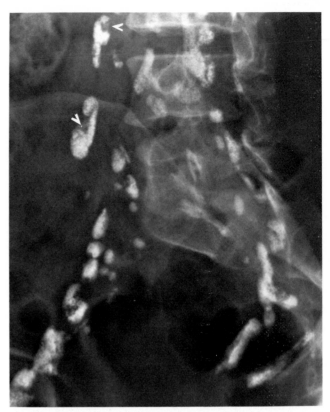

Fig. 5-21. Bipedal lymphangiogram showing normal-sized lymph nodes with focal filling defects (*arrows*). Surgical biopsy revealed lymphocytic lymphoma. Computed tomography scan in this patient was interpreted as normal because nodes were not enlarged.

with a repeat CT scan reserved for the final phases of treatment (Fig. 5-22). Likewise, abdominal x-rays after a lymphangiogram frequently preclude the necessity of a repeat CT scan.

Radiographic follow-up of lymphoma patients also includes early diagnosis of atypical infections, hypersensitivity reactions to drugs (both acute and chronic), and postirradiation pneumonitis. Most of these problems are manifested in the lungs (Figs. 5-23 and 5-24). Extrapulmonary infection caused by atypical organisms is not common but may involve the esophagus, spleen, subphrenic regions, or retroperitoneum. Work-up is tailored to the clinical situation. Imaging modalities available for pinpointing infection sites include nuclear medicine gallium and liver-spleen scans, CT, ultrasound, and a variety of barium and plain-film examinations.

Prostate Cancer

Cancer of the prostate is the third most common form of cancer in men. In the United States each year over 85,000 new cases are diagnosed and more than 25,000 males die from the disease. The incidence of prostate carcinoma increases with age but is uncommon under age 40.

More than 95 percent of prostate cancers are adenocarcinomas. Eighty-five to ninety percent are multifocal at diagnosis and arise in the posterior portion of the prostate, which is easily accessible to digital examination. Prog-

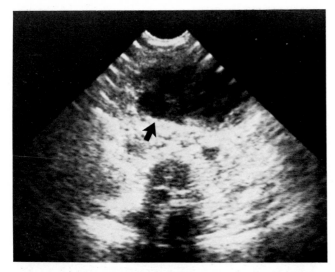

Fig. 5-22. Ultrasound easily demonstrates large mesenteric mass (*arrow*) of diffuse histiocytic lymphoma.

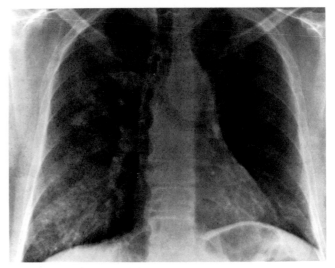

Fig. 5-24. Patchy densities caused by a hypersensitivity reaction to cytoxan.

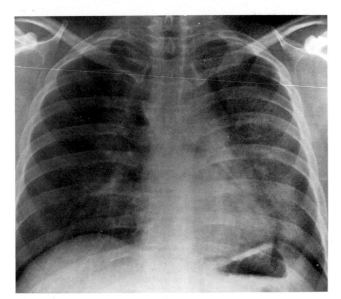

Fig. 5-23. Diffuse interstitial densities (greater on the left side) in a patient on chemotherapy for a poorly differentiated lymphoma are a typical radiographic presentation of *Pneumocystis carinii* infection.

Table 5-2. Staging of Prostate Carcinoma

Stage	Finding
A	Incidental finding by pathologist in clinically unsuspected presentation
B	Clinically palpable mass, but confined to prostate
C	Extension beyond the prostate seminal vesicles or contiguous structures
D	Metastatic disease D1 Regional lymph node metastasis D2 Distant metastasis

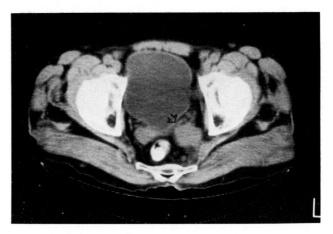

Fig. 5-25. CT staging of prostate carcinoma: The large pelvic node (*arrow*) adjacent to the pyriformis muscle was not suspected by clinical examination.

nosis is a function of histologic grade and pathologic stage of the tumor.

STAGING. Table 5-2 outlines the staging system for prostate cancer. Imaging for staging includes abdominal and pelvic CT scan to evaluate for local extension and lymphatic involvement. Computed tomography readily demonstrates extension into the seminal vesicles, proximal urethra, bladder, rectum, or to the pelvic side walls (Fig. 5-25). When lymphatic involvement produces nodal enlargement, the CT scan is diagnostic, but in up to 40 percent of patients nodes are normal in size even though they contain metastatic foci. A bipedal lymphangiogram may be required when the CT scan is negative in a patient who is at high risk for nodal involvement (i.e., large primary mass or high-grade histology) or when a lymphadenectomy is not planned. Diagnostic accuracy of an abnormal lymphangiogram is 80 to 90 percent. Of the pelvic nodal groups, only the common and external iliac nodes routinely fill with contrast, and the deep pelvic nodes are not evaluated. Occasional false-positive scans by either CT or lymphangiography are due to reactive adenopathy, an inflammatory response to the presence of the tumor.

Local extension and lymphatic spread may alternatively be evaluated by transrectal ultrasound or MRI. The results of studies using transrectal ultrasound for diagnosis of prostate cancer and for demonstration of local spread are promising, but the technique is not widely available. Ini-

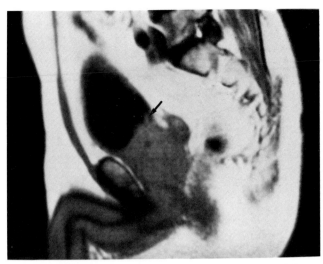

Fig. 5-26. MRI sagittal scan showing invasion of base of the
bladder by prostatic carcinoma (*arrow*).

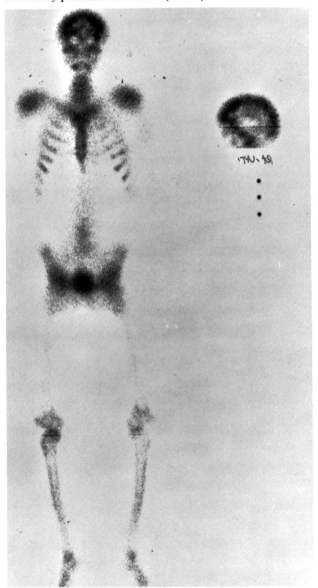

Fig. 5-27. Radionuclide bone scan suggests metastases in the
skull, but otherwise shows homogeneous uptake throughout
the skeleton. Paucity of renal uptake is indicative of diffusely
increased bony uptake.

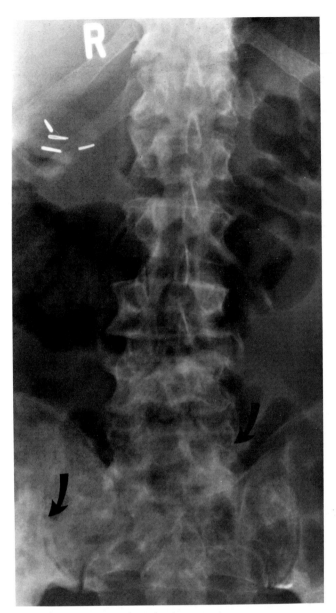

Fig. 5-28. X-ray of lower spine and pelvis reveal multiple
osteoblastic and lytic prostate carcinoma metastases
(*arrows*).

tial reports indicate that MRI may some day replace CT for
staging (Fig. 5-26) and may also have a role in diagnosis.
The advantages of MRI include direct scanning in coronal
and sagittal planes that improves detection of local spread,
and high tissue contrast that permits vessels and adjacent
lymph nodes to be readily distinguished. With MRI be-
coming more readily available, a more accurate assessment
of its role in staging of prostate carcinoma is forthcoming.

Distant metastases most often occur by hematogenous
spread, predominantly to bone. Initial staging includes a
radionuclide bone scan that may show focal areas of involvement or occasionally a diffusely increased bony uptake that can be misinterpreted as a normal bone scan. Absence of radionuclide activity in the kidneys is key to the
correct interpretation (Fig. 5-27). A radionuclide bone scan
is more sensitive than routine bone radiographs and is the
procedure of choice for following improvement or progression of bone lesions. The bony metastases have a predilection for the spine, pelvis, femurs, and ribs and frequently
show a mixed lytic and blastic radiographic pattern (Fig.
5-28). Extensive involvement of the spine may be accom-

panied by extradural masses that compress the cord and cause neurologic symptoms. Metastases to the liver, lungs, and adrenal glands may occur in advanced disease.

Bibliography

Breast cancer

El Yousef, S. J., et al. Benign and malignant breast disease: Magnetic resonance and radiofrequency pulse sequences. *A.J.R.* 145:1, 1985.

Feig, S. A., and McLelland, R. (eds.). *Breast Carcinoma: Current Diagnosis and Treatment*. New York: Mason, 1983.

Lester, R. G. The contributions of radiology to the diagnosis, management, and cure of breast cancer. *Radiology* 151:1, 1984.

Powell, R. W., McSweeney, M. B., and Wilson, C. E. X-ray calcifications as the only basis for breast biopsy. *Ann. Surg.* 197:555, 1983.

Sickles, E. A., Filly, R. A., and Gallen, P. W. Breast cancer detection with sonography and mammography. *A.J.R.* 140:843, 1983.

Tabar, L., Dean, P. B., and Pentek, Z. Galactography: The diagnostic procedure of choice for nipple discharge. *Radiology* 149:31, 1983.

Lymphoma

Blackledge, G., et al. Computed tomography in staging of patients with Hodgkin's disease. *Clin. Radiol.* 31:143, 1980.

Breiman, R. S., et al. CT-pathologic correlations in Hodgkin's disease and non-Hodgkin's lymphoma. *Radiology* 126:159, 1978.

Dooms, G. C., et al. Characterization of lymphadenopathy by magnetic resonance relaxation times: Preliminary results. *Radiology* 155:691, 1985.

Golomb, H. M. (ed.). Non-Hodgkin's lymphoma. *Semin. Oncol.* 7:221, 1980.

Kaplan, H. S. *Hodgkin's Disease* (2nd ed.). Cambridge, Mass.: Harvard University Press, 1980.

Marglin, S., and Castellino, R. Lymphographic accuracy in 632 consecutive previously untreated cases of Hodgkin's disease and non-Hodgkin's lymphoma. *Radiology* 140:351, 1981.

Prostate cancer

Grossman, I., et al. The early lymphatic spread of prostatic adenocarcinoma. *Radiology* 120:673, 1974.

Peeling, W. B., and Griffiths, G. J. Imaging of the prostate by ultrasound. *J. Urol.* 132:217, 1984.

Spernals, J. P., and Renick, M. I. Clinical staging of prostate cancer: New modalities. *Urol. Clin. North Am.* 11:231, 1984.

Williams, R. D., and Hricak, H. Magnetic resonance imaging in urology. *J. Urol.* 132: 641, 1984.

6. Bone and Joint Disease

Robert O. Cone III

Arthritis

RADIOGRAPHIC APPROACH TO ARTHRITIS. Plain radiography is an important tool in the diagnosis and evaluation of many types of arthritis. Important factors to consider when evaluating radiographs of arthritis patients are the age of the patient, the presence of known preexisting diseases, and the distribution of abnormalities, as well as the particular radiographic appearance of the patients' abnormalities. The most common variety of arthritis is degenerative osteoarthritis, while the most common inflammatory arthropathy is rheumatoid arthritis. Mastery of the radiographic appearance and distribution of these two disorders provides a firm bases for evaluating any arthropathy.

RHEUMATOID ARTHRITIS. Rheumatoid arthritis is a polyarticular arthropathy characterized by inflammation and proliferation of synovial tissue (pannus formation), leading to destruction of synovial articulations. The characteristic roentgenographic findings in rheumatoid arthritis consist of soft-tissue swelling, osteoporosis, intraarticular erosions, joint space narrowing, and articular deformities as well as a striking tendency toward symmetry of distribution (Figs. 6-1, 6-2).

Juxta-articular soft-tissue swelling is the earliest roentgenographic feature of rheumatoid arthritis. Osteoporosis is typical, first appearing in a band-like distribution on either side of an involved articulation (Fig. 6-1A) and later assuming a more generalized distribution (Fig. 6-1B). In advanced rheumatoid arthritis, osteoporosis may be severe enough to predispose to pathologic fracture. Intraarticular erosions are first noted at the margins of involved joints where synovial tissue is in contact with bone without an intervening layer of articular cartilage. Marginal erosions initially appear as minute interruptions in the subchondral bone plate (dot-dash pattern). As the disease progresses, discrete marginal erosions that enlarge toward the center of the articulation may be identified. The most common sites where erosions may be identified early in the course of the disease are the second and third metacarpal heads, the ulnar styloid process, and the first and fifth metatarsal heads (Figs. 6-1, 6-2). In large joints, such as the knee or hip, joint space narrowing may be prominent without identifiable erosions (Figs. 6-3, 6-4). Subchondral cysts tend to be small in most instances, although they may occasionally become very large (i.e. > 5 cm). These giant rheumatoid cysts are usually located about the knee, hip, elbow, or wrist and are often associated with pathologic fracture (Fig. 6-5).

Joint space narrowing in rheumatoid arthritis results from the progressive destruction of articular cartilage and occurs in synchrony with erosions. The presence of intraarticular erosions without concurrent joint space narrowing should suggest another diagnosis, especially gouty arthritis (see Fig. 6-25). Joint space narrowing in rheumatoid arthritis involves all segments of an articulation

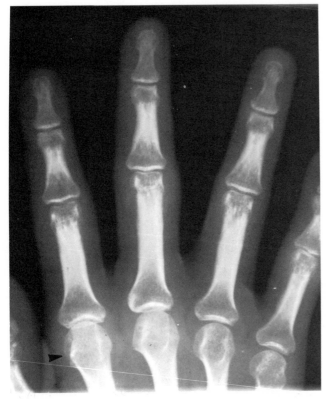

A

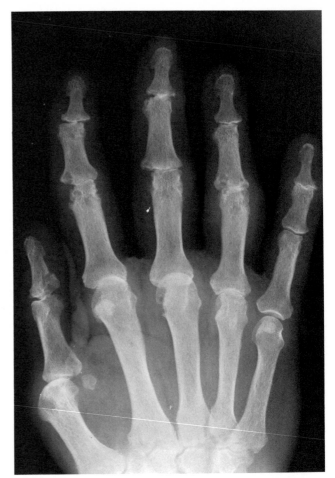

B

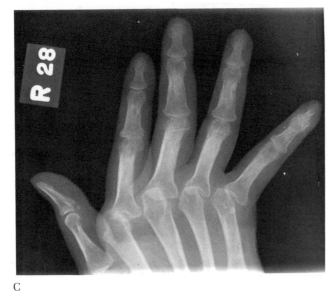

C

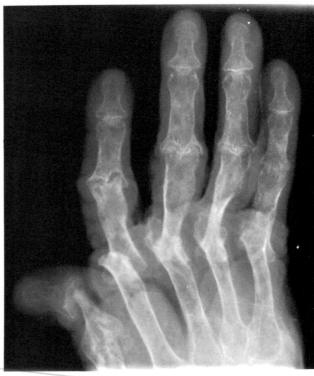

D

Fig. 6-1. Characteristic radiographic spectrum of increasingly severe rheumatoid arthritis involving the hands. A. Hand-like pattern of juxtaarticular osteoporosis and soft tissue swelling with a minimal degree of joint space narrowing and erosive change (*arrowhead*). B. Generalized osteoporosis with multiple areas of joint space narrowing and prominent marginal erosions. C. Marked ulnar deviation and palmar subluxation at the metacarpophalangeal joints. D. Virtually complete destruction of the metacarpophalangeal articulations with advanced change at the proximal interphalangeal joints.

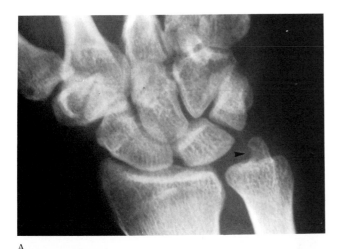

A

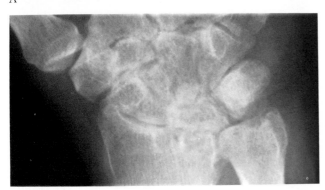

B

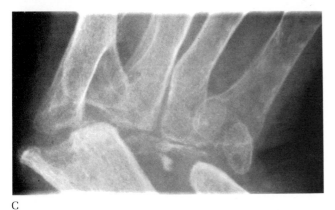

C

Fig. 6-2. Spectrum of radiographic changes of rheumatoid arthritis involving the wrist. A. The only radiographic findings are the presence of osteoporosis and a subtle erosion at the base of the ulnar styloid process (*arrowhead*). **B.** Diffuse osteoporosis, pancompartmental joint space narrowing and multiple erosions. **C.** Destruction of the wrist articulation is virtually complete.

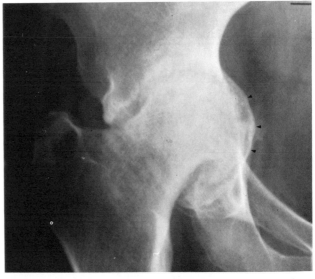

Fig. 6-3. Rheumatoid Arthritis. Concentric narrowing of the hip joint space with medial migration of the medial wall of the acetabulum (*arrowheads*) (protrusio acetabuli).

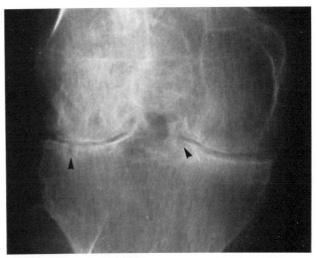

Fig. 6-4. Rheumatoid arthritis. Symmetric involvement of the knee joint with narrowing of both the medial and lateral compartments. Diffuse osteoporosis is present as well as numerous small erosions (*arrowheads*).

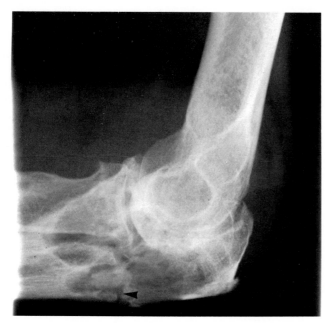

Fig. 6-5. Lateral radiograph of the elbow of a patient with rheumatoid arthritis shows a large cystic lesion in the proximal ulna, which is complicated in this instance by a pathologic fracture (*arrowhead*).

RA: No ankylosis

equally, in contrast to some other arthropathies (e.g., osteoarthritis, CPPD) in which joint space narrowing tends to occur in stressed segments of an articulation (compare Figs. 6-4 and 6-35). Intraarticular bony ankylosis is not a common feature of rheumatoid arthritis and when encountered is almost always localized to the intercarpal and intertarsal articulations.

Articular deformities are common in advanced rheumatoid arthritis and result from a combination of destruction of the articular surfaces and juxta-articular soft tissue supporting structures. The boutonniere deformity (PIP hyperflexion and DIP hyperextension), swan neck deformity (PIP hyperextension and DIP hyperflexion), and ulnar deviation and palmar subluxation of the metacarpophalangeal joints (see Fig. 6-1C) are the most characteristic of these abnormalities. In the hip, long-standing rheumatoid arthritis may result in medial migration of the medial wall of the acetabulum to such an extent that the femoral heads appear to be within the pelvis (protrusio acetabuli deformity) (see Fig. 6-3). Of particular importance in patients with rheumatoid arthritis are the instabilities that involve the cervical spine (Fig. 6-6). Lateral radiographs of the cervical spine often reveal a characteristic "stair step" deformity, in which each cervical vertebra is mildly subluxed on the vertebra beneath it. Laxity or destruction of the transverse atlantoaxial ligament may result in atlantoaxial subluxation, in which the odontoid process of the second cervical vertebra protrudes posteriorly into the upper cervical spinal canal on flexion of the head. In some individuals destruction of the lateral atlantoaxial and atlantooccipital articulations results in vertical atlantoaxial subluxation, in which the base of the skull and brainstem "settles down" over the upper cervical spine and results in brainstem compression. Pathologic fractures of the odontoid process due to large erosions are also relatively common.

JUVENILE CHRONIC ARTHRITIS. Juvenile chronic arthritis refers to a group of childhood arthropathies previously re-

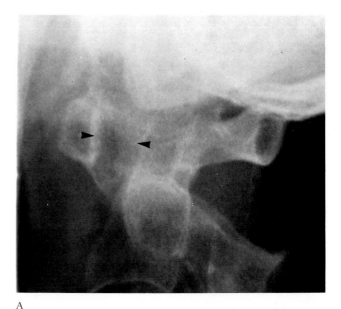

A

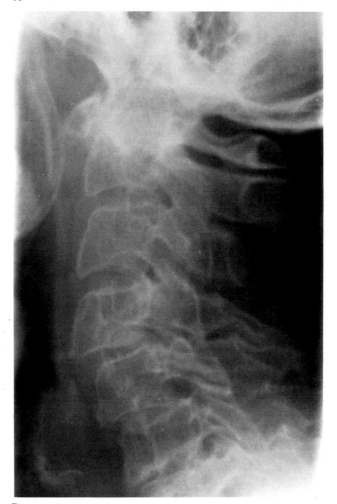

B

Fig. 6-6. Rheumatoid arthritis involving the cervical spine. A. Atlanto-axial subluxation with an abnormally increased distance (*between arrowheads*) between the odontoid process and the anterior arch of the atlas. B. Characteristic "stair-step" deformity of the cervical spine with mild subluxation of the cervical vertebra at multiple levels. Also present is vertical atlantoaxial subluxation with diminution in the space between the posterior elements of the atlas and the axis as well as between the atlas and the base of the skull.

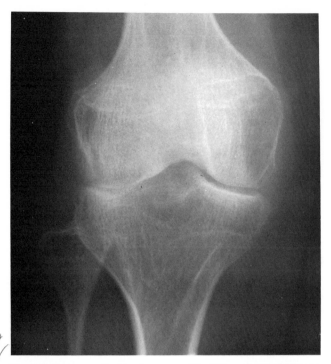

Fig. 6-9. Severe arthritic changes with diffuse osteoporosis at both hip joints in a patient with juvenile chronic arthritis.

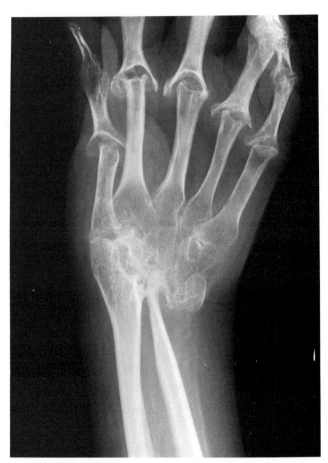

Fig. 6-11. Advanced juvenile chronic arthritis in the wrist and hand. Growth disturbances as well as intra-articular ankylosis at the intercarpal articulations and the interphalangeal joint of the thumb are prominent. Severe destructive erosive changes of the radiocarpal and metacarpophalangeal joints are also present.

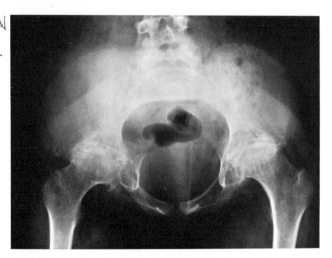

Fig. 6-10. Prominent growth deformity about the knee with overgrowth of the epiphyses of the distal femur and proximal tibia in a patient with long-standing juvenile chronic arthritis. Symmetric joint space narrowing of both the medial and lateral compartments of the knee is present without erosive change.

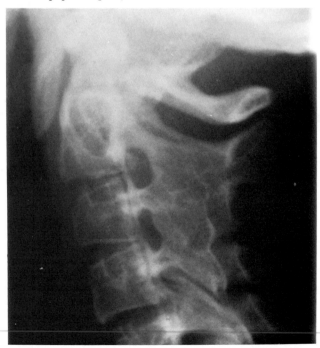

Fig. 6-12. Intervertebral ankylosis between the posterior elements of the second through fourth cervical vertebrae in a patient with juvenile chronic arthritis. In some patients ankylosis between the vertebral bodies may also occur.

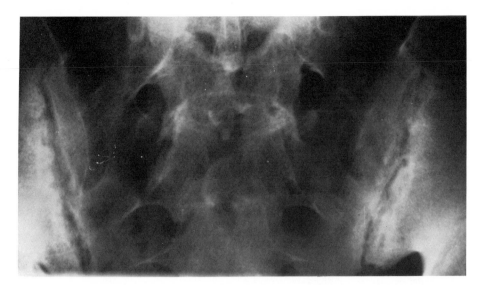

A

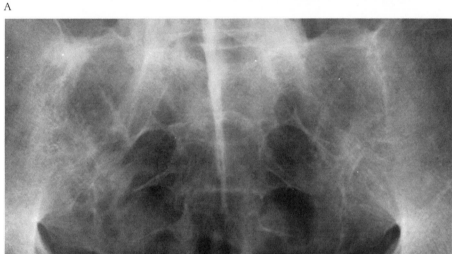

B

Fig. 6-13. A. Active sacroiliitis with apparent widening of the sacroiliac joints due to the presence of multiple marginal erosions. Note the vague, ill-defined band of sclerosis, which is most prominent on the iliac side of the articulation. B. Complete intra-articular bony ankylosis of the sacroiliac joints, a finding indicative of longstanding disease.

in the hands, wrists, feet, and cervical spine (Figs. 6-11, 6-12).

The most common sites of involvement in juvenile chronic arthritis are the hands, wrists, feet, hips, knees, ankles, and cervical spine. The hips and knees are involved much more frequently than in adult rheumatoid arthritis. Sacroiliitis and spondylitis may be seen in children with juvenile-onset seronegative spondyloarthropathies but tend to occur later in the course of the disease than they do in adults.

SERONEGATIVE SPONDYLOARTHROPATHIES. The seronegative spondyloarthropathies are a family of disorders that include ankylosing spondylitis, Reiter's syndrome, psoriatic arthritis, and the spondyloarthropathies associated with inflammatory bowel disease. The latter group includes Crohn's disease, ulcerative colitis, Whipple's disease, and infectious enteritis (e.g., Salmonella, Shigella, or Yersinia). Patients with previous intestinal bypass surgery are also at increased risk for this disorder. These disorders share common radiographic tendencies, including spondylitis, sacroiliitis, peripheral arthropathy, and inflammation at sites of tendon and ligament insertion (enthesitis).

Ankylosing Spondylitis. Ankylosing spondylitis is most common in men, usually in association with the presence of the HLA-B27 histocompatability antigen. The sacroiliac joints are the earliest sites involved, typically in a bilateral and symmetrical fashion. The earliest radiographic changes consist of apparent widening of the sacroiliac joints due to the presence of multiple small erosions of the subchondral bone plate with an ill-defined zone of sclerosis, which is most prominent on the iliac side of the articulation. As the disease progresses, larger erosions become evident in association with narrowing of the joint space (Fig. 6-13A). The final stage of disease consists of intraarticular bony ankylosis of the joint (Fig. 6-13B).

Spinal involvement typically begins at the lumbosacral junction and progresses in a cephalad direction. The earliest radiographic abnormality consists of sclerosis and loss of definition of the anterosuperior or anteroinferior margin of the vertebral body where the annulus fibrosis of the intervertebral disk inserts into the vertebral body. As the process progresses the normal concavity of the anterior margin of the vertebral body is lost, resulting in a square appearance on lateral radiographs (Fig. 6-14A). This is followed by progressive ossification of the outermost layers of the intervertebral disk (annulus fibrosis), resulting in the formation of slender, vertically oriented bony bridges that extend from the corner of one vertebra to the corner

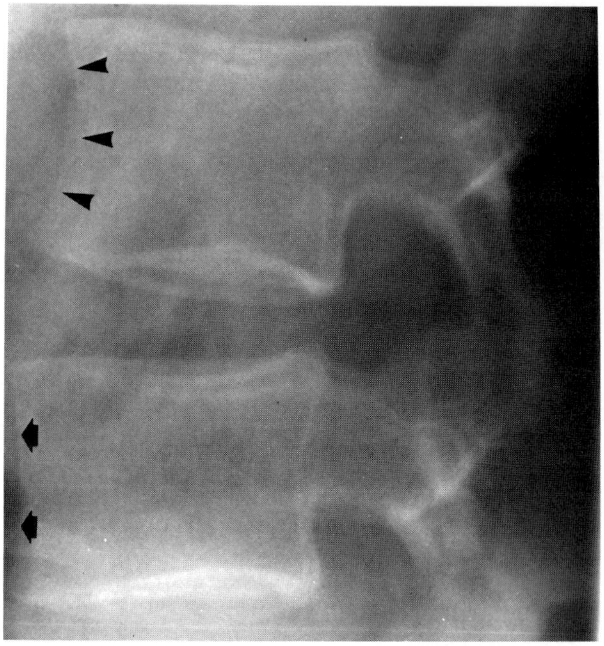

A

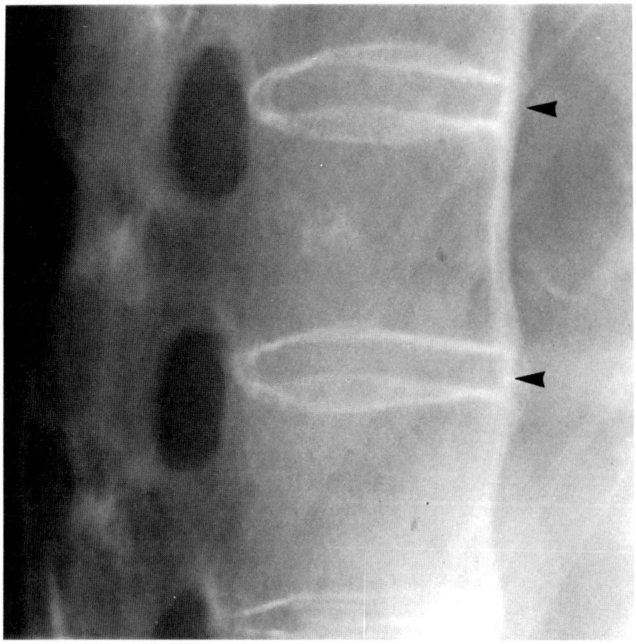

B

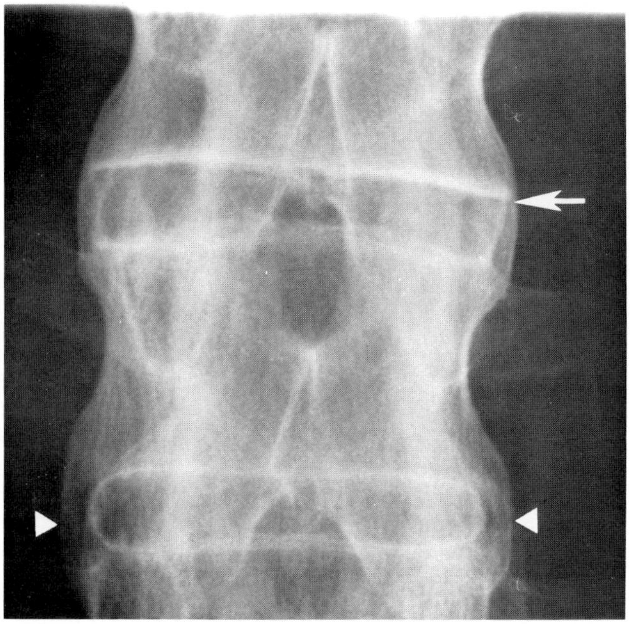

C

Fig. 6-14. A. One of the earliest findings of spinal involvement in ankylosing spondylitis is loss of the normal concave shape (*arrows*) of the anterior border of the inferior lumbar vertebral body ("squaring") as compared to the adjacent vertebra (*arrowheads*). Lateral projection (B) and anteroposterior projection (C) show mature syndesmophytes (*arrowheads*) manifested as slender osseous bars that bridge the intervertebral disk space. Note that these lesions arise from the corner of the vertebral body (*arrow*), a useful point in differentiating syndesmophytes from osteophytes and other spinal proliferative lesions.

Ankylosing Spondylitis
Squaring of Vert bodies
Bamboo spine

of the adjacent vertebra (syndesmophytes). These bridges result in bony ankylosis of adjacent vertebra (see Figs. 6-14B, C; 6-24). Syndesmophytes are present in virtually all cases of ankylosing spondylitis and in some cases of psoriatic spondyloarthritis and Reiter's syndrome. Ossification also occurs in the interspinal ligaments and capsular tissue of the spinal apophyseal joints, eventually resulting in the classic appearance of an osteoporotic and solidly fused spinal column ("bamboo spine"). Pathologic fractures are the major complications of long-standing ankylosing spondylitis, frequently occurring through the ossified intervertebral disk space and frequently associated with pseudarthrosis formation (Fig. 6-15). In other patients, relatively minor degrees of trauma may result in bizarre fractures involving multiple contiguous spinal levels, which resemble spiral fractures that occur in long, tubular bones.

Peripheral arthropathy is less commonly encountered in ankylosing spondylitis than in Reiter's syndrome and psoriatic arthritis. When present it is usually localized to the large proximal joints (hip, shoulder) and is relatively uncommon in more peripheral sites. In the hip, the arthritis of ankylosing spondylitis is characterized by bilaterality, osteoporosis, and progressive joint space narrowing, with or without erosions. In some cases medial migration of the acetabulum (protrusio acetabuli deformity) may be identified, while intraarticular ankylosis may occur in other patients. Patients with ankylosing spondylitis who undergo joint replacement surgery, especially in the hip, demonstrate a striking tendency toward the formation of large amounts of heterotopic bone in the juxta-articular soft tissues, which may result in eventual extraarticular ankylosis about the prosthetic joint (Fig. 6-16).

Enthesitis refers to inflammation and bone production that occur at sites of attachment of tendons and ligaments into bone (entheses). This is an important feature of ankylosing spondylitis and the other seronegative spondyloarthropathies. The most common sites of enthesitis include the sites of pelvic ligament attachment, the femoral trochanters, the poles of the patella, and the posterior and

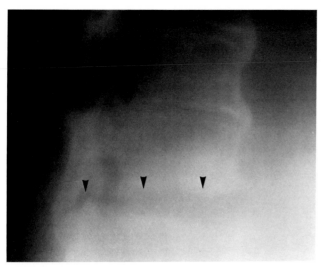

Fig. 6-15. Pathologic fracture with pseudarthrosis. This lateral tomogram of the spine of a patient with longstanding ankylosing spondylitis demonstrates an unstable fracture (*arrowheads*), which passes through the previously fused intervertebral disk space and posterior elements.

posteroinferior surfaces of the calcaneus. The radiographic appearance of inflammatory enthesitis consists of the presence of erosive and proliferative changes, which result in the formation of bony spurs with a spiculated appearance (Fig. 6-17). This must be differentiated from the degenerative enthesopathy common in elderly patients, in which there are coarse, well-defined deposits of bone at these sites.

Spondyloarthritis with Inflammatory Bowel Disease. The spondyloartl ropathy associated with a variety of inflammatory bowel diseases is identical clinically and radiographically to ankylosing spondylitis and is probably the same disorder. The radiographic features previously described for ankylosing spondylitis are also applicable to these disorders.

Psoriatic Arthritis. Arthritis is estimated to occur in 2 to 6 percent of patients with psoriasis. In terms of arthropathy distribution there is no single, typical pattern of psoriatic arthritis. Involvement may be localized to the peripheral articulations or to the articulations of the axial skeleton, or may present with a combination of the two. In terms of its radiographic appearance it does tend to share certain general tendencies with the other seronegative spondyloarthropathies, as well as other features that are relatively specific to this disease.

When axial skeletal involvement is present, sacroiliitis is usually a prominent feature. The specific changes are similar radiographically to those of ankylosing spondylitis except that involvement tends not to be as symmetric. Another differential feature is that in psoriatic sacroiliitis bony ankylosis of the articulations is not as common as in ankylosing spondylitis, although it is more common than in Reiter's syndrome.

When spine involvement is present, 15 to 20 percent of patients demonstrate a radiographic picture identical to that of ankylosing spondylitis with syndesmophyte formation and spinal bony fusion. However the majority of patients demonstrate a different pattern that is characterized by the formation of curvilinear bony deposits, which may be identified first in the soft tissues adjacent to the

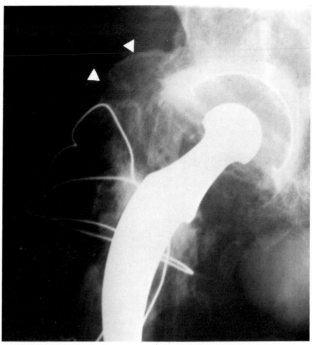

Fig. 6-16. Prominent heterotopic bone formation (*arrowheads*) in a patient with longstanding ankylosing spondylitis and a prior total hip arthroplasty. Formation bridges the lateral margin of the articulation resulting in complete extra-articular ankylosis of the hip joint.

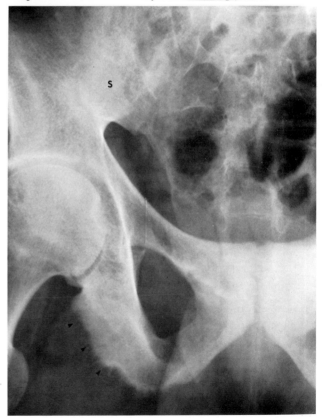

Fig. 6-17. Spiculated bony proliferation (*arrowheads*) at the inferior margin of the ischial ramus in a patient with ankylosing spondylitis. This is the appearance of inflammatory enthesitis and may be seen in the other seronegative spondyloarthropathies as well. Note also the erosive change on either side of the symphyseal articulation, as well as complete intra-articular bony ankylosis of the sacroiliac joint (S).

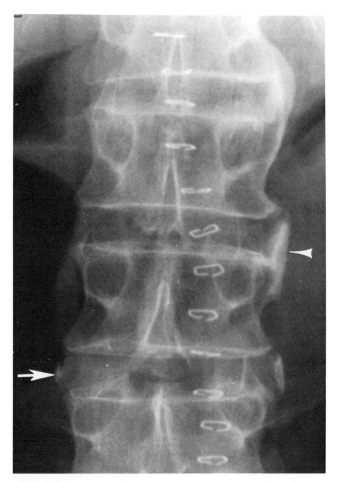

Fig. 6-18. This frontal radiograph of the lumbar spine of a patient with psoriatic spondyloarthritis demonstrates the characteristic paravertebral ossifications, which may be seen in this disorder as well as in Reiter's syndrome. Note the slender, crescenteric shaped, bony outgrowths that arise from the lateral margin of the vertebral body at some levels (*arrowhead*) and adjacent to the intervertebral disk space (*arrow*) at other levels.

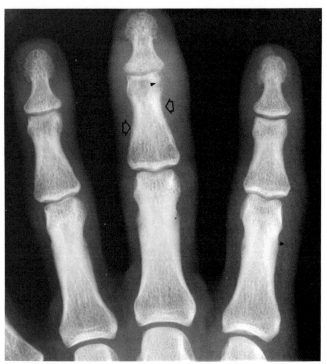

Fig. 6-19. Diffuse soft tissue swelling of the middle digit ("sausage digit"), as well as erosions at the margins of the distal interphalangeal articulation (*arrowhead*), in a patient with peripheral arthropathy of psoriatic arthritis. Periosteal new bone formation (*arrows*) along the medial and lateral margins of the middle phalanx of the third digit, as well as deformity of the nail of the second digit, can be identified.

Psoriasis: Pencil-in-cup

outer layers of the intervertebral disc. With progression, these bone deposits appear as claw-shaped bony excrescences that attach to the vertebral body adjacent to, but distinct from, the discovertebral junction (Fig. 6-18). These lesions have been termed paravertebral ossifications, parasyndesmophytes, or nonmarginal syndesmophytes by various authors. Such lesions do not represent syndesmophytes since the annulus fibrosis of the intervertebral disk is not involved in their formation (see Fig. 6-24). The lesions are irregularly and asymmetrically distributed throughout the involved spinal segment. Cervical spine involvement may be quite prominent in psoriatic spondyloarthritis, even in the presence of minimal thoracolumbar disease, and is often associated with atlantoaxial subluxation.

The peripheral arthropathy of psoriatic arthritis is characterized radiographically by soft-tissue swelling, periostitis, acroosteolysis, erosions, joint space narrowing, articular deformity and ankylosis, and enthesitis. Soft-tissue swelling may occur in a juxta-articular distribution similar to that of rheumatoid arthritis, or may be more diffuse, resulting in the appearance of diffuse swelling of an entire digit ("sausage digit") (Fig. 6-19). Abnormalities of the nails as well as resorption of the terminal tufts of the pha-

langes (acroosteolysis) can often be identified on radiographs of the hands and feet. In the hand and wrist the earliest sites of involvement tend to be the proximal and distal interphalangeal articulations. Marginal erosions, which progress centrally, occur frequently and result in a whittled or "pencil-in-cup" deformity. Periosteal new bone formation is common, especially along the diaphyseal portions of the phalanges, metacarpals, metatarsals, distal radius, and distal tibia. In some instances diffuse circumferential periosteal new bone formation about the distal phalanges of the hand or foot result in increased radiodensity, termed *ivory phalanx*. Osteoporosis is usually absent in psoriatic arthritis, except in some patients with acute exacerbations of disease. The presence of periostitis, the absence of osteoporosis, and the tendency toward distal interphalangeal joint involvement are important characteristics in differentiating psoriatic arthritis in the hands and feet from rheumatoid arthritis. In the late stages of peripheral psoriatic arthritis, articular destruction may be so severe as to result in disorganization of the joints (arthritis mutilans) (Fig. 6-20). Intraarticular ankylosis in psoriatic arthritis may involve any articulation, in contrast to its limited distribution to the carpal and tarsal regions in rheumatoid arthritis. Enthesitis is also a common and important diagnostic feature of psoriatic arthritis (Fig. 6-21). The appearance and distribution of enthesitis is identical to that previously described for ankylosing spondylitis.

Reiter's Syndrome. Reiter's syndrome is a relatively uncommon disease characterized by the clinical triad of urethritis, arthritis, and conjunctivitis. The disease is most common in young men and may be associated with sexual

(+) Periostitis
(-) Osteoporosis

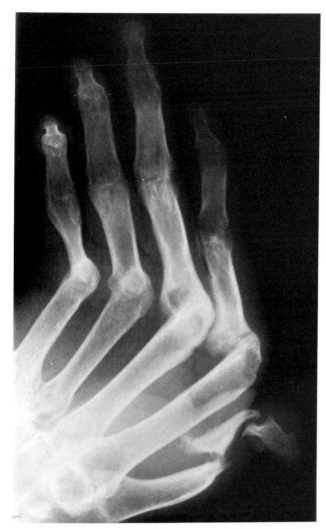

Fig. 6-20. Gross destructive changes at multiple articulations, which superficially simulates rheumatoid arthritis, in a patient with long-standing psoriatic arthritis. The presence of intra-articular ankylosis of all of the interphalangeal joints of the fingers suggests arthritis mutilans, the correct diagnosis.

psori
psoriasis → arthritis mutilans

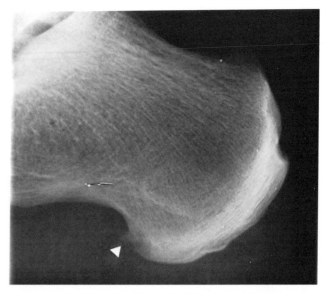

Fig. 6-21. This lateral radiograph of the heel of a patient with psoriatic arthritis demonstrates an ill-defined, eroded, calcaneal spur (*arrowhead*). This is a manifestation of inflammatory enthesitis and may be seen in any of the seronegative spondyloarthropathies.

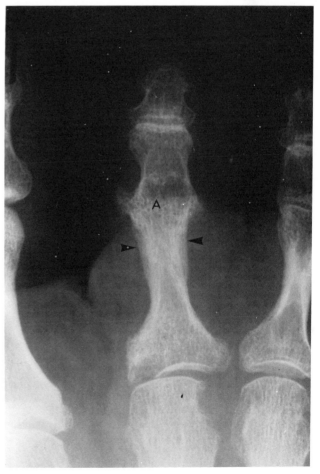

Fig. 6-22. Erosions and subluxation of Reiter's syndrome at the second metatarsophalangeal joint mimic rheumatoid arthritis, but the presence of periosteal new bone formation (*arrowheads*) along the diaphysis of the proximal phalanx and bony ankylosis (A) of the proximal interphalangeal joint suggest the proper diagnosis.

transmission or epidemic dysentery. Radiographic alterations are present in 60 to 80 percent of patients with Reiter's syndrome and in most instances are virtually indistinguishable from those of psoriatic arthritis. Synovial and cartilagenous articulations as well as entheses may be involved, usually in the lower extremity and usually bilaterally and asymmetrically.

The most commonly involved peripheral articulations are the small joints of the feet, followed in frequency by the ankle and knee, with involvement of the hip and upper extremity articulations being relatively unusual. In the axial skeleton sacroiliac and spine involvement are common. Enthesitis is also common, especially at the posterior and posteroinferior surfaces of the calcaneus.

The radiographic features of Reiter's syndrome in the peripheral articulations are similar to those of psoriatic arthritis, with interphalangeal joint involvement being most common and associated with soft-tissue swelling, marginal erosions, joint space narrowing, and periostitis (Fig. 6-22). The nails appear normal, in contrast to their appearance in psoriatic arthritis. Intraarticular bony ankylosis is relatively common in long-standing disease, espe-

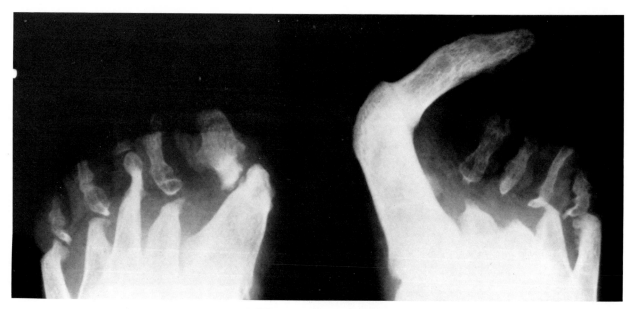

Fig. 6-23. This patient with a 31-year history of unremitting Reiter's syndrome demonstrates the arthritis mutilans pattern of joint destruction. While more typical of psoriatic arthritis, these changes may occasionally be encountered in Reiter's syndrome, as this case illustrates.

cially in the interphalangeal articulations of the foot. In most cases Reiter's syndrome is not as destructive as psoriatic arthritis, although occasionally a patient may develop a severe destructive arthropathy of the arthritis mutilans pattern (Fig. 6-23).

In the sacroiliac joints involvement tends to be bilateral and asymmetrical, resembling the changes of psoriatic arthritis with the exception that intraarticular ankylosis is even less common. In the spine paravertebral ossifications (Fig. 6-24) are the characteristic lesions as they are in psoriatic spondyloarthritis, although cervical spinal involvement in Reiter's syndrome is relatively rare.

CRYSTAL-INDUCED ARTHROPATHIES. The crystal-induced arthropathies include a relatively nonhomogenous group of disorders that share the common feature of being related to the intraarticular or juxta-articular deposition of crystals. The members of this family include gouty arthritis, calcium pyrophosphate dihydrate crystal deposition disease (CPPD), hydroxyapatite crystal deposition disease (HADD), hemochromatosis, Wilson's disease, and ochronosis. Due to a relative paucity of common features these disorders are discussed separately.

Gouty Arthritis. In the great majority of patients with gout, radiographs are normal or remarkable only for soft-tissue swelling about the involved articulations. However, in long-standing disease the deposition of monosodium urate crystals in articulations and juxtaosseous soft tissues may lead to distinctive roentgenographic changes.

The most frequent radiographic finding in gouty arthritis is soft-tissue swelling about the involved articulation that usually resolves after resolution of the acute attack. In more chronic disease, soft-tissue nodules (tophi) may be identified, most commonly near the feet, hands, ankles, elbows, or knees. Erosions are common in advanced gouty arthritis and are usually noted initially at the margins of an articulation as a "punched out" lesion, frequently with a characteristic overhanging lip of bone at its margin (Fig. 6-25). Until late in the disease the joint space is of normal width, even in the presence of prominent erosions. This is an important differential diagnostic point that is in marked contrast to the synchrony of erosions and joint space narrowing in most other inflammatory arthropathies. Another unique feature of gouty arthritis is the frequent presence of intraarticular and extraarticular erosions (Fig. 6-26).

Osteoporosis is not a prominent feature in gouty arthritis, although focal areas of demineralization adjacent to tophi may be noted. In some patients a proliferative response may occur in involved bones that results in enlargement of a segment of bone adjacent to a tophus. This enlargement is most commonly identified at the heads of the phalanges, metacarpals, metatarsals, and at the ulnar styloid. In long-standing disease the severity of destructive changes may become such that complete disorganization of an involved articulation occurs, simulating neuroarthropathy or infection. Calcification of cartilagenous structures (chondrocalcinosis) has been reported in association with gouty arthritis; however, it is not common.

Gouty arthritis is characterized by asymmetric polyarticular disease and most commonly occurs in the feet, hands, wrists, elbows, knees, and ankles. However it must be noted that any articulation may be involved, and indeed the presence of destructive arthritis at an unusual location may suggest the diagnosis. The single most characteristic site for involvement in gouty arthritis is the first metatarsophalangeal joint of the foot (podagra) (see Fig. 6-25), where erosions are most commonly noted on the dorsomedial aspect of the metatarsal head.

Calcium Pyrophosphate Dihydrate Crystal Deposition Disease. Calcium pyrophosphate dihydrate crystal deposition disease (CPPD) is a common disorder most often seen in middle-aged and elderly patients. Several terms that require some explanation are used in association with this disorder. *Pseudogout* is a clinical syndrome seen in some patients with CPPD characterized by acute intermittent episodes of arthritis, which simulate those of gout and do not connote a specific radiographic pattern. *Chondrocalcinosis* refers to calcification of hyaline or fibrocartilage that may be seen in patients with CPPD as well as in patients with some other disorders. *Pyrophosphate arthropathy* re-

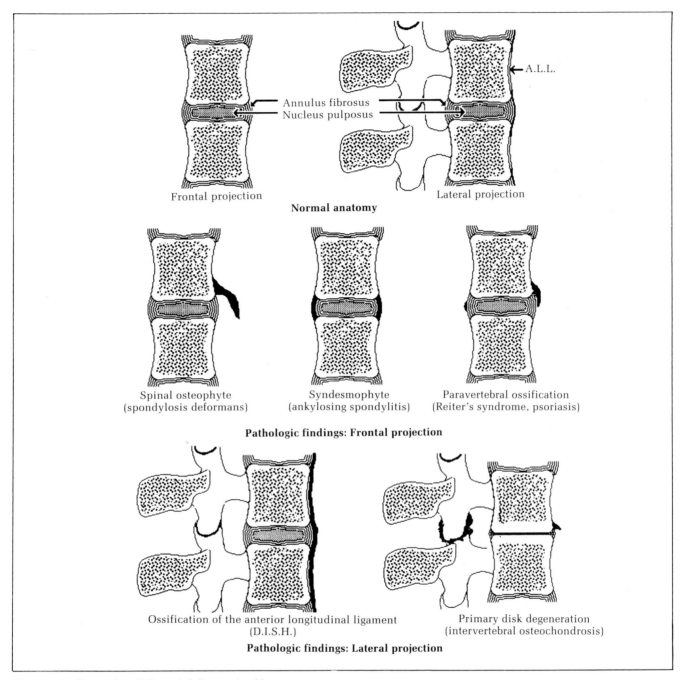

Normal anatomy

Frontal projection

Lateral projection

A.L.L.

Annulus fibrosus
Nucleus pulposus

Spinal osteophyte
(spondylosis deformans)

Syndesmophyte
(ankylosing spondylitis)

Paravertebral ossification
(Reiter's syndrome, psoriasis)

Pathologic findings: Frontal projection

Ossification of the anterior longitudinal ligament
(D.I.S.H.)

Primary disk degeneration
(intervertebral osteochondrosis)

Pathologic findings: Lateral projection

Fig. 6-24. Radiographic differential diagnosis of bony outgrowth of the spine.

fers to structural joint changes in patients with CPPD that may or may not be accompanied by the pseudogout syndrome or chondrocalcinosis.

The most characteristic radiographic feature of CPPD is calcification of hyaline or fibrocartilage, which can be demonstrated radiographically in the majority of patients with the disorder (Fig. 6-27). The most common sites of chondrocalcinosis are the fibrocartilagenous menisci of the knee, the triangular fibrocartilage of the wrist, and the symphysis pubis. Calcification of hyaline articular cartilage is somewhat less common and may be seen in any articulation. Calcification of the juxtaarticular soft-tissue structures, including synovium, articular capsules, tendons, ligaments, and bursae, may also be seen in some patients. The most common structural alterations in pyro-

phosphate arthropathy consist of narrowing of joint space with subchondral sclerosis and prominent cyst formation. This pattern may superficially resemble that of osteoarthritis; however the number and size of subchondral cysts and the variability of osteophyte formation may help to differentiate these disorders in the absence of chondrocalcinosis. Osteoporosis and periostitis are not radiographic features of CPPD.

Pyrophosphate arthropathy is most common at the knee, hip, shoulder, elbow, wrist, and metacarpophalangeal joints of the hand (Fig. 6-28). The presence of arthropathy at sites such as the shoulder and elbow, which are uncommonly involved in degenerative joint disease, may represent useful differential diagnostic features.

The radiographic progression of CPPD is widely variable. In some patients asymptomatic chondrocalcinosis may be the only identifiable manifestation. In others epi-

Fig. 6-25. Bilateral involvement of the metatarsophalangeal joints of the great toe in a patient with a long history of gout. Note the soft tissue masses medial to the articulations, which represent tophi as well as prominent erosive change with sparing of the joint space. Several of the erosions demonstrate the overhanging lip (*arrowheads*) that is characteristic of gouty arthritis.

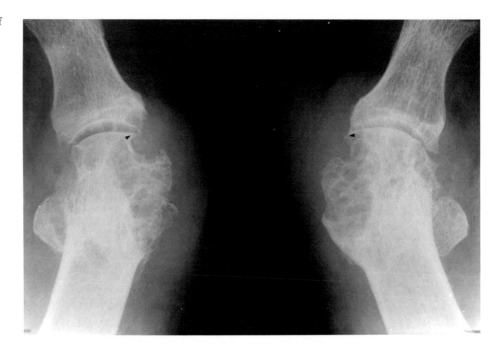

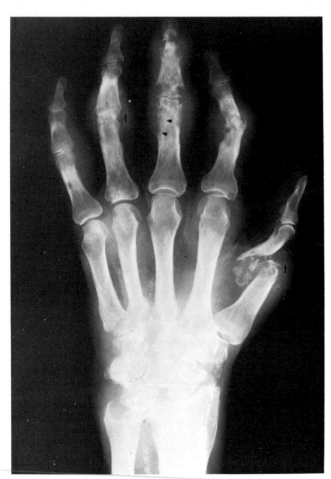

Fig. 6-26. Severe destructive articular change in a patient with advanced gouty arthritis. In particular note the soft tissue nodules (tophi) (t), erosions with overhanging lips, and the extraarticular erosion (*arrowheads*) along the ulnar border of the third proximal phalanx.

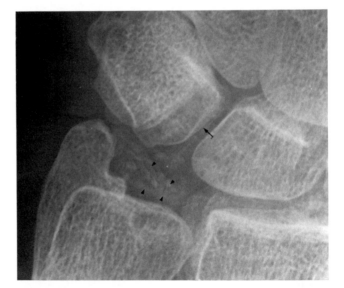

A

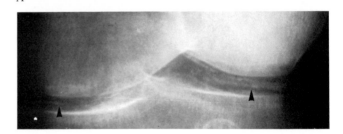

B

Fig. 6-27. This frontal radiograph of the wrist (A) of a patient with CPPD demonstrates calcification (*arrowheads*) of the triangular fibrocartilage of the wrist as well at the hyaline articular cartilage between the lunate and triquetral bones (*arrow*). B. Frontal radiograph of the knee of another patient demonstrates chondrocalcinosis involving the fibrocartilagenous menisci of the knee (*arrowheads*).

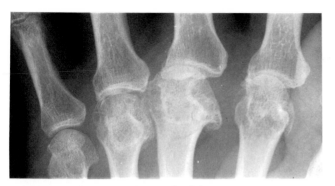

Fig. 6-28. This frontal radiograph of the metacarpophalangeal articulations of a patient with CPPD shows typical joint space narrowing and osteophyte formation with the greatest involvement at the second and third MCP joints.

sodic exacerbations of disease may be accompanied by slowly progressive arthropathy. In some patients CPPD is a rapidly progressive arthropathy that results in rapid destruction of an articulation simulating infection or neuroarthropathy (Fig. 6-29). In most cases this occurs in association with the rapid formation of large subchondral cysts that undermine the subchondral bone plate, resulting in its collapse with subsequent destruction of the joint.

Hydroxyapatite Crystal Deposition Disease. Hydroxyapatite crystal deposition disease (HADD) is primarily a disorder of juxta-articular soft tissues manifested by calcification occurring in tendons, ligaments, and capsular and fibrous tissue. On roentgenograms hydroxyapatite crystals demonstrate a smooth, cloud-like appearance in contrast to the linear deposits characteristic of calcium pyrophosphate. The most common site of HADD is within the musculotendinous rotator cuff of the shoulder (peritendinitis calcarae, calcific tendinitis) (Fig. 6-30). The supraspinatus tendon is most frequently involved, although the other components of the rotator cuff and the bicipital tendon may also be involved. Other less common sites include the soft tissue structures around the elbow, hand, wrist, pelvis, hip, knee, ankle, and heel. Occasionally intraarticular crystal deposition may lead to structural joint abnormalities that resemble degenerative joint disease and are accompanied by joint effusions and radiodense intraarticular deposits, which may mimic loose bodies (joint mice).

Hydroxyapatite crystals may be encountered in disorders other than primary HADD. These include hyperparathyroidism, hypoparathyroidism, sarcoidosis, milk-alkalai syndrome, scleroderma, dermatomyositis, tumoral calcinosis, and Ehlers-Danlos Syndrome. Dystrophic calcification secondary to burns, frost bite, trauma, and fat necrosis may also simulate HADD.

Hemochromatosis. Hemochromatosis is a disorder of iron metabolism in which arthropathy is usually a late and slowly progressive manifestation of the disease. The radiographic appearance of hemochromatosis is similar to that of CPPD, with chondrocalcinosis, joint space narrowing, subchondral sclerosis, and cyst formation being the predominant findings (Fig. 6-31A). However several features help in differentiating these disorders roentgenographically. In contrast to CPPD, hemochromatosis demonstrates a lesser incidence of chondrocalcinosis, as well as progressive and severe osteoporosis. A particularly characteristic feature of hemochromatosis arthropathy is the formation of peculiar hook-like osteophytes (Fig. 6-31A),

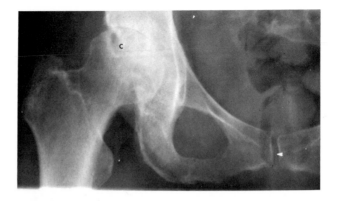
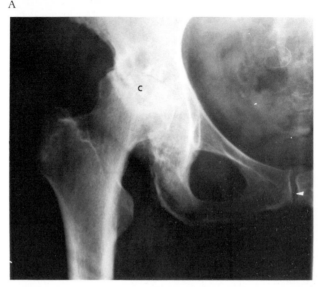

Fig. 6-29. A. Frontal radiograph of the hip of a patient with CPPD demonstrates narrowing of the superior portion of the joint space with large subchondral cysts (c) within the humeral head. The absence of large osteophytes and the presence of calcification within the articular disk of the symphysis pubis (*arrowhead*) suggest the diagnosis. B. A follow-up radiograph six months later, after the patient's symptoms grew suddenly worse, demonstrates collapse of the large femoral subchondral cyst (*arrowhead*) (c) as well as other large cysts within the acetabulum. In some patients this type of rapid progression of articular destruction may mimic septic arthritis or neuroarthropathy.

usually along the radial margins of the metacarpal heads. Periostitis as well as osteonecrosis of the femoral and humeral heads have been reported in some patients with hemochromatosis.

The distribution of radiographic abnormalities varies and almost any peripheral articulation as well as the spine may be involved in hemochromatosis. However the most frequent and characteristic abnormalities occur at the metacarpophalangeal joints of the hand. In contrast to CPPD, the disease tends to be insidious in onset with slowly progressive radiographic changes.

Wilson's Disease (Hepatolenticular Degeneration). Wilson's disease is a rare, inherited disorder that is characterized radiographically by osteoporosis, arthropathy, and rarely by chondrocalcinosis. The arthropathy of Wilson's disease

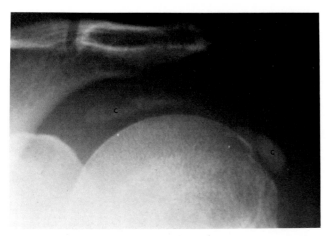

Fig. 6-30. This frontal radiograph of the shoulder of a patient with hydroxyapatite crystal deposition disease (HADD) demonstrates "cloud-like" calcific deposits (c) adjacent to the superior margin of the humeral head, secondary to the deposition of hydroxyapatite crystals within the musculotendinous rotator cuff of the shoulder.

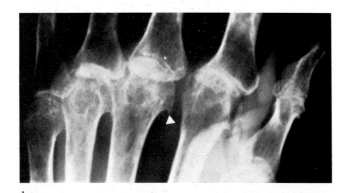

A

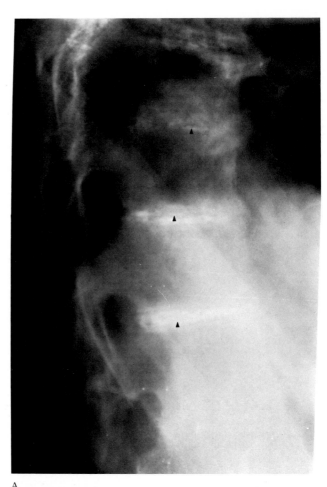

A

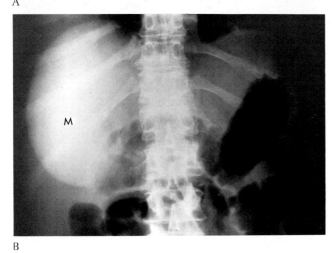

B

Fig. 6-31. A. Radiograph of the hand of a patient with hemochromatosis reveals joint space narrowing with subchondral cyst formation involving the second through fourth metacarpophalangeal joints. Note the small "hook-like" osteophytes (*arrowhead*) and severe generalized osteoporosis, which are characteristic of this disorder. B. Frontal radiograph of the upper abdomen demonstrates a large radiodense mass (M) in the right upper quadrant. This mass proved to be the patient's liver with the density due to iron deposition within the hepatic parenchyma.

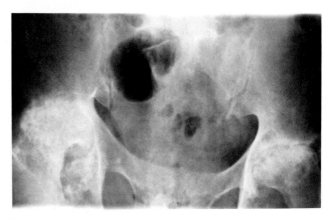

B

Fig. 6-32. A. Lateral radiograph of the lower thoracic spine of a patient with ochronosis demonstrates narrowing and dense calcification of the intervertebral disks (*arrowheads*) as well as severe osteoporosis. B. Frontal radiograph of the pelvis reveals diffuse osteoporosis and severe destructive change of both hip joints.

resembles that of osteoarthritis and CPPD, with joint space narrowing, subchondral sclerosis, and cyst formation. Osteoporosis is prominent and may be quite severe. In some patients typical changes of rickets or osteomalacia may be seen. In addition there are several other radiographic features unique to Wilson's disease. Frequently, fragmentation of the articular surface of involved joints may result in a sawtooth appearance; in other cases, larger and more localized areas of fragmentation resembling osteochondritis dissecans may be identified. Another unique radiographic feature of this disorder is a tendency toward the formation of smooth, corticated ossicles about articulations, particularly the wrist. Enthesitis may be present in some patients with fine, spiculated new bone formation occurring at sites of tendon and ligament insertion into bone (entheses). Irregularity of the normal contour of vertebral bodies, resembling the radiographic findings of Scheuermann's disease, has also been reported in patients with Wilson's disease.

Radiographic abnormalities associated with structural arthropathy are most commonly noted in the hand, wrist, knee, hip, shoulder, elbow, and foot. Osteoporosis tends to be most prominent in the hands, feet, and spine, with other areas having relatively normal mineralization.

Ochronosis. Ochronosis (alkaptonuria) is a rare, hereditary metabolic disorder characterized by the abnormal accumulation of homogentisic acid in a variety of tissues, including articular cartilage. The most characteristic abnormalities occur in the spine and are manifested by osteoporosis and calcification of the intervertebral disks (Fig. 6-32A). With progression of the disease, ossification of the disks may produce intervertebral ankylosis, or degeneration of the calcified disk may occur with formation of intradiscal radiolucent gas collections (vacuum phenomenon) in association with progressive narrowing to the disk space. Spinal osteophytes are small or absent.

Extraspinal involvement resembles degenerative joint disease with joint space narrowing and subchondral sclerosis, but with small or absent osteophytes. Collapse of articular surfaces with intraarticular loose body formation is common (Fig. 6-32B). The hip, knee, and shoulder are the most common peripheral joints involved, while involvement of the hands, feet, elbows, and ankles is uncommon.

DEGENERATIVE JOINT DISEASE. Degenerative joint disease is the most common articular abnormality. Degenerative joint disease involving a synovial articulation is termed *osteoarthritis* (OA). Degenerative joint disease may also involve nonsynovial articulations, such as the intervertebral disks of the spine or sites of ligament or tendon insertion into bone (degenerative enthesopathy).

Osteoarthritis. Osteoarthritis is a mono- or polyarticular, noninflammatory arthropathy that may be considered as having two major forms. *Idiopathic osteoarthritis* is a common disorder with a predisposition to certain articulations, which is not associated with a history of prior trauma or preexisting joint disease. *Secondary osteoarthritis* is a degenerative process that occurs in articulations at which prior trauma (acute or repetitive) or preexisting disease has damaged the articulation or altered the normal dynamic stresses across the articulation.

The major roentgenographic features of osteoarthritis are similar, regardless of its origin. These include joint space narrowing, subchondral sclerosis and cyst formation, and osteophyte formation. Joint space narrowing in osteoar-

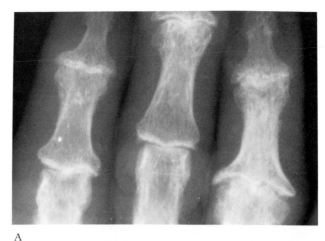

A

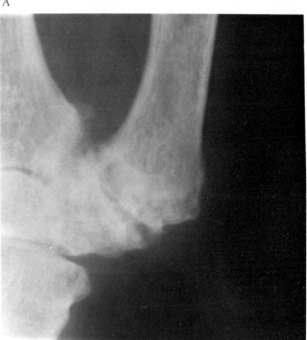

B

Fig. 6-33. A. Frontal radiograph of the fingers of a patient with primary idiopathic osteoarthritis demonstrates joint space narrowing and multiple articulations with prominent marginal osteophyte formation. **B.** Subchondral sclerosis and cyst formation are present at the first carpometacarpal articulation. These findings represent the characteristic changes of primary osteoarthritis involving the hands.

thritis varies in appearance depending on its location. In the small joints of the hands, joint space narrowing in osteoarthritis involves the entire articular surface (Fig. 6-33), while in the major weight-bearing joints, such as the hip or knee (Figs. 6-34, 6-35), joint space narrowing tends to occur in the stressed segments of the articulation and spares segments exposed to relatively less stress. In the hip, joint space narrowing tends to occur in the superior portion of the articulation, while the medial portion of the joint space tends to be spared. In the knee, osteoarthritis tends to involve the medial femorotibial compartment to a much greater degree than either the lateral femorotibial or patellofemoral compartments.

Subchondral sclerosis (eburnation) tends to be quite prominent in OA, appears on radiographs as a zone of in-

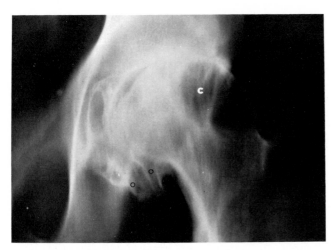

Fig. 6-34. Frontal tomographic section of the hip in a patient with advanced osteoarthritis demonstrates a large subchondral cyst (c) in the superior aspect of the humeral head, asymmetric joint space narrowing, and prominent osteophytes (o) along the medial margin of the femoral head and adjacent acetabulum.

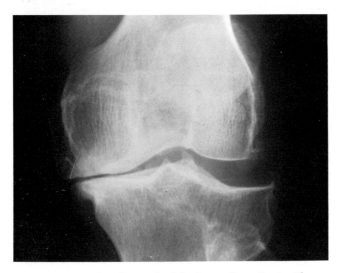

Fig. 6-35. Frontal radiograph of the knee of a patient with osteoarthritis demonstrates severe narrowing of the medial compartment with subchondral sclerosis (eburnation) and osteophyte formation. Lateral subluxation and medial angulation (genu vara) of the tibia are also present.

creased radiodensity adjacent to the subchondral bone plate, and tends to be most prominent in areas of joint space narrowing in stressed segments of the articulation. Subchondral cystic lesions are also frequently identified in osteoarthritis and appear as small, multiple, radiolucent lesions adjacent to the subchondral bone plate. In most instances these lesions are quite small, although in some regions, such as the lateral aspect of the acetabulum of the hip joint, they may attain a relatively large size.

Osteophyte formation is the single most characteristic feature of osteoarthritis. Osteophytes are bone excrescences arising either from islands of metaplastic cartilage or from capsular tissue in osteoarthritic joints. Thus osteophytes tend to be located at the margins of joints as well as at the articular surface of low-stress regions of a joint. In osteoarthritis of the hip, prominent osteophytic change is often noted along the medial surface of the femoral head in association with joint space narrowing and subchondral

sclerosis of the superior aspect of the articulation. When osteophytes arise from apposing articular surfaces they tend to present an interdigitating appearance, as if they had been broken apart and then fit back together.

Loose bodies (joint mice) are common in advanced osteoarthritis and originate from small pieces of cartilage broken loose from the articular surface. These may implant into synovial tissue and grow or be nourished by joint fluid. Joint mice, if free in the articulation, limit joint motion as well as exacerbate the degree of joint destruction. Several other features are notable for their absence in typical osteoarthritis. These include joint effusions, erosions, periostitis, and intraarticular bony ankylosis. The presence of any of these abnormalities suggests another diagnosis as being either partially or completely responsible for the patient's abnormalities.

The distribution of osteoarthritis depends to a major degree on its etiology. Secondary osteoarthritis occurs in joints where prior trauma has occurred or which preexisting disease has altered. Primary osteoarthritis is most common at the interphalangeal joints of the hand and the first carpometacarpal joint. Metacarpophalangeal joint involvement may be seen, usually in association with interphalangeal joint disease. Osteoarthritis is also common in the hip and the knee without a specific predisposing cause being identifiable. However it is easy to postulate that in these articulations chronic trauma is probably the etiology. Primary osteoarthritis is very rare in the shoulder articulation. In virtually every case osteoarthritis in this articulation is secondary to trauma (fracture or dislocation), chronic rotator cuff tear, or preexisting disease.

Erosive Osteoarthritis. Erosive (inflammatory) osteoarthritis (EOA) refers to a specific arthropathy of unknown etiology that is virtually limited to middle-aged and elderly women. EOA consists of the radiographic pattern of primary osteoarthritis of the hands with a clinical pattern of acute inflammation. In this disorder typical osteoarthritic changes (joint space narrowing, subchondral sclerosis, and osteophyte formation) are present at the interphalangeal joints of the hand, often in association with disease at the first carpometacarpal joint. In many instances no other alterations are present and the diagnosis must be based strictly on clinical criteria. However there are two radiographic features of EOA that, when present in combination with other typical features of osteoarthritis, allow a radiographic diagnosis of this disorder to be suggested (Fig. 6-36). The first abnormality is the presence of central erosions at one or more interphalangeal articulations. These lesions are quite distinctive in their appearance as a large radiolucent defect in the subchondral portion of the bone that communicates with the articular space by a wide or narrow neck. The second diagnostic feature of EOA is the presence of intraarticular bony ankylosis in association with degenerative changes.

Degenerative Joint Disease of the Spine. The spine is a complex collection of synovial, fibrous, and cartilaginous articulations, any of which may be subject to degenerative alterations. Degenerative joint disease of the spine may be further subdivided into several specific entities based on the structures primarily involved in the degenerative process. These include spondylosis deformans, intervertebral osteochondrosis, diffuse idiopathic skeletal hyperostosis, and spinal apophyseal joint osteoarthritis.

Spondylosis Deformans. Spondylosis deformans (spinal osteophytosis) (Fig. 6-37) is a relatively common disorder seen in elderly patients that is characterized by the pres-

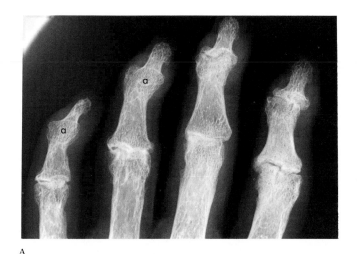

A

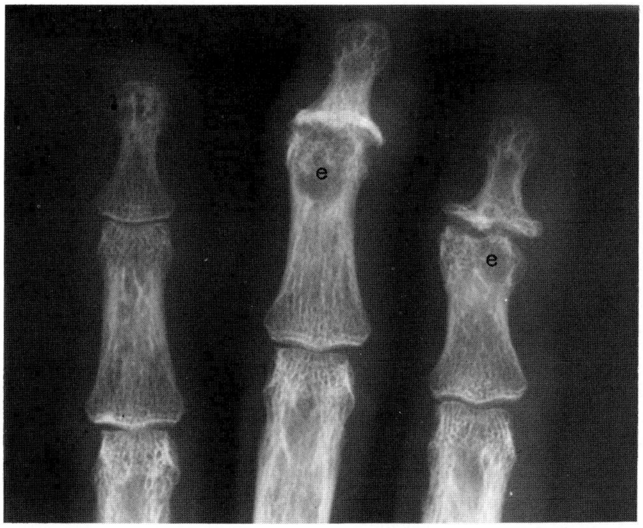

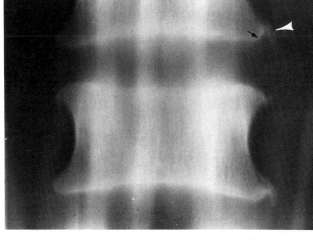

A

B

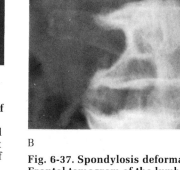

B

Fig. 6-36. A. Frontal radiograph of the fingers demonstrates the typical joint space narrowing and osteophyte formation of osteoarthritis; however, the presence of complete intraarticular bony ankylosis (a) of the distal interphalangeal articulations of the fourth and fifth digits suggests the correct diagnosis. B. Large central erosions (e) of the distal aspects of the middle phalanges of the second and third digits, in combination with typical osteoarthritic changes, are characteristic of erosive osteoarthritis.

Fig. 6-37. Spondylosis deformans (spinal osteophytosis). A. Frontal tomogram of the lumbar spine demonstrates the appearance of early spinal osteophyte formation (*arrowhead*). Note that the small bony escresences arise from the side of the vertebra rather than from the rounded corner (*arrow*), which represents the discovertebral junction, differentiating these lesions from syndesmophytes. B. Frontal radiograph of the spine demonstrates advanced spondylosis deformans with numerous large, laterally oriented, osteophytes.

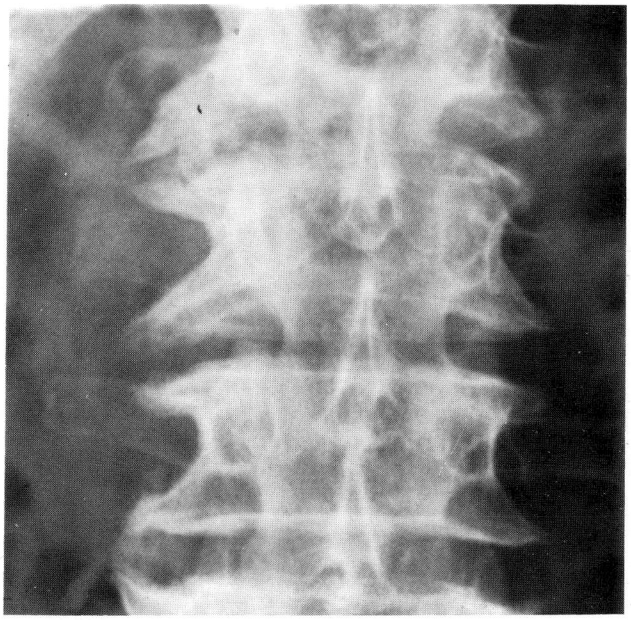

[Handwritten annotations:]

O A
(+) osteophytes
(+) subchondral sclerosis
(+) joint narrowing
(–) effusion
(–) erosion
(–) periostitis
(–) ankylosis

Fig. 6-38. Intervertebral osteochondrosis. Lateral radiograph of the lower lumbar spine demonstrates narrowing of the intervertebral disk space at L4–5 with a vacuum phenomenon (*arrowheads*), subchondral sclerosis, and small triangular osteophytes. These are the radiographic manifestations of primary intervertebral disk degeneration.

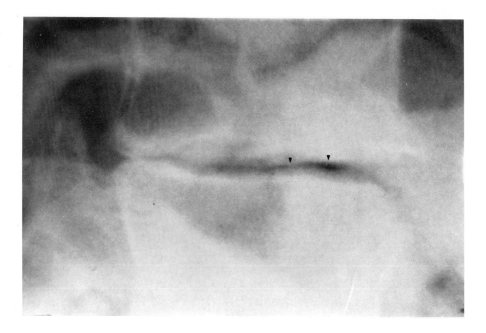

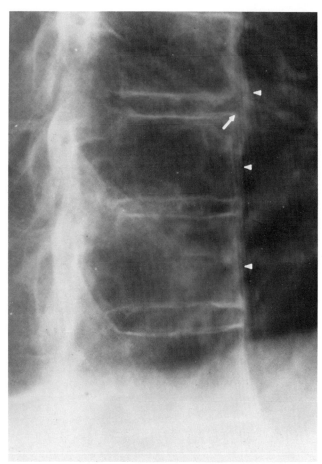

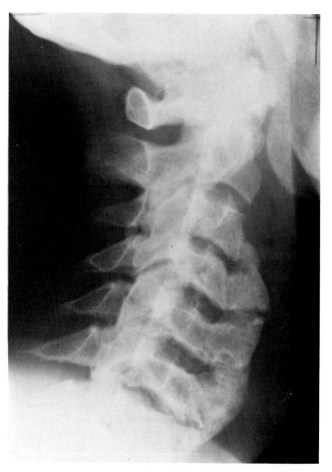

Fig. 6-39. Diffuse idiopathic skeletal hyperostosis (DISH). Lateral radiograph of the thoracic spine demonstrates the flowing ossification of the anterior longitudinal ligament of the spine (*arrowheads*), which characterizes this disorder. Also note that the corners of the vertebral bodies (*arrow*) are spaced, in contrast to the syndesmophytes of ankylosing spondylitis.

Fig. 6-40. Lateral view of the cervical spine in a patient with DISH who complained of dysphagia demonstrates a large, shell-like deposit of bone adjacent to the anterior margin of the lower cervical spine. This is typical of DISH involving the cervical spine and may also be seen in sternocostoclavicular hyperostosis.

ence of numerous, large, bony outgrowths (osteophytes) arising from the margins of vertebral bodies (see Fig. 6-24). Actually the term *osteophyte* is a misnomer in this circumstance, since true osteophytes arise in relation to synovial articulations while spinal "osteophytes" actually arise at points of fibrous tissue insertion into vertebral bodies (entheses) and thus are more accurately termed *enthesophytes*. However, in accordance with the broadly accepted terminology, the term osteophyte is used here to refer to these and related enthesophytes arising from the spine. In spondylosis deformans large osteophytes arise from the margins of vertebral bodies adjacent to, but distinct from, the point of insertion of the annulus fibrosis of the intervertebral disk into the vertebra. Initial growth is laterally oriented, but as the osteophytes enlarge the growth of the osteophyte tends to change to a more vertical orientation. Thus a mature spinal osteophyte has a laterally directed proximal segment and a cephalically or caudally directed distal segment. Often osteophytes at adjacent levels meet at their most distal extents but usually do not fuse. Spinal osteophytes in the thoracic and upper lumbar spine are virtually always more prominent on the right border of the vertebral column, presumably being inhibited on the left side by the pulsations of the adjacent thoracic and abdominal aorta. Spondylosis deformans is usually an incidental radiographic diagnosis that is not associated with symptoms or other radiographic abnormalities.

Intervertebral Osteochondrosis. Intervertebral osteochondrosis (Fig. 6-38) refers to primary degenerative joint disease of the intervertebral disks of the spinal column. The earliest manifestation in many cases is a linear, radiolucent gas collection (vacuum phenomenon) that may be identified in the midportion of an intervertebral disk space on spinal radiographs. Narrowing of the disk space follows with sclerosis (eburnation) of the adjacent vertebral endplates. Often small, triangular osteophytes may be identified arising from the margins of adjacent vertebral bodies (see Fig. 6-24). That the presence of the roentgenographic changes of intervertebral osteochondrosis implies degeneration of the intervertebral disk, but not necessarily disk herniation, must be considered.

Diffuse Idiopathic Skeletal Hyperostosis. Diffuse idiopathic skeletal hyperostosis (DISH) is a disorder characterized by the presence of ossification and calcification of the anterior longitudinal ligament of the spine and osseous proliferation at peripheral sites of ligament and tendon insertion (enthesopathy). The spinal manifestations of this disorder have long been known under the names Forrestier's disease and ankylosing hyperostosis of the spine. Changes are most common in the lower thoracic spine, followed in frequency by changes in the lumbar and cervical segments. In a typical case, changes are most apparent on the lateral radiograph of the spine and consist of smooth, flowing bridges of bone deposited along the anterior margins of the vertebra and bridging the intervertebral disk space (Fig. 6-39). This appearance may be suggestive of ankylosing spondylitis; however closer examination of the radiograph reveals several differences (see Fig. 6-24). First, a bony shell can be identified adjacent to the anterior margin of the vertebral body that is usually separated from it by a thin, radiolucent line. Second, the corner of the vertebral body, into which the annulus fibrosis of the intervertebral disk inserts, is spared and the bony bridges flow around the disk space rather than involve the outer layers of the disk. The spinal apophyseal joints and the sacroiliac joints are not involved in DISH.

In the lumbar spine, DISH may demonstrate changes

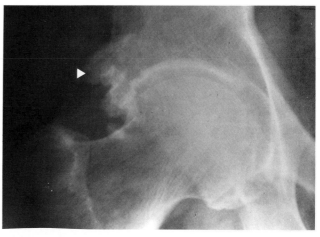

Fig. 6-41. Frontal view of the hip in a patient with DISH demonstrates coarse bony proliferation (*arrowhead*) along the anterolateral aspect of the acetabulum. This finding is typical of degenerative enthesopathy, which is common in DISH, and may be identified at a number of peripheral sites of tendon and ligament insertion.

identical to those of spondylosis deformans, with numerous, large, laterally directed osteophytes. In the cervical spine, large, thick plates of bone may be deposited anterior to the cervical vertebral bodies. In some instances these deposits may be large enough to interfere with swallowing, resulting in patient complaints of dysphagia (Fig. 6-40). The extraspinal manifestation of DISH consists of bony proliferation at sites of tendon and ligament insertion (enthesopathy) that appear as coarse deposits of bone (Fig. 6-41). These findings are identical to those of degenerative enthesopathy and are most prominent at tendon and ligament insertion sites of the pelvis, proximal femurs, patella, and calcaneus. The diagnosis of DISH is based on radiographic changes and, at present, requires typical flowing ossifications and calcifications, which bridge the intervertebral disk space at four contiguous spinal levels.

Apophyseal Joint Osteoarthritis. The synovial apophyseal joints of the spine are common sites of degenerative joint disease. Radiographic changes are most typical in the mid- and lower cervical spine, the midthoracic spine, and the lower lumbar spine. These changes are identical to those of peripheral osteoarthritis, with joint space narrowing, subchondral sclerosis, and cyst and osteophyte formation. In severe cases, compression of intraspinal neural structures may occur in association with large osteophytes or facet joint subluxation (Fig. 6-42).

NEUROARTHROPATHY. Neuroarthropathy (Charcot's joint) refers to the changes that occur in articulations deprived of proprioceptive or pain sensation and thus of normal protective mechanisms. A number of disorders are associated with neuroarthropathy (Table 6-1).

The radiographic appearance of neuroarthropathy can be summarized by four descriptive terms: (1) effusion, (2) sclerosis, (3) fragmentation, and (4) disorganization (Fig. 6-43). None of these features is diagnostic in and of itself, but together these features constitute a characteristic pattern. Joint effusions are virtually always present in a neuropathic joint and frequently attain massive size. In most instances a very large joint effusion is the earliest finding in neuroarthropathy and frequently dissects into adjacent

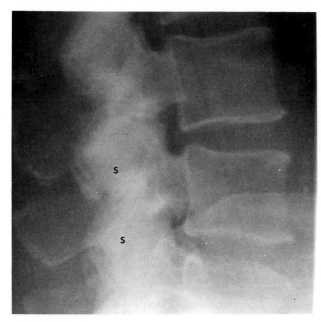

A

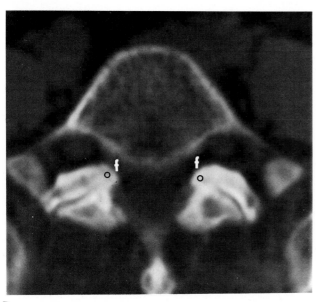

B

Fig. 6-42. Spinal apophyseal osteoarthritis. A. Lateral view of the lumbar spine demonstrates dense sclerosis (s) and proliferative changes at the spinal apophyseal articulations, posterior to the vertebral bodies resulting in a significant narrowing of the lumbar spinal canal at this level. B. In another patient, a computed tomographic section through the L5–S1 apophyseal joint level demonstrates prominent degenerative arthritis with joint space narrowing and osteophyte formation (o), which has narrowed the neural foramina (f) at this level.

Table 6-1. Disorders Associated with Neuroarthropathy

Central (upper motor neuron) Lesions
  Syphilis (tabes dorsalis)
  Syringomyelia
  Meningomyelocele
  Charcot-Marie tooth syndrome
  Spinal trauma
  Multiple sclerosis
Peripheral (lower motor neuron) Lesions
  Diabetes mellitus
  Alcoholism
  Amyloidosis
  Tuberculosis
  Familial dysautonomia (Riley-Day syndrome)
  Congenital indifference to pain
  Steroid therapy
  Fanconi's anemia

soft-tissue planes, resulting in massive soft-tissue swelling about the articulation. The next most significant finding consists of sclerosis of the juxta-articular bone with rapid diminution in the diameter of the joint space, followed by fragmentation of the articular surface that results in the presence of numerous fragments of osseous debris within the joint capsule. In the final phase complete destruction of the articulation occurs, with disruption of the supporting soft tissue structures resulting in subluxation, dislocation, or collapse of the articulation. In some instances this process may be so severe that it is difficult to tell what articulation is shown on the radiograph.

The lower extremities are more commonly involved in neuroarthropathy than the upper extremities. The ankle and foot are the most common sites of abnormality in diabetes, alcoholic neuroarthropathy, congenital indifference to pain, meningomyelocele, and leprosy. Tabes dorsalis tends to involve the spine, hip, knee, or ankle most commonly, while syringomyelia tends to involve the joints of the upper extremities, especially the shoulders and elbows.

Metabolic Bone Diseases

OSTEOPOROSIS. Osteoporosis refers to an abnormal diminution in the mass of structurally normal bone. It may be encountered in a large number of disorders as a generalized, regional, or localized process (Table 6-2).

The major radiographic finding in osteoporosis is osteopenia; there is an abnormal degree of radiolucency of the involved osseous structures. In osteoporosis the cortex of involved bones is diminished in thickness, with relative widening of the medullary space. The margins of the cortex in osteoporosis are quite sharp and distinct (pencilled), in contrast to the indistinct cortical margins in osteomalacia and the subperiosteal cortical erosions and widened haversian canals (cortical tunneling) in hyperparathyroidism. There is a diminution in the number of medullary trabeculae, characteristically with resorption of secondary (low-stress) trabeculae and preservation of primary (high-stress) trabeculae. This finding is most prominent in the vertebral bodies (Fig. 6-44), where selective resorption of horizontally oriented secondary trabeculae results in abnormal prominence of the remaining vertically oriented primary trabeculae. In the proximal femur the arc-shaped primary trabeculae also tend to be prominently accentuated.

osteoporosis
pencilled cortices

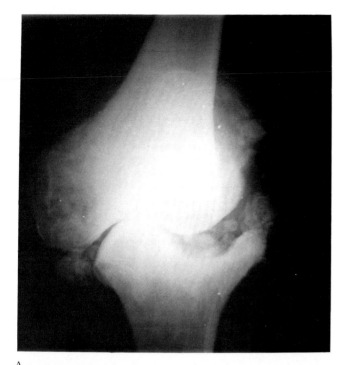

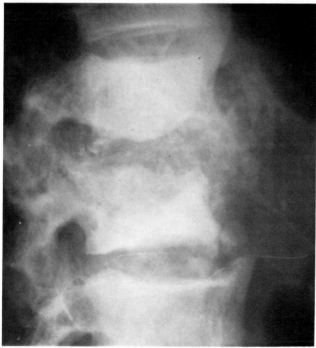

Fig. 6-43. Neuroarthropathy (Charcot's joint). A. Frontal radiograph of the knee of a patient with tabes dorsalis demonstrates three of the characteristic radiographic features of neuroarthropathy: bony sclerosis, articular fragmentation, and articular disorganization. B. Lateral radiograph of the spine of another patient with tabes dorsalis also demonstrates the typical findings of neuroarthropathy.

Table 6-2. Disorders Associated with Osteoporosis

Generalized	Localized
Endocrine disorders	Immobilization
Cushing's syndrome	Disuse
Hyperparathyroidism	Reflex sympathetic dystrophy
Hypoparathyroidism	syndrome
Post menopausal	Septic arthritis
Turner's syndrome	Regional migratory
Acromegally	osteoporosis
Malnutrition	Transient osteoporosis of the
Vitamin C deficiency	hip
Idiopathic	Arthritis (Multiple)
Hypovitaminosis A	
Neoplasms	
Myeloma	
Leukemia	
Hepatoblastoma	
Chronic liver disease	
Iatrogenic	
Heparin	
Steroid	
Congenital	
Arthritis	
Rheumatoid arthritis	
JRA	
Hemochromatosis	
Pregnancy	
Lactation	
Anemia and marrow disease	
Gaucher's disease	
Thalassemia	
Sickle cell disease	

In some forms of osteoporosis, especially the varieties associated with the reflex sympathetic dystrophy syndrome (RSDS) (Fig. 6-45) or immobilization, a more localized, aggressive pattern of osteoporosis may be encountered. In these patients the radiographic changes of osteoporosis may be characterized by band-like radiolucent zones traversing the metaphysis or paralleling the epiphyseal subchondral bone plate, or by a patchy pattern consisting of numerous, small, ill-defined cystic lesions. In this latter form the changes may resemble those of diffuse metastatic disease, myeloma, or infection.

The most common complication of osteoporosis is fracture, usually following minimal trauma (see Fig. 6-44). Osteoporotic fractures are common in the spine and may consist of anterior compression fractures of the vertebral body, rounded compression of the vertebral end plates (fish vertebra), or focal herniations of disk material through the vertebral end plate (Schmorl's nodes). Fractures of the femoral neck, distal radius, and humeral neck are also common in osteoporotic patients and may be more difficult to visualize on radiographs because of the osteoporosis.

OSTEOMALACIA AND RICKETS. Osteomalacia is deficiency of mature mineralized bone relative to the amount of unmineralized osteoid. Rickets specifically refers to osteomalacia in the immature skeleton. Some common causes of osteomalacia are listed in Table 6-3. Although basically the same disease process, the radiographic manifestation of adult osteomalacia and childhood rickets are distinct enough that they should be considered separately.

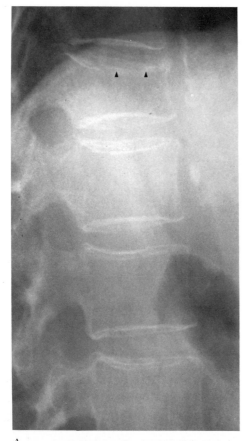

A

B

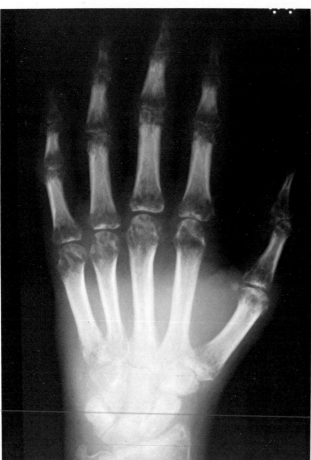

Fig. 6-44. Osteoporosis. A. Lateral radiograph of the spine demonstrates diffuse demineralization of the vertebral bodies. Note the thin, pencilled cortical margins, loss of radiographic density, and prominent vertical striations in the lower vertebral body. An anterior compression fracture (*arrowheads*), typical of osteoporosis, is also present. **B.** Frontal radiograph of the hip demonstrates advanced osteoporosis with marked cortical thinning and a pathologic fracture through the intertrochanteric portion of the femur.

Osteomalacia. Osteomalacia, like osteoporosis, is characterized by osteopenia and resorption of secondary trabeculae; however, in contrast to osteoporosis the remaining trabeculae and cortical margins are coarse, with indistinct margins. In some areas, particularly in areas of high stress, excessive deposition of poorly mineralized osteoid may result in areas of cortical thickening with relative osteosclerosis. Looser's zones (pseudofractures) are characteristic of osteomalacia and consist of radiolucent defects oriented at right angles to the cortex of the bone, which most typically involve the concave border of a long bone. This is in contrast to stress fractures and the pseudofractures of Paget's disease, in which the radiolucent defects are characteristically found on the convex border of the bone. The most typical sites of Looser's zones are the outer (concave) borders of the scapula, ribs, pubic rami, proximal femur, and proximal ulna. In some instances a complete pathologic fracture may complicate these lesions. Gross skeletal deformities with bowing of long bones, spinal scoliosis, and

Fig. 6-45. Osteoporosis in a predominantly juxtaarticular pattern in a patient with reflex sympathetic dystrophy syndrome (RSDS, Sudek's atrophy). Note the patchy, mottled appearance of the demineralization, which may mimic tumor in some instances.

Osteoporosis: concave pseudofracture
Osteomalacia: convex pseudofracture

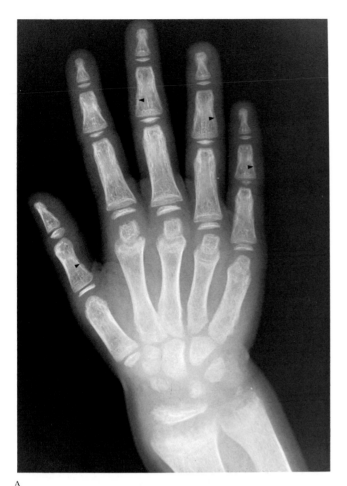

A

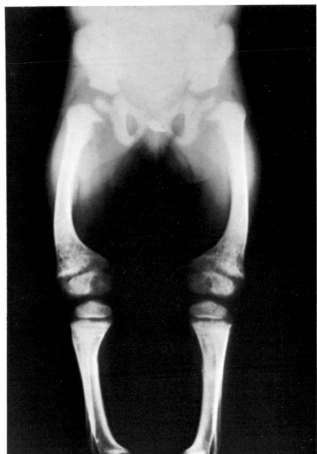

B

Fig. 6-46. A. This frontal radiograph of the hand of a child with rickets demonstrates characteristic cupping and fraying of the metaphyses of the distal radius and ulna. Also note the diffuse osteopenia and subperiosteal bony resorption (*arrowheads*), most prominent along the diaphyseal regions of the middle phalanges. B. This frontal radiograph of the lower extremities in a child with longstanding rickets reveals bowing deformities of the long bones and metaphyseal irregularities.

basilar invagination of the skull may accompany longstanding osteomalacia due to the abnormal softening of osseous structures.

Rickets. Rickets (Fig. 6-46) is characterized by the changes of osteomalacia as well as by abnormalities of bone growth and maturation. The most characteristic radiographic changes relate to the epiphysis, cartilaginous growth plate, and the adjacent metaphysis. Early in the disorder, slight widening of the growth plate with radiolucency of the zone of provisional calcification on the metaphyseal side of the growth plate may be seen. With progression the growth plate becomes markedly widened, while the adjacent metaphysis assumes a concave shape with a spiculated border (cupping and fraying of the metaphysis). Demineralization and loss of definition of the epiphyseal ossification center occurs, and in some patients the epiphysis may disappear entirely. Bowing deformities of long bones are common, especially in the lower extremity where a bowleg (genu varum) deformity is quite common. Enlargement of the costochondral junctions of multiple ribs results in the rachitic rosary, while resorption at the

Table 6-3. Common Causes of Osteomalacia and Rickets

Vitamin D deficiency
GI malabsorption syndromes
   Sprue
   Crohn's disease
   Scleroderma
   GI surgery
Hepatic disease
Benign neoplasms
   Nonossifying fibroma
   Osteoblastoma
   Giant cell tumor
Anticonvulsant drugs
   Phenobarbital
   Phenytoin (Dilantin)
Renal osteodystrophy
Hereditary rickets (vitamin D-dependent)
Renal tubular disease (vitamin D-resistant)
Fibrous dysplasia
Atypical axial osteomalacia
Hypophosphatasia
Parathyroid gland disorders

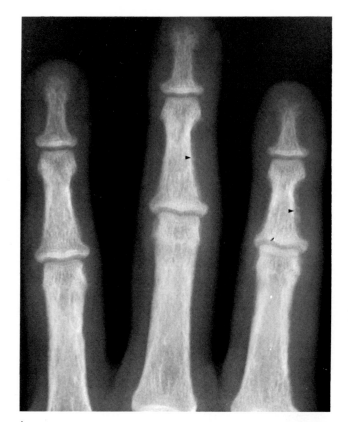

A

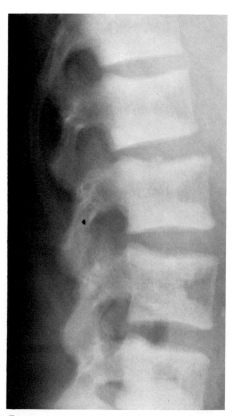

B

Fig. 6-47. Hyperparathyroidism. A. Frontal radiograph of the fingers demonstrates loss of definition of the terminal tufts of the distal phalange as well as subperiosteal resorption (*arrowheads*), which is most prominent along the radial margins of the middle phalanges. B. Lateral radiograph of the lumbar spine in patient with chronic renal failure (renal osteodystrophy) demonstrates broad osteosclerotic bands paralleling the vertebral endplates (Rugger-Jersey spine). C. Frontal radiograph of the hand in a patient with primary hyperparathyroidism demonstrates typical subperiosteal resorptive changes and osteopenia as well as radiolucent defects (brown tumors) (t) in the medullary cavity of the third metacarpal and fifth proximal phalanx.

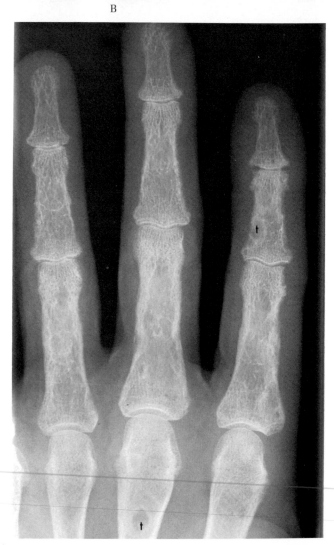

C

costal insertion of the diaphragm results in Harrison's groove.

In the United States the most common cause of rickets is pediatric renal disease, which may be either congenital or acquired. Nutritional rickets is very uncommon in industrialized countries. When changes of rickets of unusual severity are encountered, two other causes should be kept in mind. *Hypophosphatasia* is a rare autosomal recessive disorder that is due to the inability of osteoblasts to produce alkaline phosphatase. The radiographic changes of this disorder are a cross between severe rickets and osteogenesis imperfecta. Another possibility to be considered in children with severe rachitic change is *iatrogenic rickets*, which occurs primarily in children with seizure disorders being treated with phenytoin (Dilantin).

HYPERPARATHYROIDISM. Hyperparathyroidism (HPTH) is a disorder caused by abnormally elevated circulating levels of parathormone, which may relate to intrinsic abnormalities of the parathyroid glands (e.g., primary HPTH, osteitis fibrosa cystica), overstimulation of the glands due to renal functional abnormalities (e.g., secondary HPTH, renal osteodystrophy), or autonomous hyperfunction of the glands following prolonged hyperstimulation (e.g., tertiary HPTH). In general, the radiographic appearance of all types of HPTH is similar regardless of their etiologies; however some differences exist that may assist in differentiation of primary and secondary HPTH.

The osseous changes of HPTH result from parathormone activation of osteoclasts and osteocytes (osteocytic osteoclasis), resulting in a markedly elevated rate of bone resorption that far exceeds capacity for repair. Thus resorption is the key word to remember when considering the skeletal manifestations of this disorder. The classic early finding in HPTH is osseous resorption involving the outer cortical margin (subperiosteal resorption) of a tubular bone (Fig. 6-47A). Early in the process there is a subtle loss of sharpness of the outer cortical margin, followed by a lacy and finally spiculated appearance. The earliest sites where subperiosteal resorption can be identified are typically along the radial margins of the middle phalanges of the second and third digits of the hand. Other characteristic sites of bony resorption include the terminal tufts of the distal phalanges, the medial border of the proximal tibia, the distal aspects of the clavicles, and the lamina dura that surrounds the roots of the teeth. Intracortical osseous resorption of bone is centered around the haversian canals of cortical bone, resulting in a radiographic appearance of thin, linear radiolucent bands that parallel the long axis of the involved bone. This finding is noted earliest in the cortex of the metacarpals especially the second of the hand, and is unusual in the phalanges. Endosteal resorption of cortical bone results in a loss of definition of the inner cortical surface of a bone. Osseous resorption also occurs at sites of tendon and ligament insertion into bone (entheses), resulting in a frayed and whiskered appearance that may simulate those seen in the seronegative spondyloarthropathies.

Brown tumors (osteoclastomas) (Fig. 6-47C) are single or multiple, well-defined, osteolytic lesions that are frequently eccentrically located in bones of the axial or appendicular skeleton. Pathologically these lesions consist of collections of osteoclasts and fibrous tissue and have no malignant potential. Brown tumors are more common in primary HPTH, although they may be noted occasionally in secondary HPTH. Osteosclerosis may be encountered in some patients and is more common in secondary HPTH. The most characteristic osteosclerotic changes occur in the spine, with a characteristic radiographic appearance consisting of thick, osteosclerotic bands that parallel the upper and lower vertebral end plates (Rugger jersey spine) (Fig. 6-47B). Far less common is the presence of diffuse osteosclerosis of the ribs, pelvis, or peripheral skeleton. Chondrocalcinosis due to the deposition of calcium pyrophosphate crystals in fibrocartilage and hyaline cartilage is common in primary HPTH and less common in secondary HPTH. Soft-tissue and vascular calcification is most common in renal osteodystrophy. In particular the presence of prominent vascular calcification in the hands should bring this possibility to mind. Occasionally large deposits of calcific material (secondary tumoral calcinosis) may be encountered adjacent to, but distinct from, the joints. Osteonecrosis, especially of the femoral head, is common in renal osteodystrophy and may be related to corticosteroid therapy in many cases.

In children the radiographic changes of primary or secondary HPTH are the same as those of rickets and include osteopenia, widening and irregularity of the growth plates, cupping and fraying of the metaphysis, and bowing deformities. Slipped epiphyses are common in these patients and occur most commonly at the capital femoral epiphysis, although other sites may be involved.

HYPOPARATHYROIDISM, PSEUDOHYPOPARATHYROIDISM, AND PSEUDOPSEUDOHYPOPARATHYROIDISM. Hypoparathyroidism is a deficiency of parathormone that may be seen as a primary idiopathic disorder or secondary to trauma or surgery of the parathyroid glands. Pseudohypoparathyroidism and pseudopseudohypoparathyroidism (PH) (PPH) are congenital disorders characterized by end organ resistance to the effects of parathormone. They are closely related. PPH may be considered a normocalcemic form of PH.

Osteosclerosis is the most constant radiographic finding in hypoparathyroidism and may be generalized or localized. Thickening of the calvarium of the skull with narrowing of the diploic space is common. Dense transverse bands in the metaphyses of tubular bones may also be seen. When onset occurs during childhood there is a generalized abnormality of skeletal maturation that includes hypoplasia and late appearance of dentition, as well as premature fusion of epiphyseal plates that results in short stature. Subcutaneous soft-tissue calcification may be noted, as well as calcification of the basal ganglia of the brain on skull radiographs or computed tomography. In some cases calcification and ossification of the anterior longitudinal ligament of the spine result in radiographic changes identical to those of DISH.

Radiographically PH and PPH are similar as well. The density of osseous structures in these disorders is variable and may be increased, diminished, or normal. The single most characteristic abnormality in both is shortening of the metacarpal bones of the hand, which is present in 75 percent of patients and most frequently involves the first, fourth, and fifth digits (Fig. 6-48). Shortening of the first and fourth metatarsal bones of the foot is also a frequent finding. Hypoplasia of the distal phalanx of the thumb may also be seen. Subcutaneous soft-tissue calcification is frequent and slightly more common in PH than in PPH. Basal ganglia calcification and thickening of the calvarium is commonly seen in both disorders. Small exostoses may be seen, especially in the tubular bones of the hands and feet, that tend to originate from the midshaft of the bone and are directed at right angles to the long axis of the bone. In some patients with PH or PPH coincidental findings of HPTH may be seen.

2° HPTH: Rugger-Jersey spine

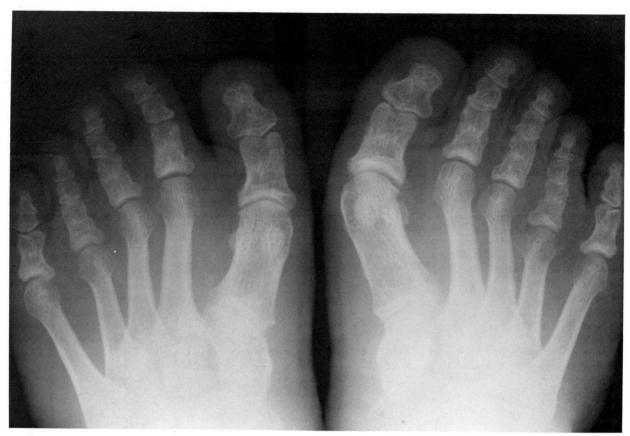

Fig. 6-48. This frontal radiograph of the feet of a patient with pseudohypoparathyroidism demonstrates shortening of the first and fourth metatarsal bones on the left and the fourth metatarsal bone on the right. Also note the small exostoses that arise from the middiaphyseal region of the medial surfaces of several of the proximal phalanges.

PAGET'S DISEASE. Paget's disease (osteitis deformans) is a metabolic bone disorder of unknown etiology characterized by abnormally rapid bone turnover and proliferation of abnormal new bone. Paget's disease is a common disorder estimated to be present in 3 percent of the population over 40 years of age and is often incidentally encountered on routine radiographs.

Both radiographically and pathologically Paget's disease may be subdivided into three phases; (1) osteolytic, (2) mixed osteolytic and osteosclerotic, and (3) osteosclerotic. The osteolytic and mixed phases represent the active, expanding phase of the disorder while the osteosclerotic phase is the terminal inactive stage.

The earliest radiographic abnormalities consist of purely osteolytic lesions involving the diploë of the skull or the medullary space of a tubular bone. These lesions tend to be sharply demarcated from adjacent normal bone, although they lack a sclerotic border. In the skull this lesion is termed *osteoporosis circumscripta* and is most common in the frontal and occipital bones, although it may involve any portion of the skull. Although the initial lesion begins in the diploë, expansion into both the inner and outer tables of the skull occurs, in contrast to fibrous dysplasia, which may have similar radiographic appearance but which usually spares the inner table. In long, tubular bones the initial lesion virtually always begins in the subchondral portion of the epiphysis and expands into the metaphysis and diaphysis, often with a characteristic wedge-shaped leading edge (the blade of grass appearance of osteolytic Paget's disease) (Fig. 6-49A). The tendency of Paget's disease to originate at one end of a long bone and progress toward the other end cannot be overemphasized, and in fact an osteolytic lesion localized to the diaphysis of a tubular bone is unlikely to be Paget's disease. In the

earliest phase of Paget's disease, trabeculae cannot be identified within the lesion and the internal architecture has a hazy or ground glass appearance. As the disease progresses, coarse, thickened, osteosclerotic trabeculae appear in association with marked thickening of the cortex and an overall increase in size of the affected bone. This represents the mixed phase of Paget's disease, in which osteolytic and osteosclerotic areas are interspersed. In the skull circular radiodense lesions appear superimposed on the larger osteolytic lesion, resulting in a characteristic radiographic appearance that is often termed the cotton wool skull (Fig. 6-50). In vertebral bodies bone condensation may parallel the outer margins of the vertebra, with a radiolucent central region that results in the picture frame vertebra that is virtually pathognomonic of Paget's disease (Fig. 6-51). The final phase of Paget's disease consists of dense, homogenous osteosclerosis and overall enlargement of the involved bone. This stage provides the most characteristic roentgenographic appearance. Involved bones are markedly radiodense, with coarse and thickened trabeculae, cortical proliferation, and narrowing of the medullary space (Fig. 6-49B).

Radionuclide bone scintigraphy is markedly abnormal in all phases of Paget's disease with an extremely increased uptake in the involved bones. In diffuse Paget's disease the diseased bone may take up virtually all of the radionuclide, causing uninvolved osseous structures to not be visualized. In most cases the use of radionuclide scintigraphy is limited in this disease because the plain

Fig. 6-49. A. Lateral radiograph of the tibia of a patient with
Paget's disease reveals the characteristic features of this
disorder in tubular bones. The abnormality begins in one end
of the bone (proximal tibia) with the older areas of disease
demonstrating dense osteosclerosis associated with
thickening and expansion of both the cortical surfaces and
individual trabeculae. In the mid-tibia the mixed phase is
evident with a combination of osteosclerotic and osteolytic
changes. In the distal tibia the osteolytic configuration is
present with the characteristic flame-shaped advancing edge
(*arrowheads*). B. Frontal radiograph of the hip of another
patient with Paget's disease demonstrates prominent
thickening of the cortex and trabecular structures. The linear
radiolucent defects perpendicular to the outer cortex of the
femur (*arrowheads*) represent pseudofractures.

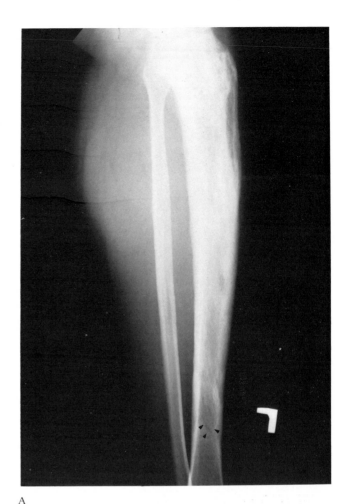

A

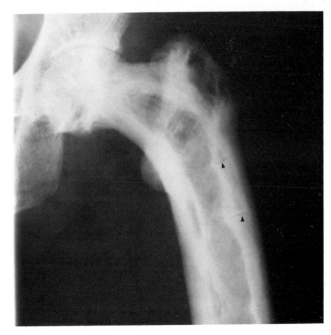

B

radiographic changes are more characteristic. However, in
some cases of early Paget's disease a markedly abnormal
radionuclide bone scan may precede the presence of plain
roentgenographic abnormalities.

The enlarged, radiodense bone in Paget's disease gives
the appearance of great structural strength; however the
bone in actuality is quite soft, with significantly decreased
structural integrity. Bowing and deformity of weight-bearing bones is common, especially around the hip where a
shepherd's crook deformity (coxa vara) of the proximal femur may be seen. Softening of the acetabulum may result
in a protrusio acetabuli deformity in which the femoral
head sinks into the softened pagetic acetabulum. In the
spine compression of the softened vertebral end plate by
the intervertebral disc may result in a biconcave fish vertebra similar to that seen in osteoporosis. Fractures are
common in Paget's disease, either as incomplete pseudofractures (see Fig. 6-49B) that tend to involve the convex
surface of a long bone, or as complete, usually transverse,
fractures that tend to heal with exuberant callus formation.
Neoplasms complicating Paget's disease are uncommon
but giant cell tumors and sarcomas occur with increased
frequency in these patients, especially those with widely
disseminated disease.

Hemoglobinopathies and Anemias

Anemia associated with hemoglobinopathy, as well as anemia from other causes, commonly affects the skeletal system. In general osteoarticular manifestations relate to one
of three main mechanisms: (1) marrow hyperplasia, (2) hyperemia, or (3) vascular occlusion. The radiographic manifestations of these disorders are therefore somewhat nonspecific, although the severity and distribution of changes
often suggest the diagnosis.

SICKLE CELL DISEASE. Homozygous sickle cell anemia (Hb
S-S) is a relatively common disorder, frequently accompanied by striking roentgenographic findings. Marrow hyperplasia is characterized by osteopenia, expansion of the
medullary space, and thinning of the cortex of affected
bones. The distribution of changes varies to a large degree
with the age of presentation of the disorder. In infants and
children peripheral and axial skeletal involvement is typical, while in adults changes tend to be most prominent in
the axial skeleton and proximal long bones. In the skull a
coarse granular pattern involves the convexity of the calvarium with widening of the diploë and thinning of both

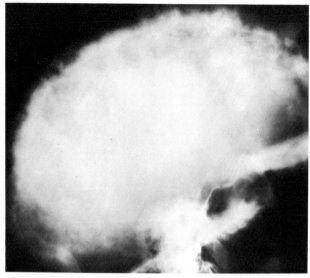

Fig. 6-50. Lateral radiograph of the skull of a patient with Paget's disease demonstrates a mottled appearance due to the presence of numerous osteoblastic lesions. This constitutes the cotton wool skull of Paget's disease.

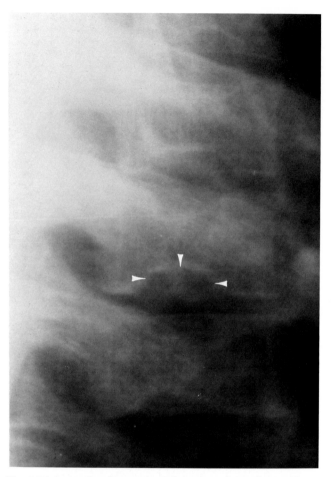

Fig. 6-52. Lateral radiograph of the spine of a patient with homozygous sickle cell anemia reveals the characteristic squared indentations (*arrowheads*) of the vertebral end plates, which result in the H-vertebra characteristic of this disorder.

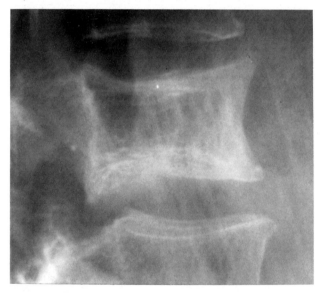

Fig. 6-51. Lateral radiograph of a lumbar vertebra in a patient with Paget's disease demonstrates the characteristic picture frame appearance that is virtually pathognomonic of this disorder.

the inner and outer tables. Vertebral osteoporosis is common, as is a characteristic deformity of the vertebral bodies in which a squared depression is present in the midportion of the vertebral end plate (H-vertebra) (Fig. 6-52). In other patients, smooth, rounded, biconcave depressions identical to those seen in osteoporosis (fish vertebra) may be present in the vertebral end plates. In the peripheral skeleton medullary bone infarctions and avascular necrosis of epiphyseal centers are common. Sickle cell dactylitis (hand-foot syndrome) is seen in young children (age 6 mo–2 yr) due to osteonecrosis of the small tubular bones of the hands and feet. Soft-tissue swelling is the earliest radiographic feature, followed by periosteal new bone formation and patchy radiolucencies of the shafts of affected metacarpals, metatarsals, and phalanges. This appearance may be indistinguishable from osteomyelitis, which is also a frequent complication in these patients. Growth disturbances other than the previously mentioned H-vertebra that may be present include epiphyseal overgrowth, V-shaped physeal plates, and abnormal angulation of the ankle joint (tibiotalar slant).

Complications of sickle cell disease include osteomyelitis and septic arthritis, often with *Salmonella* as the pathogenic organism. In severe cases of sickle cell disease, secondary hyperuricemia due to hemolysis may result in radiographic and clinical findings of gouty arthritis.

Sickle cell trait (Hb A-S) is usually not associated with radiographic abnormalities. Sickle cell-hemoglobin C

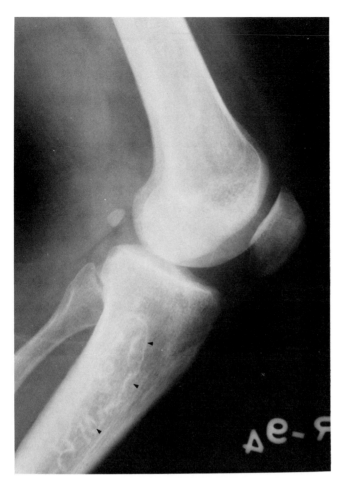

Fig. 6-53. Medullary bone infarction (*arrowheads*) in the proximal tibia in a patient with hemoglobin S-C disease. This finding, along with epiphyseal avascular necrosis, is the most characteristic finding in this disorder.

disease (Hb S-C) is often associated with radiographic changes that are similar to sickle cell disease, although peripheral medullary bone infarctions appear to be more common, while spinal abnormalities tend to be less prominent (Fig. 6-53).

THALASSEMIA. Thalassemia (also called Cooley's anemia and Mediterranean anemia) is a family of disorders associated with an inherited abnormality of production of alpha globin chains (alpha thalassemia) or beta globin chains (beta thalassemia). It may be manifested as a homozygous (thalassemia major) or heterozygous (thalassemia minor) form.

Radiographic changes related to marrow hyperplasia and growth disturbances form the cornerstone for the radiographic diagnosis of thalassemia major, while vascular occlusive changes (e.g., bone infarction, avascular necrosis) are not prominent. Marrow hyperplasia in thalassemia major is severe, resulting in profound osteopenia with medullary expansion, extreme cortical thinning, and a lacework pattern of the remaining trabeculae (Fig. 6-54). Pathologic fractures are common and may involve virtually any bone. In the skull, expansion of the diploë, thinning of the tables, and "hair-on-end" periosteal new bone formation are marked and much more prominent than in sickle cell anemia. Biconcave (fish) vertebra are typical, but H-vertebra similar to those seen in sickle cell anemia are encountered only occasionally. Extramedullary hema-

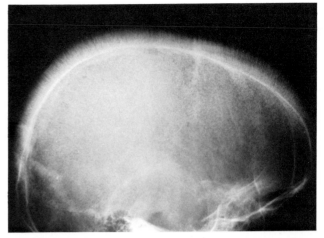

A

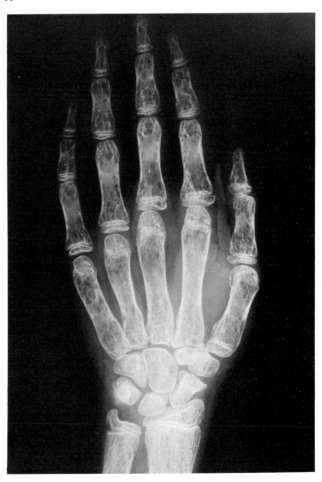

B

Fig. 6-54. A. This lateral radiograph of the skull of a patient with thalassemia major demonstrates the hair-on-end appearance of the calvarium that is seen in severe anemias. B. Frontal radiograph of the hand demonstrates severe osteopenia with expansion of the medullary cavities of the tubular bones due to markedly increased hematopoietic activity.

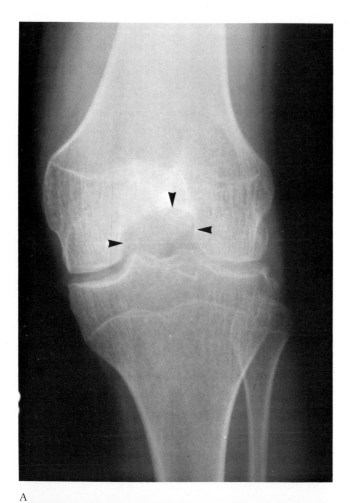

A

B

Fig. 6-55. A. Frontal radiograph of the knee of a patient with hemophilia demonstrates severe demineralization, widening of the intercondylar notch (*arrowheads*) of the distal femur, and epiphyseal overgrowth. **B.** Sunrise projection of the same knee demonstrates large erosive defects (e) in the anterior femur related to multiple episodes of intraosseous hemorrhage.

topoiesis may be profound, resulting in massive soft-tissue masses that may mimic tumor or infection, especially in the paraspinal regions. The most common growth disturbance is a modeling deformity of the ends of the long bones that is characterized by flaring of the metaphysis and epiphyseal overgrowth resulting in the Erlenmeyer flask deformity. Premature epiphyseal plate fusion is common and may involve the entire growth plate or only a segment. Secondary hemochromatosis due to repeated transfusions may complicate thalassemia, resulting in arthropathy associated with chondrocalcinosis. Secondary hemochromatosis due to repeated transfusions may complicate thalassemia, resulting in arthropathy associated with chondrocalcinosis. Secondary gouty arthritis due to massive hemolysis may be seen, as in sickle cell anemia. Thalassemia intermedia and thalassemia minor demonstrate similar findings but tend to be considerably less severe.

IRON-DEFICIENCY ANEMIA. Radiographic changes in iron-deficiency anemia are most commonly identified in infants and young children, and only rarely in adults. The most prominent radiographic changes are in the skull, where a granular pattern associated with widening of the diploic space is most typical. The hair-on-end pattern is rare, although it may be seen in especially severe cases.

OTHER ANEMIAS. Hereditary spherocytosis and the nonspherocytic hemolytic anemias usually are not associated with radiographic changes in the skeletal system. In rare instances when skeletal abnormalities are present, they are usually localized to the skull and resemble those of iron-deficiency anemia.

HEMOPHILIA. Hemophilia is an x-linked, recessive bleeding diathesis caused by a functional deficiency in factor VIII (antihemophilic factor). Skeletal radiographic abnormalities are typically centered around joints and consist of growth disturbances that occur because it is congenital, as well as destructive changes secondary to intraosseous and intraarticular hemorrhage.

The earliest radiographic change is soft-tissue swelling around the involved articulations due to hemarthrosis or juxta-articular hemorrhage into the soft tissues. Joint effusions are large and frequently abnormally dense on radiographs, due to hemosiderin deposition in the synovium. Osteoporosis is common and is frequently in a juxta-articular distribution. Epiphyseal overgrowth is common, resulting in a radiographic appearance similar to that of juvenile rheumatoid arthritis (Fig. 6-55A). Squaring of the inferior pole of the patella and abnormal angulation of the ankle joint (tibiotalar slant) may also be seen. Subchondral cysts and erosions, initially without associated joint space narrowing, occur due to intraosseous hemorrhage (Fig. 6-55B). Widening of the intercondylar notch of the distal femur is often present and probably relates to hemorrhage at the insertions of the cruciate ligaments. Cartilage destruction with obliteration of the joint space is a late manifestation and frequently involves the entire articular surface. In the late stages of the disease severe destructive changes of the joints are present, with collapse of the articular surfaces and secondary degenerative changes.

Hemophiliac pseudotumors are radiolucent lesions resembling primary bone neoplasms that are due to chronic repetitive intraosseous hemorrhage. These lesions may attain massive size and are most commonly found in the pelvic bones, femur, and tibia. Hemophiliac arthropathy most

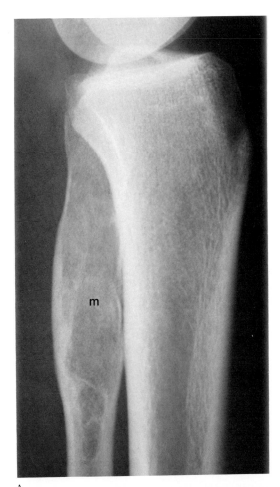

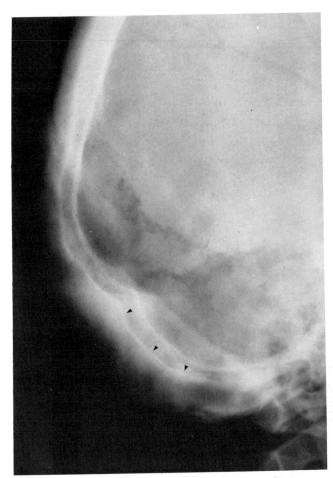

A   B

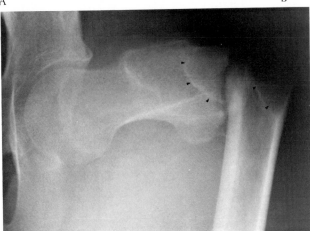

C

Fig. 6-56. Fibrous dysplasia. A. Lateral radiograph of the proximal tibia and fibula demonstrates an expansile lesion (m) within the proximal fibular metaphysis and diaphysis. Note that the lesion has a multilocular appearance with the characteristic ground glass radiographic appearance of the matrix. B. Lateral radiograph of the skull demonstrates expansion of the calvarium, which involves the diploic space and outer table with sparing of the inner table (*arrowheads*). Note the combination of osteosclerotic and osteolytic lesions. C. Frontal radiograph of the proximal femur in a patient with sudden onset of left hip pain demonstrates a transverse subtrochanteric pathologic fracture of the proximal femur. Careful examination reveals that the fracture passes through a sclerotic bordered lesion (*arrowheads*) with the characteristic ground glass internal matrix of the fibrous dysplasia.

commonly affects the knee, ankle, and elbow articulations, although any joint may be involved.

Disorders of Unknown Origin

FIBROUS DYSPLASIA. Fibrous dysplasia is a nonhereditary, skeletal developmental abnormality that may be seen in monostotic (solitary) or, less commonly, polyostotic (multiple) forms. In some patients polyostotic fibrous dysplasia may be associated with cutaneous and endocrine abnormalities (McCune-Albright syndrome). This disorder usually affects young females and consists of unilateral polyostotic fibrous dysplasia, café au lait spots, and precocious puberty.

The most common sites of fibrous dysplasia are the proximal femur, tibia, ribs, skull, and facial bones. Radiographically the peripheral skeletal lesions tend to be located in the diametaphyseal, and rarely the epiphyseal, portions of the bone and are usually well-defined within the medullary cavity, with a distinct sclerotic margin. Periosteal reaction is not present around an uncomplicated lesion. The internal structure of the lesion is quite characteristic, with a hazy appearance similar to ground glass (Fig. 6-56A). Large lesions in weight-bearing bones tend to result in bowing deformities, most typically the shepherd's crook deformity of the proximal femur. Spontaneous fracture through a lesion is common and is in fact the most common clinical presentation (Fig. 6-56C). Rib

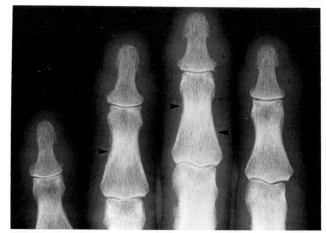

A

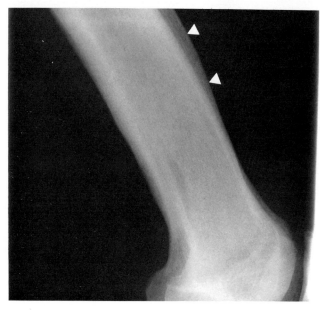

C

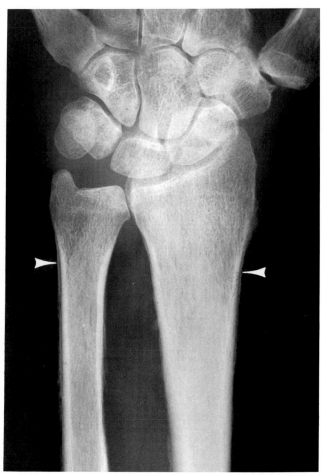

B

Fig. 6-57. Hypertrophic osteoarthropathy. A. Frontal radiography of the fingers of a patient with bronchogenic carcinoma demonstrates swelling (s) of the distal soft tissues (clubbing) as well as periosteal new bone formation (*arrowheads*) along the diaphyses of the middle phalanges. B. Periosteal new bone formation (*arrowheads*) along the distal cortical surfaces of the radius and ulna. These are the typical radiographic findings of secondary hypertrophic osteoarthropathy. C. Lateral radiograph of the distal femur in a patient with primary hypertrophic osteoarthropathy (pachydermoperiostosis) demonstrates a thick zone of periosteal new bone formation (*arrowheads*).

lesions are similar to peripheral skeletal lesions with the characteristic ground glass appearance but are frequently markedly expansile. In the skull and facial bones the lesions may be radiolucent, osteosclerotic, or mixed. Radiolucent lesions originate in the diploë of the calvarium, producing expansion of the outer table with sparing of the inner table (Fig. 6-56B). Sclerotic lesions are most common in the skull base and in the sphenoid wings. In some cases gross deformity of the skull may occur. Radionuclide bone scans demonstrate increased activity in fibrous dysplastic lesions.

HYPERTROPHIC OSTEOARTHROPATHY. Hypertrophic osteoarthropathy (HOA) is a clinical syndrome characterized by digital clubbing, pain, swelling, and osseous proliferation. Two forms of the disease may be encountered. *Primary hypertrophic osteoarthropathy* (pachydermoperiostosis) is a rare inherited disorder most often seen in black males. *Secondary hypertrophic osteoarthropathy* is a common disorder that may be seen in association with a number of visceral diseases and malignancies. The most common etiology associated with HOA is bronchogenic

carcinoma; because of its frequency, however, pleural mesotheliomas actually demonstrate the strongest association with HOA. Other disorders that may be accompanied by HOA include pulmonary abscesses, bronchiectasis or emphysema, inflammatory bowel disease, cirrhosis, congenital heart disease, neoplasms of the GI tract, liver, and nasopharynx, and metastatic lesions to the lung.

The most common sites of radiographic abnormality in HOA are the proximal and distal diaphyses of the tibia, fibula, ulna, and radius. Less commonly the femur, humerus, metacarpals, metatarsals, and proximal phalanges are involved. The earliest radiographic abnormalities involve the sift tissues. Soft-tissue proliferation at the distal ends of the digits results in the radiographic counterpart of digital clubbing (Fig. 6-57A). Periosteal bone deposition follows and is characterized by the deposition of smooth layers of bone adjacent to the involved cortical surfaces (Fig. 6-57B). Early in the course of the disorder the patient may have clinical complaints without radiographic changes. In these instances a radionuclide bone scan usu-

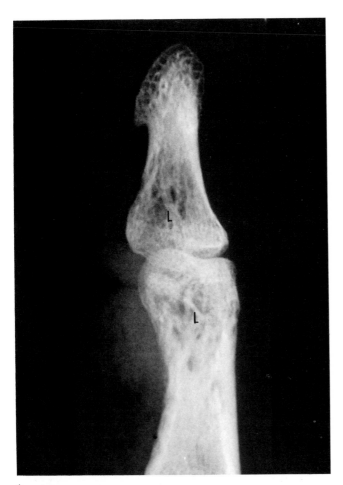

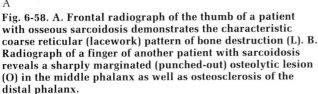

A

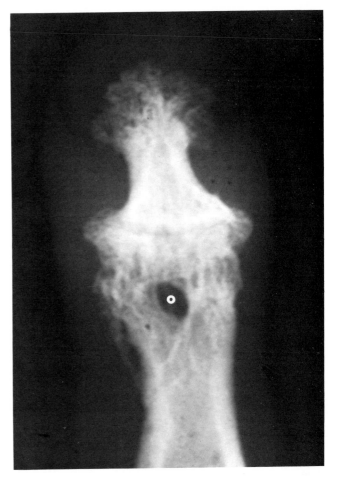

B

Fig. 6-58. A. Frontal radiograph of the thumb of a patient with osseous sarcoidosis demonstrates the characteristic coarse reticular (lacework) pattern of bone destruction (L). B. Radiograph of a finger of another patient with sarcoidosis reveals a sharply marginated (punched-out) osteolytic lesion (O) in the middle phalanx as well as osteosclerosis of the distal phalanx.

ally demonstrates a distinctive pattern, with markedly increased uptake along the cortical margins of involved long bones creating a railroad track sign. The radiographic abnormalities in primary HOA (pachydermoperiostosis) are similar to those of the secondary form, except that the periosteal new bone deposits tend to be larger and coarser (Fig. 6-57C).

SARCOIDOSIS. Sarcoidosis is a multisystem disease of unknown etiology characterized pathologically by the formation of noncaseating granulomata in a number of body tissues. Skeletal involvement occurs in approximately 5 percent of patients and most commonly involves the hands, and less commonly the wrists or feet. Involvement of the long tubular bones and axial skeleton is uncommon. Three main radiographic patterns of osseous sarcoidosis may be seen (Fig. 6-58). The first of these is osteopenia, with a coarse reticular or lacework trabecular pattern of the involved bone a common finding. The second, osteolytic lesions, may be noted at other sites either centrally or eccentrically located in the bone with a sharply marginated (punched out) appearance. The third appearance is focal or generalized osteosclerosis. Focal nodular densities

may be noted in the medullary cavities of involved bones or in the terminal phalanges (acroosteosclerosis). Rarely, generalized osteosclerosis may be identified, usually in the axial skeleton or proximal long bones. In long-standing sarcoidosis a destructive arthritis may be seen most commonly in the hands, wrists, shoulders, ankles, or knees. This disorder appears to be secondary to collapse of the articular surface into adjacent destructive lesions.

Osteonecrosis

Osteonecrosis (avascular necrosis) refers to the ischemic death of the cellular components of osseous and marrow tissue. An important point to remember concerning osteonecrosis is that cell death does not alter the radiographic appearance of bone. Therefore, the radiographic changes that we can see are secondary manifestations and may require several months to become visible on radiographs. Radionuclide studies are more sensitive than plain radiography in detecting the ischemic and early reactive changes of osteonecrosis. Magnetic resonance imaging (MRI), which has not as yet been fully evaluated, offers great potential. A variety of processes may be associated with osteonecrosis (Table 6-4).

Radiographically there are two distinct patterns of osteonecrosis, depending on its location in either the juxta-articular (epiphyseal) portion of the bone or the metadiaphyseal (marrow cavity) region. Epiphyseal osteonecrosis

Table 6-4. Causes of Osteonecrosis

Steroids
    Endogenous (Cushing's disease)
    Exogenous
Occlusive vascular disease
Trauma
Hemoglobinopathies
    Sickle Cell Anemia
    S-C disease
Gaucher's disease
Dysbaric disorders (Caisson's disease, astronaut's disease)
Radiation therapy
Idiopathic (Legg-Calvé-Perthes disease, spontaneous
    osteonecrosis)
Fat embolism
    Alcoholism

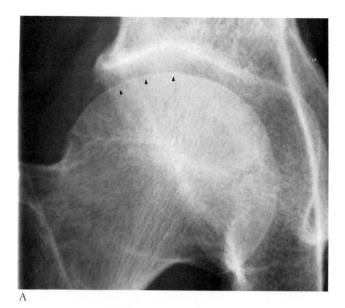

A

follows a characteristic radiographic pattern of progression. Early after the vascular insult (up to several months) no radiographic changes are demonstrable, although scintigraphic abnormalities may be identified on radionuclide bone scans (Fig. 6-59). The earliest radiographic abnormality is hyperemic osteoporosis of the area adjacent to the infarction, resulting in apparent radiodensity of the infarcted zone. Remodelling around the margins of the necrotic zone results in deposition of dense new bone at the margin of the infarction. With continued stress a characteristic fracture develops separating the subchondral bone plate from the subjacent necrotic segment. This finding constitutes the crescent sign and is diagnostic of epiphyseal osteonecrosis. In the later stages collapse and deformity of the articular surface occurs, often with secondary degenerative changes.

Bone infarctions in the metaphyseal and/or diaphyseal segment of a tubular bone follow a similar evolution, except that stress is considerably less than at a subarticular location and fractures and compression do not occur. These infarcts are most commonly identified on radiographs as mottled lesions within the medullary cavity of the involved bone in which patchy radiolucent areas are interspersed with numerous, thin, serpiginous, osteosclerotic bands that resemble wisps of smoke (Fig. 6-60). In severe cases, especially in sickle cell anemia, an entire segment of bone may be involved, including the cortex, which assumes a bone within a bone appearance following reparative changes.

In general metadiaphyseal bone infarcts are most common in the proximal and distal shafts of the femur, proximal tibia, and proximal humerus. Epiphyseal osteonecrosis is most common in the femoral head and condyles, followed in frequency by the humeral head. Certain sites are especially susceptible to osteonecrosis following trauma. These include the femoral and humeral heads, the talar dome, the proximal pole of the carpal scaphoid, the

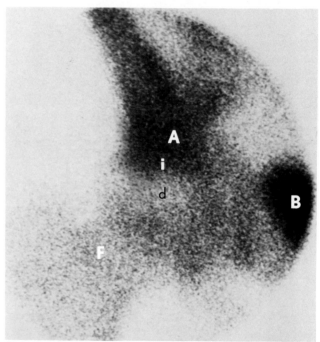

B

Fig. 6-59. A. Frontal radiograph of the hip of a patient with early epiphyseal osteonecrosis demonstrates a subtle radiolucent line (*arrowheads*) paralleling the subchondral bone plate of the femoral head. B. Radionuclide bone scan performed at the same time reveals areas of diminished activity (necrosis) (d) and increased activity (reactive bone formation) (i) within the femoral head. C. Frontal radiograph of the same hip ten months later demonstrates advanced changes with flattening of the femoral head and an epiphyseal fracture (*arrowheads*). F = femur, A = acetabulum, B = urinary bladder.

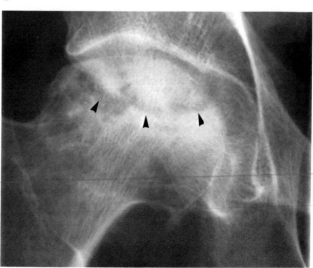

C

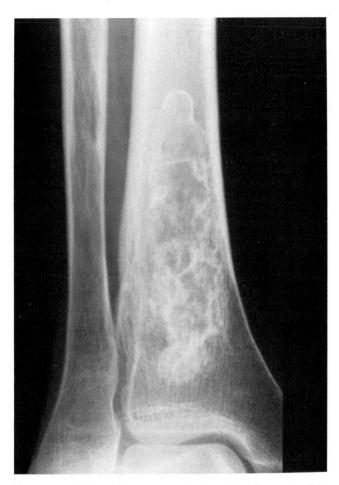

Fig. 6-60. Diaphyseal osteonecrosis. Frontal radiograph of the distal tibia of a patient with a bone infarction demonstrates a typical mottled lesion in the distal tibia containing radiolucent and sclerotic areas surrounded by a thin calcified shell.

carpal lunate, the patella, and the heads of the metatarsals and metacarpals. Idiopathic spontaneous osteonecrosis is most common in the femoral head in males and in the femoral (especially medial) condyles in females, and is rare in the metadiaphyses of long bones in either sex.

Bone and Joint Infections

Bone and joint infections are common disorders whose specific radiographic features vary with (1) age of the patient, (2) location of infection, (3) infective organism, and (4) predisposing factors. In most instances the identity of the infective organism cannot be determined by radiographic changes. These disorders are considered here based on the location of infection as well as on the major families of infective organisms.

PYOGENIC HEMATOGENOUS OSTEOMYELITIS. Hematogenous bacterial osteomyelitis is more common in children than adults. The typical site of implantation of pathogenic organisms varies with the age of the patient, due to differences in the vascular supply to osseous structures. In infants less than one year old and in adults (over 16 yr) there is communication between metaphyseal and epiphyseal blood vessels; thus, in these age groups epiphyseal localization of infection is common and often associated with spread to the adjacent articulation (septic arthritis). In children between the ages of 1 and 16 years the metaphyseal vessels are end vessels and epiphyseal involvement and septic arthritis are rare. The long tubular bones are most frequently involved in infants and children, while involvement of the axial skeleton and small bones of the hands and feet are relatively uncommon. In adults the axial skeleton is the most common site of involvement, followed in frequency by the small bones of the hands and feet, with long tubular bone involvement least common. These features are summarized in Table 6-5.

In early osteomyelitis the plain radiograph is relatively insensitive and may actually be misleading, since a normal radiographic examination does not by any means exclude the possibility of early osteomyelitis. Radionuclide bone scintigraphy is a far more sensitive indicator of early infection and is invariably positive prior to demonstrable radiographic changes (Fig. 6-61). In fact, in the ideal circumstance osteomyelitis may be diagnosed, treatment instituted, and recovery made without any plain radiographic abnormalities ever being present. However, an understanding of the radiographic manifestations of osteomyelitis is necessary (Fig. 6-62).

The earliest finding in pyogenic hematogenous osteomyelitis is deep soft-tissue swelling, which may take up to three days to appear. This is followed in several days by more generalized soft-tissue swelling with obliteration of the soft-tissue planes. One to two weeks after onset, the infection changes appear in the involved bone, initially as a faint, ill-defined area of radiolucency in the medullary portion of the bone, with adjacent periostitis. As the infection progresses, a larger destructive lesion can be seen spreading away from the metaphysis, usually in association with prominent periosteal new bone formation. In the infant lack of ossification of the epiphysis may make recognition of the changes in this region very difficult; however, the presence of a joint effusion in combination with the adjacent metaphyseal changes should imply epiphyseal involvement. In the adult the first manifestation is often the presence of a joint effusion followed by the appearance of erosions, joint space narrowing, and increased radiolucency of the adjacent epiphysis. *Sequestrum* refers to a radiodense fragment of bone that becomes isolated from its blood supply by the infectious process and undergoes necrosis. The presence of sequestra (Fig. 6-63) is associated with an increased risk of chronic osteomyelitis, and surgical sequestrectomy may be required in these

Table 6-5. Features of Pyogenic Hematogenous Osteomyelitis

Feature	Infant (< 1 yr)	Child (1–16 yr)	Adult (> 16 yr)
Location	Metaphysis and epiphysis	Metaphysis	Epiphysis
Distribution	Long bones, axial skeleton, small bones	Long bones, axial skeleton, small bones	Axial skeleton, small bones, long bones
Septic arthritis	Common	Rare	Common

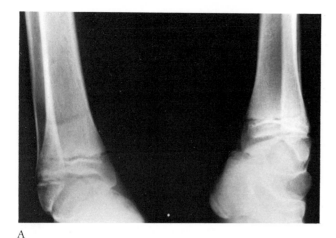

A

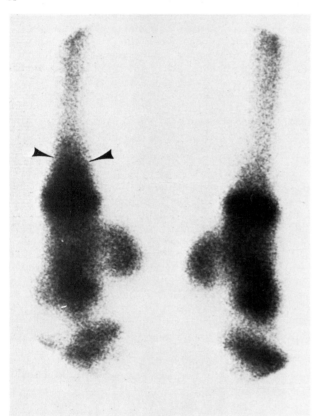

B

Fig. 6-61. A. Frontal radiograph of the ankles of a child with staphylococcal pyogenic osteomyelitis shows no radiograph abnormalities. B. Radionuclide bone scan performed at the same time demonstrates markedly increased activity in the right tibial metaphysis (*arrowheads*).

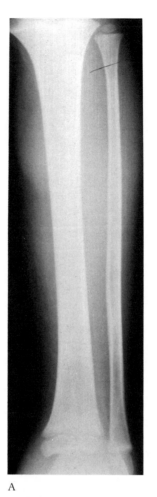

A

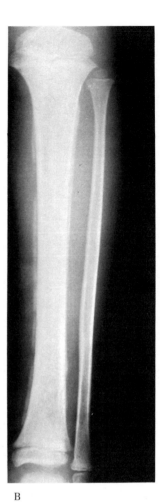

B

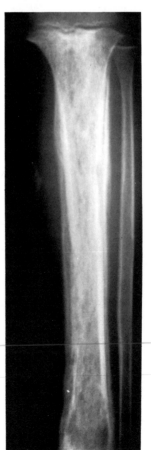

C

Fig. 6-62. The spectrum of radiographic findings in staphylococcal pyogenic osteomyelitis is documented in this series of radiographs. In the initial radiograph (A) the only radiographic abnormality is deep soft tissue swelling, which is most prominent adjacent the medial border of the distal tibia. Two weeks later (B) a mottled osteolytic defect is present in the distal tibial metaphysis with prominent periosteal new bone formation. Six weeks after the initial radiograph (C) diffuse osteolytic destructive change is present with a thick layer of periosteal new bone (involucrum).

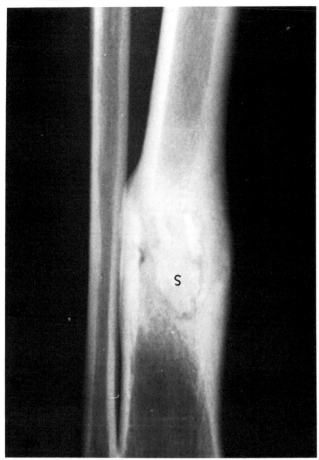

Fig. 6-63. In this patient with chronic osteomyelitis a large isolated fragment of infected, necrotic bone (sequestrum) (S) is seen within the medullary cavity of the distal tibia. This finding is virtually pathognomonic of chronic osteomyelitis.

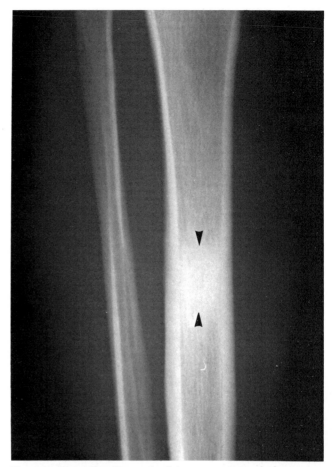

Fig. 6-64. Frontal radiograph of the upper tibia of a patient with sclerosing osteomyelitis demonstrates an ill defined area of bony sclerosis (*arrowheads*) within the medullary cavity. Thickening of the adjacent cortex is present without periosteal new bone formation.

cases. *Involucrum* refers to an exuberant sheath or cloak of periosteal new bone surrounding the shaft of an infected bone. This finding is more common in infants and children than in adults and results in a distinctive bone-within-a-bone appearance on radiographs. Sclerosing osteomyelitis is a form of chronic osteomyelitis in which the only radiographic finding is an ill-defined area of bony sclerosis within the medullary cavity of the involved bone (Fig. 6-64).

Brodie's Abscess. Brodie's abscess (Fig. 6-65) is a focal form of subacute or chronic osteomyelitis characterized by the presence of one or more circumscribed radiolucent defects, usually located in the metaphyseal portion of a long bone. Brodie's abscess is most common in males and in children, and is usually of staphylococcal origin. Radiographically a well-defined, circular or oval, radiolucent lesion measuring 1 to 4 cm in diameter that may be surrounded by a dense band of reactive bone is present. The lesion may be impossible to differentiate from osteoid osteoma, a benign neoplasm that is common in this age group.

PYOGENIC SEPTIC ARTHRITIS. Bacterial contamination of an articulation may occur by means of primary hematogenous implantation, direct extension from an adjacent area of infection (i.e., osteomyelitis or soft tissue abscess), or by direct implantation (e.g., postoperative infection, trauma). The general radiographic features of septic arthritis, in order of occurrence, consist of effusion, soft-tissue swelling, osteoporosis, erosions, and joint space narrowing (Fig. 6-66). In some articulations, such as the knee, elbow, and ankle, joint effusions can be recognized on conventional radiographs. At other articulations, such as the adult hip and the shoulder, joint effusions cannot be reliably identified. In infants and small children hip joint effusions may be identified by noting an increased width (> 2 mm) of the medial portion of the joint space, between the medial border of the femoral head and the acetabular teardrop, as compared to the normal side (Fig. 6-67). Displacement of juxta-articular fat planes, which is often described as a radiographic sign of pediatric hip joint effusions, actually relates to the position of mild external rotation in which the child tends to hold a painful hip. Erosions may be noted at any location but tend to occur first at the margins of the involved articulation. Destruction of articular cartilage occurs rapidly in pyogenic septic arthritis, resulting in rapidly progressive joint space narrowing. In the final stage complete destruction of the articular surfaces occurs, often leading to late fibrous or bony ankylosis.

In contrast to pyogenic septic arthritis, fungal or tubercular infections often demonstrate prominent juxta-articular osteoporosis and relatively slow progression with erosions often preceding joint space narrowing by weeks to

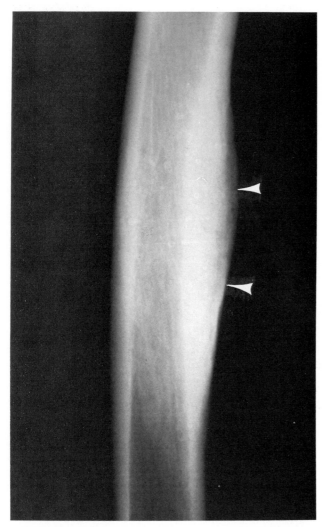

Fig. 6-65. Frontal radiograph of the midportion of the femur of a patient with Brodie's abscess demonstrates a sclerotic lesion associated with cortical thickening (*arrowheads*). The major differential diagnostic possibility in this circumstance is osteoid osteoma.

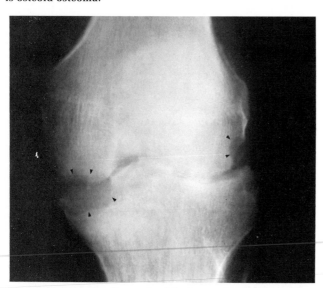

Fig. 6-66. Frontal radiograph of the knee of a patient with staphylococcal septic arthritis demonstrates soft tissue swelling and large irregular erosions (*arrowheads*) in the distal femoral and proximal tibial articular surfaces.

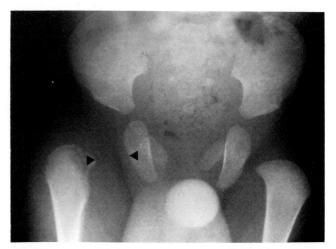

Fig. 6-67. Frontal radiograph of the pelvis in a four-week-old infant reveals loss of the normal fat planes about the right hip and lateral displacement of the femoral head (*arrowheads*), due to the presence of a large joint effusion. An osteolytic lesion is present in the medial portion of the proximal femoral metaphysis. These findings suggest infantile osteomyelitis and pyogenic septic arthritis.

months. In some cases septic arthritis may quite closely resemble the changes of an inflammatory arthropathy.

Another radiographic sign useful in the diagnosis of joint sepsis is the presence of a radiolucent gas collection within the joint of a trauma patient. In the absence of joint instrumentation, this suggests an open communication with the skin and a high likelihood of sepsis unless appropriately treated.

Any synovial or fibrous joint may be involved in septic arthritis; however, some generalizations as to its usual distribution may be useful. In most instances pyogenic septic arthritis is a monoarticular process that is most common in the knee in adults and in the hip or the knee in infants and children. Prior joint instrumentation, surgery, or prosthetic joint replacement predisposes to septic arthritis, often with unusual organisms. Intravenous drug users and other immunosuppressed patients tend to have infections at unusual locations, such as the sacroiliac, acromioclavicular, or sternoclavicular articulations, and often with unusual pathogens (i.e., *Serratia*, *Pseudomonas*, or *Proteus sp.*).

PYOGENIC INFECTIOUS SPONDYLITIS. As with other forms of skeletal infection, spinal infections may originate from hematogenous spread, spread from contiguous foci, direct implantation, and microorganisms. In the last two instances the cause and site of infection are frequently evident. However, pyogenic spondylitis of hematogenous origin is frequently difficult to diagnose in its early stages because radiographic signs of infection may be absent or very subtle. As previously mentioned for osteomyelitis, the radionuclide bone scan plays a very important role in the early diagnosis of these disorders and demonstrates abnormalities prior to their appearance on conventional radiographs. Computed tomography is often more sensitive than plain radiography in identifying the changes of infection and is much better at delineating the extent of pathologic changes (Fig. 6-68).

In hematogenous infections of the spine, the site of origin of the infectious focus depends on the age of the patient. In children and young adults (up to the age of ap-

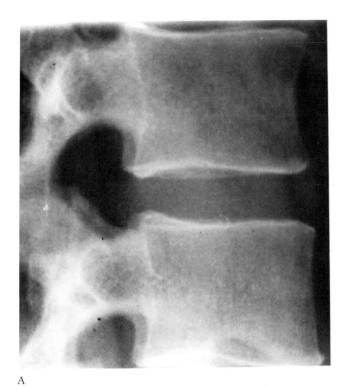

A

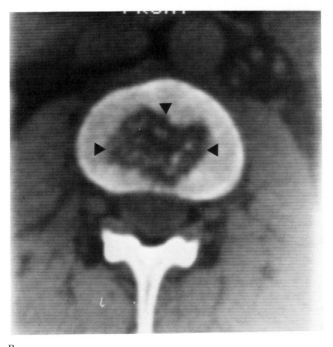

B

Fig. 6-68. A. Lateral radiograph of the second and third lumbar vertebra appears normal. A radionuclide bone scan performed at the same time, however, demonstrated increased accumulation of radionuclide at the L2–3 level. **B.** Computed tomographic section demonstrates a destructive lesion (*arrowheads*) in the inferior aspect of the second lumbar vertebral body with numerous small central bone fragments.

proximately 20), vascular channels perforate the vertebral end plate to supply the intervertebral disk. In older patients these communications are lost, and the intervertebral disk is avascular. Thus in infants, children, and young adults primary infection of the intervertebral disk (diskitis) is most likely, while in older adults the infectious process almost always starts in the vertebral body adjacent to

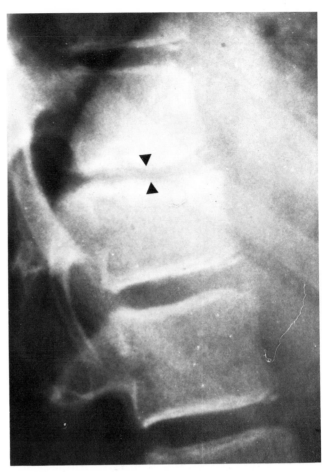

Fig. 6-69. Pyogenic diskitis. Lateral radiograph of the thoracic spine of a nine-year-old patient demonstrates characteristic irregularity of the vertebral end plates (*arrowheads*) of two contiguous thoracic vertebra as well as diminution in the intervertebral disk space.

the end plate and spreads to involve the adjacent intervertebral disk (vertebral osteomyelitis).

The radiographic findings in infectious spondylitis are similar regardless of the primary focus of bacterial implantation. During the first week of infection prominent clinical symptoms are accompanied by normal spinal radiographs. It is in this period that radionuclide bone scintigraphy may be diagnostic. After the first week the patient with diskitis is noted to have a loss of the normal intervertebral disk height at the affected level followed by irregularity and loss of definition of the adjacent vertebral end plates (Fig. 6-69). In vertebral osteomyelitis irregularity of the vertebral end plate slightly precedes or occurs simultaneously with disk space narrowing. These changes are usually best demonstrated by computed tomography, which also may be used to direct percutaneous aspiration of the involved area for bacterial culture. With progression of the infection irregular radiolucent destructive lesions appear in the vertebral body, leading to vertebral collapse. In the late stages (10-12 wk), reparative changes become prominent, with sclerosis and new bone formation at involved segments. In some patients paravertebral or psoas abscess formation may complicate the process, appearing as soft-tissue masses adjacent to the spine on plain radiographs and as low-density areas on computed tomographic studies.

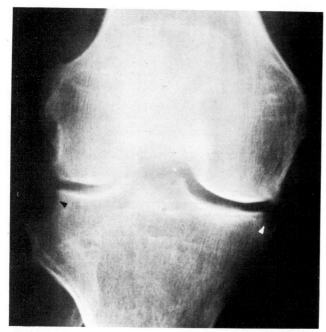

Fig. 6-70. Frontal radiograph of the knee of a patient with tuberculous septic arthritis demonstrates preservation of the joint space with marginal erosions (*arrowheads*) present on both sides of the articulation and juxtaarticular osteoporosis.

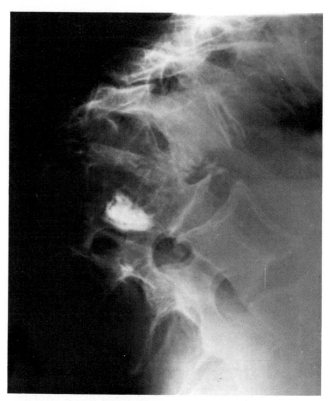

Fig. 6-71. Lateral radiograph of the lumbar spine of a patient with long-standing tuberculous spondylitis. There is a marked kyphotic angular deformity of the spine with ankylosis and collapse of several contiguous vertebrae.

Pyogenic spondylitis is most common in the lumbar spine, followed in frequency by the thoracic and cervical segments. In most cases differentiation between pyogenic and tuberculous spondylitis is not possible using radiographic criteria. One feature that may be of help is the slow and relatively indolent progression of the tuberculous process, in contrast to the rapid progression of pyogenic infections.

SKELETAL TUBERCULOSIS. Osteoarticular tuberculosis is a relatively uncommon disorder which, in the majority of cases, results through hematogenous dissemination from an extraskeletal focus, usually the lung. As in pyogenic infections skeletal tuberculosis may manifest as osteomyelitis, spondylitis, or septic arthritis. The radiographic findings of skeletal tuberculosis are similar to those of pyogenic infection, but a key feature that suggests the diagnosis is its relatively slow progression.

Tuberculous osteomyelitis may involve any bone. In long bones it tends to occur near one end of the bone and frequently spreads into an adjacent articulation. On radiographs tuberculous osteomyelitis appears as a poorly defined zone of osteolysis, often surrounded by a sclerotic border. Periosteal new bone formation is often present but is less prominent than in pyogenic infections. Occasionally a radiodense focus of sequestra may be identified within the osteolytic zone, but sequestrum formation is less prominent that in pyogenic infections. Regional osteoporosis of the adjacent uninvolved bone is typical and more prominent than in pyogenic osteomyelitis.

Tuberculous septic arthritis may occur by the primary hematogenous route or by contamination of the articulation from an adjacent focus of osteomyelitis. The earliest radiographic signs are the presence of a joint effusion and soft-tissue swelling around the articulation. Juxta-articular osteoporosis is usually quite prominent and is followed by erosive lesions, usually at the margins of the joint (Fig. 6-

70). Joint space narrowing occurs relatively late, often several months after the patient first becomes symptomatic. The differential diagnosis of tuberculous arthritis may include inflammatory arthropathy (i.e., RA); however, the monoarticular distribution and discordance of erosions and joint space narrowing provide differential points. The changes may also be identical to those of pyogenic septic arthritis; again, however, the relative indolence of the process suggests the diagnosis.

Tuberculous spondylitis occurs most frequently at the thoracolumbar junction (T-10 to L-2). In the majority of cases the initial focus of infection occurs adjacent to the subchondral bone plate within the anterior half of the vertebral body. An osteolytic destructive lesion may be initially identified, with subsequent involvement and narrowing of the intervertebral disk. The radiographic changes are similar to those of pyogenic infection except for the slower progression of destructive changes. Once the disk has been contaminated, dissemination into the adjacent paravertebral soft tissues may occur, leading to involvement of adjacent vertebra or paraspinal soft-tissue abscess formation. Psoas abscesses occur in approximately 5 percent of cases of tuberculous spondylitis, are often bilateral, and often attain massive size. On plain radiographs psoas abscesses appear as soft-tissue masses adjacent to the spine, often containing internal calcifications. Collapse of an involved vertebra is not unusual and may vary from mild anterior compression to an acute kyphotic (gibbous) angular deformity (Fig. 6-71). In the late stages ankylosis of one or more adjacent vertebrae may be seen as a reparative response.

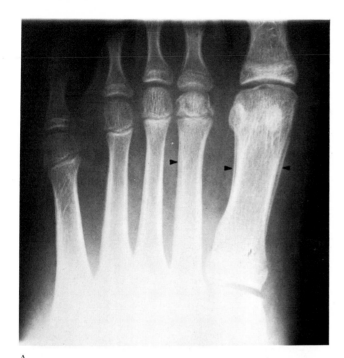

A

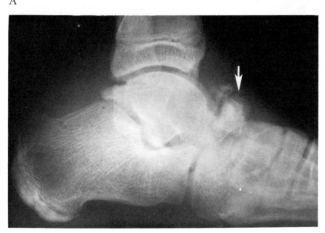

B

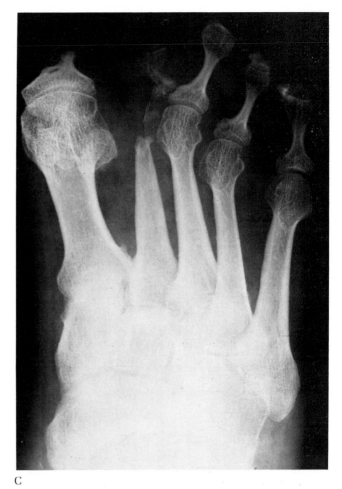

C

Fig. 6-72. Frontal (A) and lateral (B) radiographs of the foot of a 13-year-old male with leprosy demonstrate prominent soft-tissue swelling as well as periostitis (*arrowheads*) along the shafts of several of the metatarsals and proximal phalanges (leprous osteitis). Neuropathic changes are also present with fragmentation and collapse of the midfoot (*arrow*). A frontal radiograph of the foot (C) in another patient with long-standing leprosy demonstrates advanced neuropathic atrophic change in the small bones of the forefoot.

LEPROSY. Leprosy (Hansen's disease) is an infectious disease caused by *Mycobacterium leprae* that may manifest skeletal changes either through active infection or neuroarthropathy. Skeletal infection occurs in less than 5 percent of patients with leprosy and is most common in the small bones of the hands and feet and in the facial bones. Most commonly osseous infection occurs via spread from an overlying infected dermal or mucosal site. Initially on radiographs periostitis (Fig. 6-72A) is noted, followed by patchy destructive changes in the cortex (leprous osteitis) and finally in the marrow space (leprous osteomyelitis). Less commonly direct hematogenous implantation of organisms results in primary leprous osteomyelitis, in which case any bone may be involved. Symmetric periostitis of long tubular bones, especially in the leg, associated with erythema and pain (red leg) may be seen. By far the most common skeletal manifestation of leprosy is neuroarthropathy, which is seen in 70 percent of patients with chronic disease. The radiographic findings in neuroarthropathy have already been described and, in leprosy, are most common in the bones of the hands and feet (Fig. 6-72B). Cal-

cification of peripheral nerves is a well-known pathognomonic sign of leprosy, but unfortunately is extremely rare and is thus of little diagnostic value.

SYPHILIS. Skeletal changes associated with *Treponema pallidum* infections have become unusual since the advent of the modern antibiotic era, but they may be encountered occasionally. Three different syndromes relating to the musculoskeletal system may be seen in this disease: (1) congenital syphilis, (2) acquired syphilis, and (3) neuroarthropathy (tabes dorsalis). Tabes dorsalis is described in the section on neuroarthropathy and is not considered here.

Congenital Syphilis. Congenital syphilis occurs through transplacental migration of the treponeme during fetal development, with invasion of the skeletal system. At birth and in early infancy the skeletal manifestations of congenital syphilis may consist of one or more of the following: (1) osteochondritis, (2) osteomyelitis, and (3) periostitis. These changes are usually self-limited and disappear

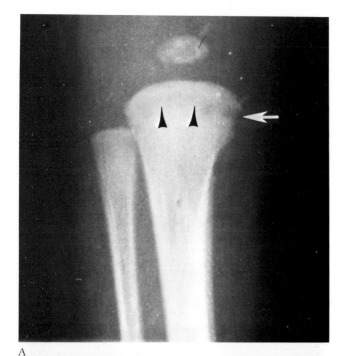

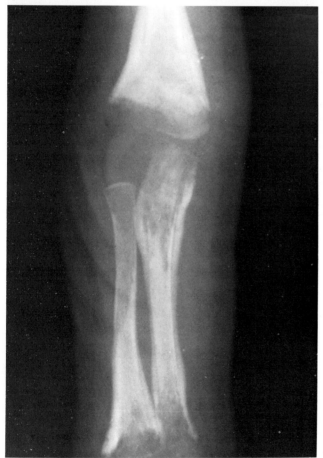

A

B

Fig. 6-73. Congenital syphilis. A. Frontal radiograph of the proximal tibia of an infant demonstrates a prominent lucent metaphyseal band (*arrowheads*) with periostitis and an erosion of the proximal medial tibial metaphysis (*arrow*) (Wimberger's sign). B. Frontal radiograph of the forearm of a child with congenital syphilis demonstrates the changes of advanced syphilitic osteomyelitis with prominent osteolytic destructive lesions and periostitis.

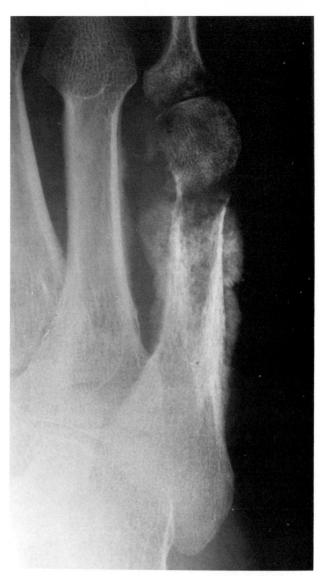

Fig. 6-74. Acquired syphilis. A frontal radiograph of the foot reveals advanced syphilitic osteomyelitis of the fifth metatarsal with prominent destructive change and periostitis as well as extension of the process into the adjacent articulation.

within weeks or years, even without specific therapy. Syphilitic osteochondritis typically involves the junction of the epiphysis and metaphysis of tubular bones and the costochondral junctions of the ribs. The earliest radiographic sign of congenital syphilis is a broad, metaphyseal, radiolucent band paralleling the metaphyseal side of the growth plate, similar to those seen in childhood leukemia and metastatic neuroblastoma. Later, erosions appear at the margins of the growth plate with the medial tibial metaphysis a particularly characteristic site (Wimberger's sign) (Fig. 6-73A). Syphilitic periostitis consists of widespread, symmetric periosteal new bone formation seen predominantly in long tubular bones. Syphilitic osteomyelitis consists of osteolytic destructive lesions, surrounded by a sclerotic reactive zone, which involve the medullary cavity and cortex of affected bones (Fig. 6-73B). These lesions are most common in the tubular bones, may be multifocal, and are often associated with localized periostitis.

Other skeletal lesions may appear late in the course of congenital syphilis. Osteomyelitis and periostitis may result in diffuse hyperostosis of tubular bones, with narrowing of the medullary cavity and bowing deformities. This narrowing is most typical in the tibia in association with anterior bowing and is referred to as the *saber shin* deformity. Osteolytic destructive lesions may involve the nasal bones and calvarium. Peg-shaped hypoplastic dentition (Hutchinson's teeth) may be identified on radiographs of the skull. Large asymptomatic joint effusions (Clutton's joints) may be encountered without other radiographic changes in older children.

Acquired Syphilis. In acquired syphilis bony abnormalities may be seen, usually in the tertiary stage of the disease. A proliferative periostitis or syphilitic osteomyelitis (Fig. 6-74) may occur; the skull is a common site of involvement. The nasal bones, maxilla, mandible, and peripheral tubular bones may also be involved. A saber shin deformity similar to that of congenital syphilis may be seen, which differs in that the medullary cavity is of normal diameter and periosteal new bone formation, rather than anterior bowing, is responsible for the deformity.

FUNGAL BONE AND JOINT INFECTIONS. Osteomyelitis or septic arthritis of fungal origin are relatively rare and in most instances radiographically resemble similar bacterial infections, although they tend in general to be more slowly progressive.

VIRAL INFECTIONS. Viral infections of bone are very rare. In many viral syndromes a self-limited arthritis may be present without radiographic findings. Actual radiographic change due to viral infection is most typical in congenital infections due to the transplacental migration of Rubella or Cytomegalovirus during the first trimester of pregnancy. Skeletal changes typically involve the long bones, especially the distal femur and proximal tibia. Metaphyseal radiolucent bands are present due to the absence of the zone of provisional calcification. Irregularity, without cupping, of the metaphysis is present and often a characteristic appearance, with alternating, longitudinally oriented zones of sclerosis and lucency that results in the celery stalk appearance is present. Epiphyseal ossification centers may have irregular margins. Periostitis is not present in these disorders in contrast to congenital syphilis, which may have a similar radiographic appearance.

Bone Tumors

RADIOLOGIC APPROACH TO BONE NEOPLASMS. Osseous neoplasms tend to be a very difficult area of diagnosis in skeletal radiology for most physicians. If we approach these lesions in a logical, stepwise manner much of the mystery can be overcome. Not all destructive skeletal lesions are neoplastic. A variety of processes may demonstrate destructive changes that resemble neoplasms. These include osteomyelitis, giant rheumatoid subchondral cysts, brown tumors of hyperparathyroidism, hemophilic pseudotumors, and sites of prior trauma or surgery. Thus the first rule when faced with a destructive osseous lesion is to consider the clinical status as well as the past medical history of the patient. These often suggest another diagnosis and spare the patient a great deal of misery as well as a costly medical work-up. A less comforting fact to consider is that destructive lesions in the medullary space of

bone may be invisible on standard radiographs until relatively far advanced. In compact cortical bone, small alterations tend to be easily visible, while in cancellous bone approximately 50 percent of the bone mass at a specific level must be destroyed before the lesion is visible on plain radiographs. Not infrequently a hot bone scan is accompanied by a normal radiograph. In these instances a careful search for subtle abnormalities on plain radiographs or utilization of more sensitive procedures (i.e., computed tomography) is indicated. Another consideration is that, in most instances, a specific pathologic diagnosis in bone neoplasms is not possible regardless of the sophistication of the clinical and radiographic work-ups. The primary purpose of the radiographic evaluation of bone neoplasms is to localize the lesion, evaluate its extent, and identify certain characteristics of the lesion that suggest a benign or malignant process. In a few instances (i.e., osteoid osteoma, nonossifying fibroma) a confident diagnosis may be based entirely on radiographic criteria; however, this is the exception rather than the rule. The age of the patient is of particular importance in evaluating radiographs of bone neoplasms. In middle-aged and elderly adults osseous neoplasms are usually metastatic from a nonosseous primary lesion, while in children and young adults such lesions usually represent a primary bone neoplasm. Quite often the most important factor in narrowing the radiographic differential diagnosis of a bone neoplasm is the age of the patient.

The position of a lesion within an involved bone is also a factor of diagnostic importance (Fig. 6-75). Most primary neoplasms in tubular bones arise within the metaphyseal segment while metastases and round cell tumors tend to arise within the diaphysis. Tumors arising within an epiphysis are extremely unusual, with the exception of chondroblastoma (see Fig. 6-79) and giant cell tumor of bone (see Fig. 6-85). The presence of certain preexisting lesions that predispose patients toward developing bone neoplasms is also important diagnostic information. These lesions include bone infarction, radiation osteonecrosis, Paget's disease, Ollier's disease, and chronic draining osteomyelitis.

The radiologic tools available for the evaluation of osseous neoplasia and their utility should be considered next. As usual, the plain radiograph is the keystone of the radiologic work-up. In some cases a confident diagnosis can be based entirely on the plain radiographic appearance of a lesion, although in most cases a more extensive evaluation is required. Radionuclide bone scintigraphy is most useful, not to evaluate a known lesion, but rather to determine the extent of a lesion and to detect multiple lesions or metastases. While radionuclide bone scintigraphy is currently the most sensitive means of detecting primary and metastatic bone tumors, it does have several shortcomings that should always be kept in mind. First of all, it is very nonspecific, so that benign and malignant neoplasms, infection, trauma, and a whole host of other processes all look the same. Second, in some cases of diffuse metastatic disease, tumor uptake may be so extensive and homogenous as to appear normal. In these cases lack of radionuclide activity in the kidneys, due to the markedly increased bone uptake, suggests the correct interpretation. Other tumors, especially myeloma, demonstrate a poor affinity for the diphosphonate radiopharmaceuticals used in bone scanning and may not be identified on bone scans.

In the past plain tomography was considered important in characterizing the internal architecture and to detect subtle cortical alterations suggesting malignancy. At this time computed tomography has almost completely supplanted plain tomography in the radiologic work-up of

epiphyseal • chondroblastoma
giant cell

Fig. 6-75. Typical sites of origin of bone neoplasms and neoplasm-like lesions.

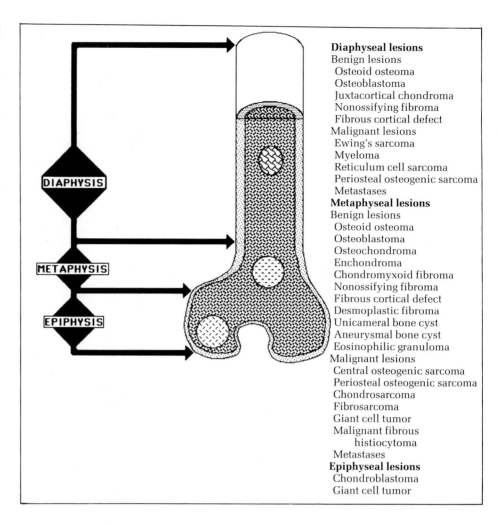

Diaphyseal lesions
Benign lesions
  Osteoid osteoma
  Osteoblastoma
  Juxtacortical chondroma
  Nonossifying fibroma
  Fibrous cortical defect
Malignant lesions
  Ewing's sarcoma
  Myeloma
  Reticulum cell sarcoma
  Periosteal osteogenic sarcoma
  Metastases
Metaphyseal lesions
Benign lesions
  Osteoid osteoma
  Osteoblastoma
  Osteochondroma
  Enchondroma
  Chondromyxoid fibroma
  Nonossifying fibroma
  Fibrous cortical defect
  Desmoplastic fibroma
  Unicameral bone cyst
  Aneurysmal bone cyst
  Eosinophilic granuloma
Malignant lesions
  Central osteogenic sarcoma
  Periosteal osteogenic sarcoma
  Chondrosarcoma
  Fibrosarcoma
  Giant cell tumor
  Malignant fibrous
    histiocytoma
  Metastases
Epiphyseal lesions
  Chondroblastoma
  Giant cell tumor

Fig. 6-76. Radiographic evaluation of bone neoplasms.

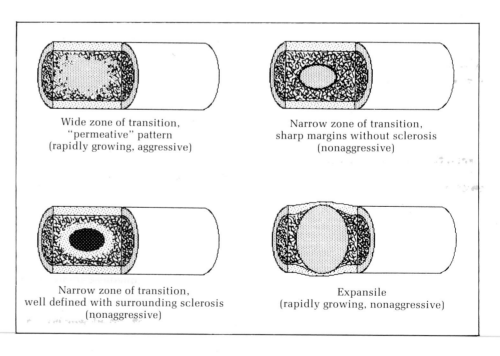

Wide zone of transition,
"permeative" pattern
(rapidly growing, aggressive)

Narrow zone of transition,
sharp margins without sclerosis
(nonaggressive)

Narrow zone of transition,
well defined with surrounding sclerosis
(nonaggressive)

Expansile
(rapidly growing, nonaggressive)

bone tumors since it has greater resolution and adds the ability to directly visualize intra- and extraosseous soft tissues. Angiography likewise has been supplanted by computed tomography in most instances, although angiography still may be useful in specific lesions. Magnetic resonance imaging (MRI) is still in its infancy but offers the potential to evaluate lesions on a physiologic basis rather than merely by density differences, as with radiographic techniques.

Several specific radiographic findings are of considerable importance in the assessment of the malignant potential of a specific lesion. The zone of transition (Fig. 6-76) of a bone neoplasm refers to the radiographic appearance of the peripheral margin and surrounding normal bone. A narrow zone of transition (geographic pattern) refers to a lesion that is sharply marginated so that its exact outline can easily be traced on the radiograph with a sharp pencil (see Fig. 6-77). This finding usually indicates a relatively slow-growing, nonaggressive lesion. A sclerotic zone due to reactive bone formation and adjacent to the outer margin of the lesion is another good radiographic sign of benignancy (see Fig. 6-78). A wide zone of transition around a lesion indicates that the precise margins of the lesion cannot be determined on the radiograph (see Fig. 6-86A). This finding indicates a more rapidly growing, aggressive lesion that cannot be contained by the normal protective and reparative processes within the bone and represents the appearance of most primary and metastatic bone neoplasms.

The internal architecture of a bone neoplasm refers to the radiographic appearance of its internal contents. Trabeculation, often resulting in a "bubbly" radiographic appearance (see Fig. 6-81), generally indicates a benign process such as fibrous dysplasia, enchondroma, nonossifying fibroma, aneurysmal bone cyst, or chondromyxoid fibroma. However, more aggressive lesions such as giant cell tumor of bone, plasmacytoma, or metastases from primary thyroid or renal malignancies may also have this appearance. Calcifications within destructive osseous lesions may be seen in neoplasms as well as in infections (sequestrations). Chondroid calcifications within a tumor appear as coarse, ring-shaped, or flocculent deposits within the central portion of the lesion (see Fig. 6-87). Identification of chondroid calcifications indicates a neoplasm of cartilaginous origin, such as enchondroma, chondroblastoma, chondrosarcoma, or rarely chondromyxoid fibroma. Calcified osteoid matrix tends to have a "fluffy" appearance on radiographs (see Fig. 6-86A) and is most typical of osteogenic sarcoma, although this appearance may be encountered in some benign lesions, such as osteoblastoma. A homogenous ground glass appearance of the matrix of a destructive lesion suggests the diagnosis of fibrous dysplasia (see Fig. 6-56A).

The effect of a lesion on the adjacent cortex is also an important consideration. Rapidly growing benign lesions tend to result in a rounded expansion of the cortex (see Fig. 6-81), which remains intact unless a pathologic fracture occurs (see Fig. 6-76). Aggressive malignant processes erode and destroy the cortex rather than expand it. The most subtle cortical change in malignant lesions is a scalloped appearance of the endosteal cortical surface, which may be focal or quite extensive. This finding indicates that bone is being destroyed and replaced and may be identified before enough medullary bone destruction has occurred to allow identification of the lesion on radiographs. Frank cortical destruction, often with an associated soft tissue mass, is an ominous sign suggesting an advanced malignant process (see Fig. 6-88). Pathologic fractures may occur in both benign and malignant lesions (see Fig. 6-

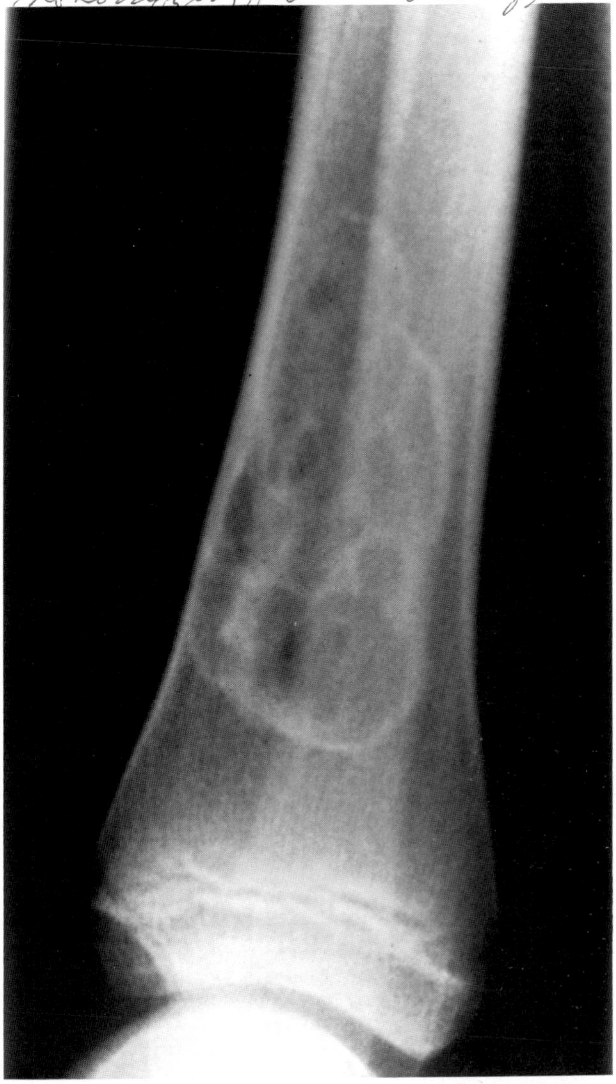

Fig. 6-77. Nonossifying fibroma. Lateral radiograph of the distal tibia with characteristic bubbly lesions with sharp sclerotic margins.

90B). The physician must be careful to identify radiographic features due to the fracture (e.g., hemorrhage, periostitis), which may simulate a malignant appearance in lesions that appear otherwise benign.

Periosteal reaction is common in a number of bone neoplasms. In malignant neoplasms presence of a discontinuous pattern of periosteal new bone formation (i.e., spiculated or lamellar) indicates an aggressive, often malignant lesion. Codman's triangle refers to a triangular focus of periosteal new bone formation that generally indicates a rapid growth. It is not specific for malignancy, however, since it is most commonly noted in association with osteomyelitis.

BENIGN NEOPLASMS OF BONE. Fibrous Cortical Defect and Nonossifying Fibroma. *Fibrous cortical defect* and *nonossifying fibroma* refer to the same histologic lesion, which is most common in males and typically is seen in the first and second decades of life. Fibrous cortical defects are small, ovoid, radiolucent lesions with a sharply marginated sclerotic border that are located within the cortex of a tubular bone. These lesions are initially located near the

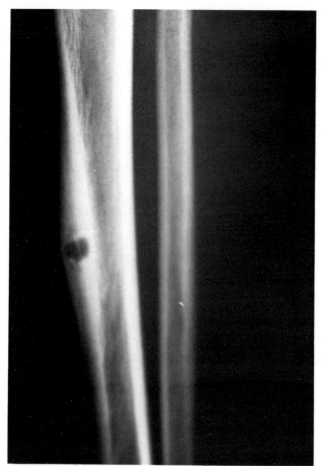

Fig. 6-78. Osteoid osteoma. Lateral radiograph of the mid-shaft of the tibia shows a radiolucent lesion in the anterior tibial cortex surrounded by a broad zone of reactive sclerosis and cortical thickening.

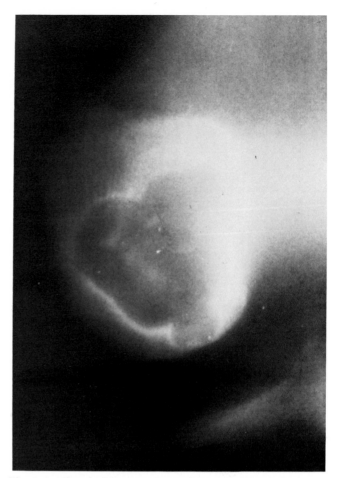

Fig. 6-79. Chondroblastoma. Frontal tomogram through the distal femur demonstrates a sharply circumscribed epiphyseal lesion in the femoral condyle, which contains internal calcifications of the chondroid type, typical of chondroblastoma.

fibrous cortical defect
grows → nonossifying fibroma

metaphysis and appear to migrate out of the diaphysis as the bone grows. In most cases the lesion is eventually obliterated and disappears; however, in some instances it may continue to grow and expand into the medullary cavity. In these instances the lesion is referred to as a *nonossifying fibroma*. On radiographs nonossifying fibromas are visualized as eccentric metaphyseal or diaphyseal lesions with a bubbly appearance and a dense sclerotic border (Fig. 6-77). Pathologic fractures are common complications of large lesions.

Osteoid Osteoma. Osteoid osteoma is a benign lesion seen in children and young adults and is associated with pain that is typically worse at night and relieved by aspirin. Radiographically the lesion has a characteristic appearance consisting of a small, round or oval, radiolucent lesion surrounded by a prominent zone of dense reactive sclerosis (Fig. 6-78). Often a small sclerotic nidus can be visualized in the center of the radiolucent zone. The radiographic appearance of these lesions is characteristic in most instances, with the primary differential diagnosis being Brodie's abscess. In the spine osteoid osteoma is typically located in the vertebral pedicle and may be associated with a painful scoliosis. Lesions adjacent to the hip joint may be quite subtle on radiographs and are often associated with widening of the medial joint space due to effusion.

Chondroblastoma
benign   sclerotic margin
epiphyseal
punctate Ca++

Chondroblastoma. Chondroblastoma is a benign neoplasm of cartilaginous origin that is most common in young males. The lesion is typically located in the epiphysis of a tubular bone in a patient with open growth plates. On radiographs the lesion is usually eccentrically located within the epiphysis, with a dense sclerotic border and a central matrix containing numerous small punctate calcifications (Fig. 6-79).

Solitary Bone Cyst. Solitary (unicameral) bone cyst is a benign, fluid-filled lesion most commonly seen in the metaphysis of a tubular bone, especially the proximal humerus and femur. The lesion is most common in the first decade of life and radiographically consists of a symmetric, radiolucent lesion of homogenous internal density, with sharply defined sclerotic borders. In some cases growth of the lesion may expand the normal bony contour. Pathologic fracture is the most common presentation of this lesion and is accompanied by a pathognomonic radiographic sign (floating fragment sign) in approximately 10 percent of cases (Fig. 6-80). The floating fragment sign consists of a fragment of cortical bone that is displaced into the fluid-filled central cavity and falls into the most dependent portion of the lesion.

Aneurysmal Bone Cyst. Aneurysmal bone cyst is a benign lesion usually discovered in the first two decades of life. It

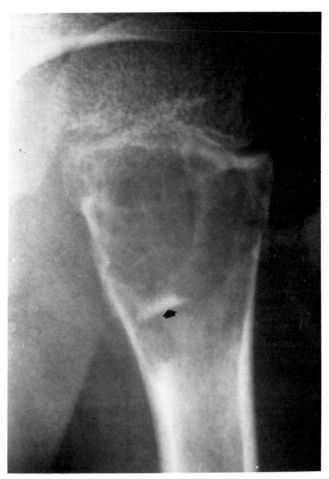

Fig. 6-80. Solitary bone cyst. Frontal radiograph of the proximal humerus in a child with the sudden onset of shoulder pain demonstrates a well-defined osteolytic lesion in the proximal humerus. Note the small fragment of bone ("floating fragment sign") (arrow) within the lesion, which represents a pathognomonic radiographic sign of this lesion.

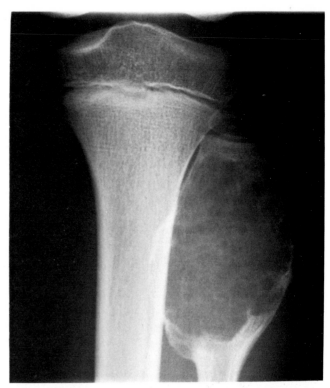

Fig. 6-81. Aneurysmal bone cyst. Frontal radiograph of the proximal tibia demonstrates an expansile lesion of the proximal fibula with a bubbly appearance.

is usually seen in long tubular bones as well as in the posterior elements of the spine. On radiographs a markedly expansile lesion of the metaphysis surrounded by a thin shell of bone is present. The internal architectural pattern is typically trabeculated or bubbly (Fig. 6-81). Presentation is usually due to the presence of a rapidly growing mass, or pain associated with a pathologic fracture. In one-third of cases the lesion appears to develop in association with a preexisting lesion, such as nonossifying fibroma, fibrous dysplasia, chondroblastoma, solitary bone cyst, or giant cell tumor. Aneurysmal bone cyst has no malignant potential, although recurrence following inadequate curettage is common.

Osteochondroma. Osteochondroma is a benign cartilaginous-capped exostosis, which probably represents a developmental defect. Any bone may be involved, but more than half of the lesions are encountered in the distal femur, proximal humerus, and proximal tibia. The lesion arises from the outer cortical surface of the metaphysis and typically grows away from the adjacent articulation. The cortex and medullary cavity of the lesion are contiguous with those of the bone of origin. The lesion may arise on a stalk (pedunculated) or from a broad flat base (Fig. 6-82). In most instances osteochondroma is a solitary lesion; however, an autosomal dominant disorder (e.g., multiple fa-

milial exostoses), characterized by the presence of large numbers of osteochondromas, which are often responsible for growth disturbances and deformity, may be seen. Malignant degeneration is rare in solitary lesions but occurs in up to 20 percent of patients with multiple familial exostoses.

Enchondroma. Enchondroma is a benign cartilaginous tumor that is most common in the small tubular bones of the hands and feet. On radiographs the lesion is usually centrally located, well-circumscribed, and osteolytic. Multiple, small, stippled internal calcifications are usually present in the central portion of the lesion (Fig. 8-83). The potential for malignancy of this lesion appears to be more accurately related to the location of the lesion rather than to its specific radiographic appearance. In the small bones of the hands and feet malignant degeneration is rare, while in the large flat bones of the pelvis many pathologists classify all of these lesions as low-grade chondrosarcomas, regardless of histologic and radiographic appearance. In the long tubular bones the malignant potential of the lesion is intermediate.

Ollier's disease is a noninherited disorder characterized by the presence of numerous enchondromata scattered throughout the skeletal system. Growth disturbances and deformity are common, and malignant transformation occurs in up to 50 percent of patients. Maffucci's syndrome is a varient of Ollier's disease, in which multiple soft tissue hemangiomas are present in addition to the enchondromas.

Eosinophilic Granuloma. Eosinophilic granuloma is a benign lesion consisting of collections of histiocytes and eosinophils. The lesions are most common in the first decade of life, with the skull, pelvis, and long tubular bones being

Osteochondroma

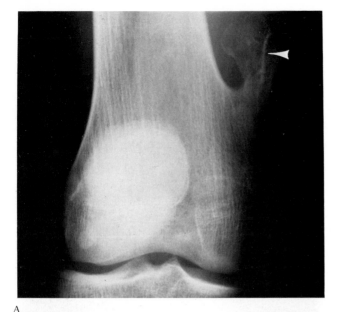

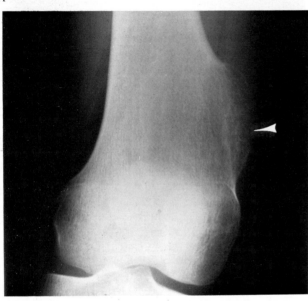

Fig. 6-82. Pedunculated (A) and sessile (B) osteochondromas. In both instances note that the lesion is contiguous with the cortex and medullary cavities of the adjacent bone and appears to be growing away from the adjacent articulation.

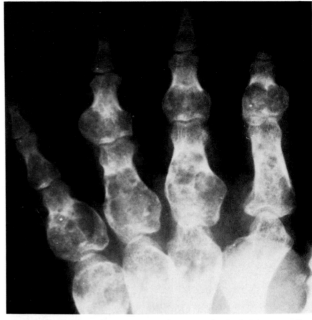

Ollier = enchondroma

Fig. 6-83. Frontal radiograph of the hand of a patient with Ollier's disease demonstrates multiple enchondromata involving virtually all of the osseous structures. Note that the lesions are sharply marginated, expansile, and contain faint stippled (chondroid) internal calcifications.

ized by the triad of calvarial eosinophilic granuloma, diabetes insipidus, and exophthalmos. Lesions at other skeletal sites as well as pulmonary interstitial fibrosis may also be present. Letterer-Siwe disease is usually fatal in infancy; however, in patients who survive the typical appearance of Hand-Schüller-Christian disease occurs.

MALIGNANT NEOPLASMS OF BONE. Giant Cell Tumor of Bone. The giant cell tumor of bone is a subject of long-standing controversy regarding its classification as a benign or malignant lesion. Because of its aggressive behavior, high rate of recurrence, and potential for metastasis, the lesion should be considered at best a low-grade malignancy. Giant cell tumor of bone is most common between the ages of 20 and 40, and virtually always involves the epiphysis of a tubular bone. Approximately 50 percent of these lesions occur around the knee, with the next most common location being the distal forearm. On radiographs a typical giant cell tumor appears as an eccentric osteolytic, epiphyseal lesion without internal calcifications (Fig. 6-85). The border of the lesion is often indistinct, without a surrounding zone of reactive sclerosis. Destruction of the cortex is common and is often associated with a surprisingly minimal degree of periosteal reaction. The internal matrix of the lesion is bland and homogenous, although a pseudotrabeculated appearance may be present due to differences in cortical erosion. It is not possible to entirely differentiate benign giant cell tumors from aggressive or even frankly malignant lesions on the basis of radiographic criteria.

Osteogenic Sarcoma. Osteogenic sarcoma (osteosarcoma) may be subdivided into three main types, (1) central, (2) parosteal, and (3) periosteal on the basis of radiologic and histologic criteria. It is best to consider these types separately, since the radiographic appearance as well as the potential for survival varies with these patterns.

the most common sites of origin. The lesion is most often solitary and nonexpansile and is located in the metaphysis or metadiaphysis. In early phases of development the lesion may demonstrate a poorly marginated ("moth-eaten") osteolytic pattern (Fig. 6-84A) with periosteal new bone formation; it is often mistaken for osteomyelitis or Ewing's sarcoma. As the lesion matures a well-defined sclerotic border develops and a benign radiographic appearance is present (Fig. 6-84B). In flat bones, especially the skull, the margins of an eosinophilic granuloma may demonstrate a characteristic beveled edge. In the spine, wafer-like collapse of an affected vertebral body is common and has previously been known as vertebra plana or Calvé's disease. Multifocal eosinophilic granuloma with extraskeletal involvement (Hand-Schüller-Christian disease) is character-

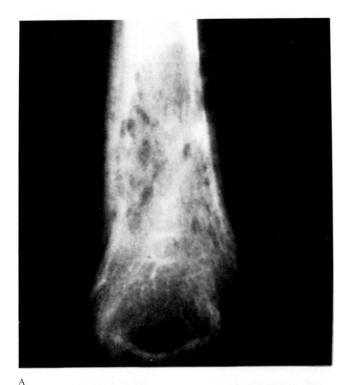

A

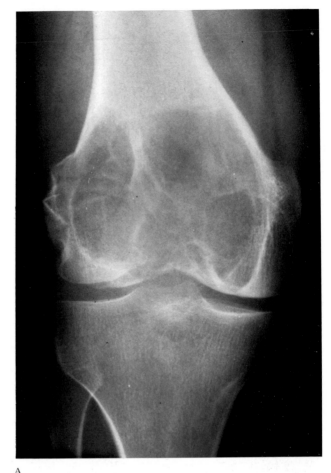

A

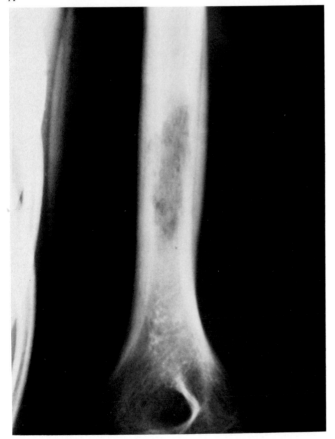

B

Fig. 6-84. Eosinophilic granuloma. Two lesions involving the distal humerus are demonstrated. In A the lesion is in an early, pseudomalignant phase of development and demonstrates a poorly marginated (moth-eaten) osteolytic pattern with prominent periosteal new bone formation. In B a more mature stage is present with a sharply marginated lesion with thick, benign appearing, periosteal new bone formation.

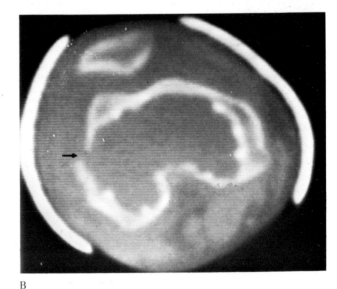

B

Fig. 6-85. A frontal radiograph (A) and a computed tomographic scan (B) demonstrate the typical appearance of giant cell tumor of bone. In the frontal radiograph note the epiphyseal involvement, indistinct borders, and lack of surrounding sclerosis. Differential erosions of the endosteal surface result in a pseudotrabeculated appearance of the lesion. In the computed tomographic scan note the homogeneous internal matrix as well as the presence of a pathologic fracture (*arrow*) of the lateral femoral cortex.

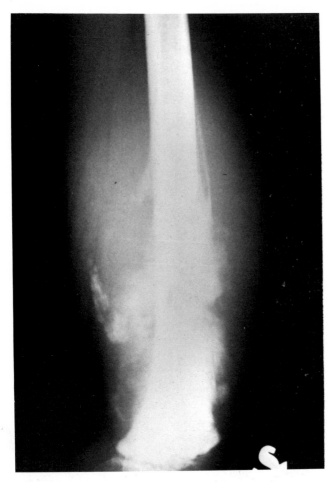

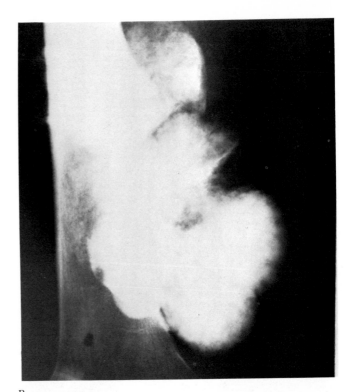

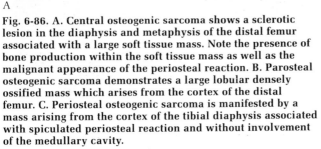

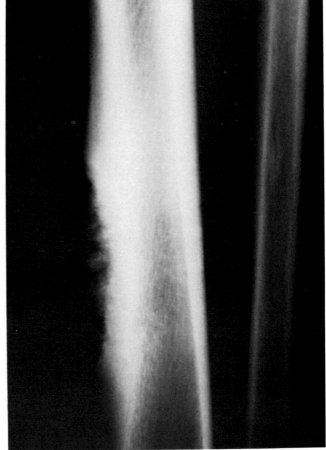

A

B

C

Fig. 6-86. A. Central osteogenic sarcoma shows a sclerotic lesion in the diaphysis and metaphysis of the distal femur associated with a large soft tissue mass. Note the presence of bone production within the soft tissue mass as well as the malignant appearance of the periosteal reaction. B. Parosteal osteogenic sarcoma demonstrates a large lobular densely ossified mass which arises from the cortex of the distal femur. C. Periosteal osteogenic sarcoma is manifested by a mass arising from the cortex of the tibial diaphysis associated with spiculated periosteal reaction and without involvement of the medullary cavity.

Central Osteogenic Sarcoma. This is a highly malignant neoplasm that arises from intramedullary bone. The neoplasm is most common in males (a ratio of 2 : 1) in the second decade of life. The tumor typically arises in the metaphysis of a long tubular bone, especially the distal femur, proximal tibia, and proximal humerus. On radiographs a poorly defined lesion is present, usually with cortical destruction, soft-tissue mass, and prominent periosteal reaction (sunburst pattern) (Fig. 6-86A). Approximately 90 percent of osteogenic sarcomas demonstrate radiographically visible bone formation within the lesion. Metastases are common, with the lungs the most frequent site. Computed tomography is quite useful in evaluating osteogenic sarcoma. In suspected osteogenic sarcoma the entire bone in which the lesion is present should be studied by computed tomography, since intramedullary skip lesions are relatively common and of great importance to the orthopedic surgeon in planning appropriate therapy.

Secondary osteogenic sarcoma may complicate a number of preexisting lesions, especially Paget's disease and prior sites of radiation therapy. Multicentric osteogenic sarcoma (osteosarcomatosis) is a rare disorder usually seen in children as densely osteoblastic lesions that are located within the metaphyseal region of multiple bones.

Parosteal (Juxtacortical) Osteogenic Sarcoma. This is a rare tumor usually seen in the third through fifth decades of life. On radiographs a large, lobulated, osteosclerotic lesion is seen that is continuous with the cortex of an adjacent bone, without evidence of medullary cavity involvement (Fig. 6-86B). The most common sites are the distal femur and proximal tibia. This neoplasm tends to be relatively indolent and can be cured in most cases by surgical resection.

Periosteal Osteogenic Sarcoma. This is a malignant lesion arising from the periosteal surface of a long bone, especially the tibia, and is often located in the diaphyseal segment. On radiographs a saucerized, destructive lesion of the outer cortical surface of the involved bone is present, usually with spiculated new bone formation that appears malignant (Fig. 6-86C). These lesions are more aggressive than parosteal osteogenic sarcoma but have a better prognosis than central osteogenic sarcoma.

Chondrosarcoma. Chondrosarcoma is most common in patients older than forty and has no sexual predilection. On radiographs (Fig. 6-87) the lesion appears as a large, ill-defined, destructive lesion with coarse internal calcifications that are often shaped like the letters C, O, or Y. A scalloped appearance of the endosteal cortical surface or frank cortical destruction with an adjacent soft tissue mass may be present. The pelvis is the most common site of origin, followed in frequency by the femur and humerus. Secondary chondrosarcoma is most common in patients with Ollier's disease, in which malignant transformation of enchondromata is frequent.

Ewing's Sarcoma. Ewing's sarcoma is a round cell tumor that arises from marrow elements and is most common in the first and second decades of life. Radiographs reveal a mottled, permeative pattern of bone destruction, typically beginning in the diaphysis of a long tubular bone (Fig. 6-88). Cortical penetration occurs rapidly and is often associated with a layered or lamellar appearance of overlying periosteal new bone formation (onion skin appearance). Metastases to the lungs are common and bone to bone metastases may occur as well.

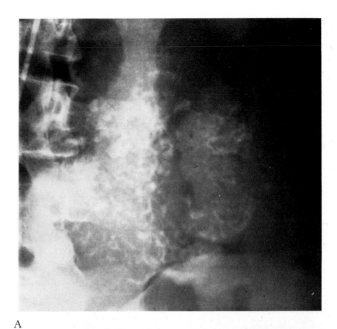

A

B

Fig. 6-87. Frontal radiograph (A) and computed tomographic scan (B) of a patient with a chondrosarcoma arising from the transverse process of the fourth lumbar vertebra demonstrates a large mass with coarse (chondroid) internal calcifications.

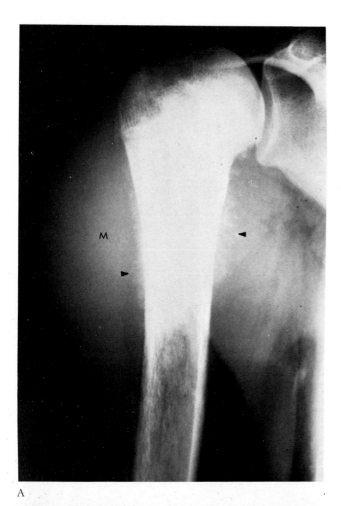

A

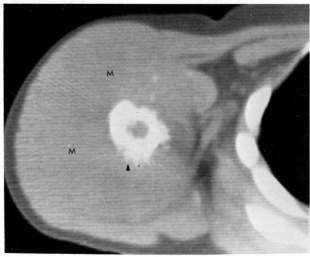

B

Fig. 6-88. Ewing's sarcoma. Frontal radiograph (A) and computed tomographic scan (B) demonstrate an osteolytic lesion arising in the proximal humerus with malignant appearing periosteal reaction (*arrowheads*) as well as a large soft tissue mass (M).

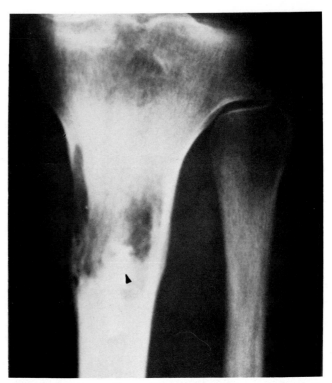

Fig. 6-89. Malignant fibrous histiocytoma. Frontal radiograph of the proximal tibia shows a poorly marginated osteolytic lesion associated with destruction of the cortex as well as a dense zone of bone infarction (*arrowhead*).

Myeloma. Myeloma is a common neoplastic disease that is most common in patients in their seventh and eighth decades, and is slightly more common in men. In most cases multiple lesions (multiple myeloma) are present, although occasionally a solitary lesion (plasmacytoma) may be encountered. Radiographically multiple myeloma is usually characterized by numerous, round or elliptical, discretely marginated, punched out lesions. Involvement tends to be more prominent in the axial skeleton, especially the skull, spine, ribs, and pelvis. In some instances the disorder may be characterized radiographically by a pattern of diffuse osteopenia that simulates osteoporosis. Solitary plasmacytoma is most common in the spine and pelvis and is characterized by an osteolytic lesion often associated with a vertebral compression fracture. Extraskeletal plasmacytomas may arise in the paranasal sinuses, nasal cavity, or upper airway. As has been previously noted, bonescanning radiopharmaceuticals demonstrate a poor affinity for myelomatous lesions, which may result in a false negative bone scan.

Reticulum Cell Sarcoma. Reticulum cell sarcoma is an uncommon malignant neoplasm seen in all age groups, with a male predominance of 2 : 1. The tumor usually arises within the medullary cavity of a tubular bone and demonstrates a permeative, osteolytic appearance on radiographs. Irregular cortical destruction is typical and a soft-tissue mass may be present.

Malignant Fibrous Histiocytoma. Malignant fibrous histiocytoma of bone is a relatively uncommon tumor that occurs in an even distribution between the second and eighth decades of life, with no sexual predominance. Any bone may be involved but the femur and tibia are the most

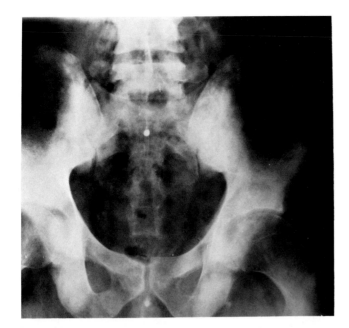

A

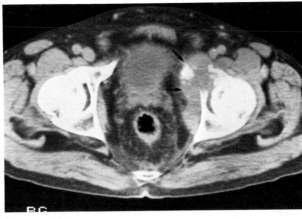

C

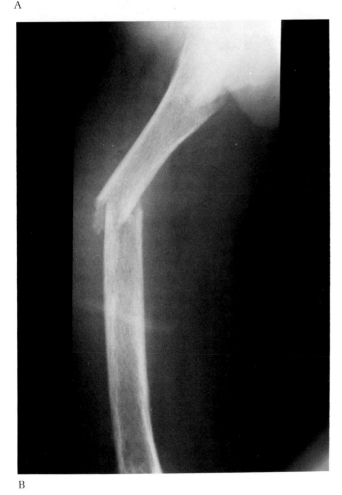

B

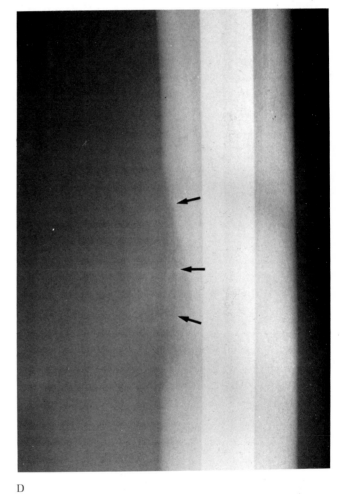

D

Fig. 6-90. Metastatic carcinoma. A. Frontal radiograph of the pelvis demonstrates diffuse osteoblastic metastases in a patient with prostatic carcinoma. B. Lateral radiograph of the femur of a patient with metastatic neuroblastoma demonstrates a diffuse infiltrative pattern of metastatic disease associated with a pathologic fracture. C. Computed tomographic scan of a patient with a known hypernephroma and equivocal plain radiographs reveals a large destructive mass (*arrows*) involving the anteromedial aspect of the acetabulum. D. Frontal radiograph of the femur in a patient with bronchogenic carcinoma reveals the characteristic saucerized ("cookie bite") cortical metastasis (*arrows*) which can be seen with this tumor.

common locations. On radiographs the lesions tend to be located in the metaphysis as an osteolytic defect with a permeative or moth-eaten appearance (Fig. 6-89). Cortical disruption with adjacent soft-tissue mass may be present. In many instances the lesion resembles a purely osteolytic osteogenic sarcoma. Malignant fibrous histiocytoma may be seen in association with preexisting medullary bone infarction. In these instances radiographs reveal typical shell-like or serpiginous calcification of a medullary bone infarction, with an ill-defined focus of destruction involving a portion of the necrotic bone.

Metastatic Carcinoma Involving Bone. A detailed review of the radiographic appearance and distribution of osseous metastases from carcinomas is beyond the scope of this text. However several generalizations can be made that are useful in suggesting the possibility of a metastatic lesion and often suggesting the likely primary source. In general, osseous metastases tend to occur in the axial skeleton (i.e., skull, spine, pelvis) and proximal long tubular bones (i.e., humerus, femur) and are rarely found distal to the elbows and knees. In tubular bones the location may be metaphyseal or diaphyseal and is only rarely epiphyseal. Periosteal new bone formation is usually minimal, and multifocal lesions are common in association with metastatic carcinoma, in contrast to most primary bone neoplasms.

The radiographic appearance of metastatic carcinoma may be osteolytic, osteoblastic, or mixed (Fig. 6-90). Carcinomas arising from the lung, kidney, breast, thyroid, and gastrointestinal tract are responsible for the majority of purely osteolytic lesions. In children metastatic neuroblastoma is the most common osteolytic metastatic lesion. Mixed osteolytic and osteoblastic metastases are most common in carcinoma of the lung, breast, prostate, and urinary bladder, as well as in childhood neuroblastoma. Adenocarcinoma of the prostate is by far the most common cause of purely osteoblastic metastases, although carcinomas arising from the breast and gastrointestinal tract, and metastatic carcinoid tumor, may also have this appearance. As can be surmised from the previous discussion, many metastatic lesions can have any of the appearances described earlier.

Several other clues may be helpful in the radiographic evaluation of skeletal metastases. Metastases distal to the knees or elbow are unusual, but when present are due to metastatic bronchogenic carcinoma in more than 50 percent of cases. Expansile radiolucent metastases, often with a soap bubble appearance, suggest metastases from carcinoma of the kidney or thyroid. Multiple discrete osteolytic lesions in the skull are common in carcinomas of the breast and lung as well as in childhood neuroblastoma and must be differentiated from multiple myeloma. Isolated metastases to the spine without involvement of other visceral organs are most common in carcinoma of the prostate or breast. In the spine most metastases occur in the pedicle or the portion of the vertebral body adjacent to the pedicle, in contrast to myeloma, in which the central portion of the vertebral body is the initial site of the lesion. The presence of an ivory vertebra may be seen with metastatic prostate carcinoma, as well as with round cell tumors (e.g., Hodgkin's disease, leukemia, lymphoma) or with Paget's disease. A saucerized excavation of the outer cortical surface of a tubular bone ("cookie bite" metastasis) is usually due to metastatic bronchogenic carcinoma (Fig. 6-90D). Diffuse dissemination of osseous metastases is most common with carcinoma of the prostate or breast.

Bibliography

Arthritis

Ansell, B. M., and Kent, P. A. Radiological changes in juvenile chronic polyarthritis. *Skel. Radio.* 1:129, 1977.

Bloch, C., Hermann, G., and Yu, T. F. A radiologic reevaluation of gout: A study of 2000 patients. *A.J.R.* 134:781, 1980.

Bonavita, J. A., Dalinka, M. K., and Schumacher, H. R., Jr. Hydroxyapatite deposition disease. *Radiology* 134:621, 1980.

Cabot, A., and Becker, A. The cervical spine in rheumatoid arthritis. *Clin. Orthop.* 131:130, 1978.

Golding, D. N., and Walshe, J. M. Arthropathy of Wilson's disease: Study of clinical and radiographic features in 32 patients. *Ann. Rheum. Dis.* 36:99, 1977.

Hirsch, J. H., Killien, C., and Troupin, R. H. The arthropathy of hemochromatosis. *Radiology* 118:591, 1976.

Kidd, K. L., and Peter, J. B. Erosive osteoarthritis. *Radiology* 86:640, 1966.

Laskar, R. H., and Sargison, K. D. Ochronotic arthropathy: A review with four case reports. *J. Bone Joint Surg.* [Br.] 52B:653, 1970.

McEwen, C., et al. Ankylosing spondylitis and the spondylitis accompanying ulcerative colitis, regional enteritis, psoriasis, and Reiter's disease: A comparative study. *Arthritis Rheum.* 14:291, 1971.

Martel, W. The pattern of rheumatoid arthritis in the hand and wrist. *Radiol. Clin. North Am.* 2:221, 1964.

Norman, A., Robbins, H., and Milgram, J. E. The acute neuropathic arthropathy: A rapid severely disorganizing form of arthritis. *Radiology* 90:1159, 1968.

Resnick, D. The patterns of migration of the femoral head in osteoarthritis of the hip: Roentgenographic-pathologic correlation and comparison with rheumatoid arthritis. *Am. J. Roentgenol.* 124:62, 1975.

Resnick, D., and Niwayama, G. Radiographic and pathologic features of spinal involvement in diffuse idiopathic skeletal hyperostosis (DISH). *Radiology* 119:559, 1976.

Resnick, D., and Niwayama, G. (eds.). *The Diagnosis of Bone and Joint Disorders.* Philadelphia: Saunders, 1981.

Resnick, D., Shaul, S. R., and Robins, J. M. Diffuse idiopathic skeletal hyperostosis (DISH): Forestier's disease with extraspinal manifestations. *Radiology* 115:513, 1975.

Resnick, D., et al. Clinical, radiographic and pathologic abnormalities in calcium pyrophosphate dihydrate deposition disease (CPPD): Pseudogout. *Radiology* 122:1, 1977.

Schaller, J., Wedgwood, R. J. Juvenile rheumatoid arthritis: A review. *Pediatrics* 50:940, 1972.

Schumacher, T. M., et al. HLA-B27 associated arthropathies. *Radiology* 126;289, 1974.

Vyhanek, L., Lavicka, J., and Blahos, J. Roentgenological findings in gout. *Radiol. Clin. North Am.* 29:256, 1960.

Metabolic bone diseases

Edeiken, J., Depalma, A. F., and Hodes, P. J. Paget's disease: Osteitis deformans. *Clin. Orthop.* 146:141, 1966.

Mankin, H. J. Rickets, osteomalacia, and renal osteodystrophy: Part I. *J. Bone Joint Surg.* [Am.] 56A:101, 1974.

Mankin, H. J. Rickets, osteomalacia, and renal osteodystrophy: Part II. *J. Bone Joint Surg.* [Am.] 56A:352, 1974.

Price, C. H. G., and Goldie, W. Paget's sarcoma of bone. *J. Bone Joint Surg.* [Br.] 51B:205, 1969.

Reynolds, W. A., and Karo, J. J. Radiologic diagnosis of metabolic bone disease. *Orthop. Clin. North Am.* 3:521, 1972.

Steinbach, H. L. The roentgen appearance of osteoporosis. *Radiol. Clin. North Am.* 2:191, 1964.

Steinbach, H. L., et al. Evolution of skeletal lesions in pseudohypoparathyroidism. *Radiology* 85:670, 1965.

Steinberg, H., and Waldron, B. R. Idiopathic hypoparathyroidism: Analysis of 52 cases, including report of new case. *Medicine* (Baltimore) 31:133, 1952.

Hemoglobinopathies and anemias

Becker, J. A. Hemoglobin S-C disease. *Am. J. Roentgenol.* 88:503, 1962.

Caffey, J. Cooley's anemia: A review of the roentgenographic findings in the skeleton. *Am. J. Roentgenol.* 78:381, 1957.

O'Hara, A. E. Roentgenographic osseous manifestations of the anemias and the leukemias. *Clin. Orthop.* 52:63, 1967.

Pettersson, H., Ahlberg, A., and Nilson, I. M. A radiologic classification of hemophilic arthropathy. *Clin. Orthop.* 149:153, 1980.

Reynolds, J. *The Roentgenological Features of Sickle Cell Disease and Related Hemoglobinopathies.* Springfield, Ill.: Thomas, 1965.

Disorders of unknown origin

Berman, B. Pulmonary hypertrophic osteoarthropathy. *Arch. Intern. Med.* 112:L947, 1963.

Grabias, S. L., and Campbell, C. J. Fibrous dysplasia. *Orthop. Clin. North Am.* 8:771, 1977.

Herman, M. A., et al. Pachydermoperiostosis: Clinical spectrum. *Arch. Intern. Med.* 227:918, 1965.

Knuttson, F. Skeletal changes in sarcoidosis. *Acta Radiol.* 51:429, 1959.

Bone and joint infections

Barnetson, J. Osseous changes in neural leprosy. *S. Afr. Med. J.* 27:827, 1953.

Cremin, B. J., and Fisher, R. M. The lesions of congenital syphilis. *Br. J. Radiol.* 43:333, 1970.

Dalinka, M. K., et al. Roentgenographic features of osseous coccidioidomycosis and differential diagnosis. *J. Bone Joint Surg.* [Am.] 53A:1157, 1971.

Gilday, D. L., Paul, D. J., and Paterson, J. Diagnosis of osteomyelitis in children by combined blood pool and bone imaging. *Radiology* 117:331, 1975.

Goldblatt, M., and Cremin, B. J. Osteo-articular tuberculosis: Its presentation in coloured races. *Clin. Radiol.* 29:669, 1978.

Miller, W. B., Murphy, W. A., and Gilula, L. A. Brodie abscess: Reappraisal. *Radiology* 132:15, 1979.

O'Conner, B. T., Steel, W. M., and Sanders, R. Disseminated bone tuberculosis. *J. Bone Joint Surg.* [Am.] 52A:537, 1970.

Resnick, D., and Niwayama, G. Osteomyelitis, Septic Arthritis, and Soft Tissue Infection: The Mechanisms and Situations. In D. Resnick and G. Niwayama (eds.), *The Diagnosis of Bone and Joint Disorders.* Philadelphia: Saunders, 1981. P. 2042.

Resnick, D., and Niwayama, G. Osteomyelitis, Septic Arthritis, and Soft Tissue Infection: The Organisms. In D. Resnick and G. Niwayama (eds.), *The Diagnosis of Bone and Joint Disorders.* Philadelphia: Saunders, 1981. P. 2155.

Rosen, R. S., and Jacobson, G. Fungus disease of bone. *Semin. Roentgenol.* 1:370, 1966.

Truog, C. P. Bone lesions in acquired syphilis. *Radiology* 40:1, 1943.

Bone tumors

Abrams, H. L., Spiro, R., and Goldstein, N. Metastases in carcinoma: Analysis of 1000 autopsied cases. *Cancer* 3:74, 1950.

Aprin, H., Riseborough, E. J., and Hall, J. E. Chondrosarcoma in children and adolescents. *Clin. Orthop.* 166:226, 1982.

Berger, P. E., and Kuhn, J. P. Computed tomography of tumors of the musculoskeletal system in children. *Radiology* 127:171, 1978.

Bonakdarpour, A., Levy, W. M., and Aegerter, E. Primary and secondary aneurysmal bone cyst: A radiological study of 75 cases. *Radiology* 126:75, 1978.

Cohen, J. Etiology of simple bone cyst. *J. Bone Joint Surg.* [Am.] 52A:1493, 1970.

Dahlin, D. C. *Bone Tumors: General Aspects and Data on 6221 Cases* (3rd ed.). Springfield, Ill.: Thomas, 1978.

Dahlin, D. C., and Coventry, M. B. Osteogenic sarcoma. *J. Bone Joint Surg.* [Am.] 49A:101, 1967.

Dahlin, D. C., Cupps, R. E., and Johnson, E. W. Giant-cell tumor: A study of 195 cases. *Cancer* 25:1061, 1970.

deSantos, L. A., et al. The radiographic spectrum of periosteal osteosarcoma. *Radiology* 127:123, 1978.

deSantos, L. A., et al. Computed tomography in the evaluation of musculoskeletal neoplasms. *Radiology* 128:89, 1978.

Destouet, J. M., Gilula, L. A., and Murphy, W. A. Computed tomography of long-bone osteosarcoma. *Radiology* 131:439, 1979.

Deutsch, A., and Resnick, D. Eccentric cortical metastases to the skeleton from bronchogenic carcinoma. *Radiology* 137:49, 1980.

Enneking, W. F., and Kagan, A. "Skip" metastases in osteosarcoma. *Cancer* 36:2192, 1975.

Henderson, E. D., and Dahlin, D. C. Chondrosarcoma of bone: A study of 288 cases. *J. Bone Joint Surg.* [Am.] 45A:1450, 1963.

Hesier, S., and Schwartzman, J. J. Variations in the roentgen appearance of the skeletal system in myeloma. *Radiology* 58:178, 1952.

Krishnamurthy, G. T., et al. Distribution pattern of metastatic bone disease. *J.A.M.A.* 237:2504, 1977.

Levine, E., et al. Comparison of computed tomography and other imaging modalities in the evaluation of musculoskeletal tumors. *Radiology* 131:431, 1979.

Lodwick, G. S. The Radiologic Diagnosis of Metastatic Cancer in Bone. *Tumors of Bone and Soft Tissue.* Chicago: Year Book, 1965.

Lodwick, G. S. The Bones and Joints. In P. J. Hodes (ed.), *Atlas of Tumor Radiology.* Chicago: Year Book, 1971.

Mcleod, R. A., and Beabout, J. W. The roentgenographic features of chondroblastoma. *Am. J. Roentgenol.* 118:464, 1973.

Pear, B. L. Skeletal manifestation of the lymphomas and leukemia. *Semin. Roentgenol.* 9:229, 1974.

Skrede, O. Non-osteogenic fibroma of bone. *Acta Orthop. Scand.* 412:369, 1970.

Spanier, S. S. Malignant fibrous histiocytoma of bone. *Orthop. Clin. North Am.* 8:947, 1977.

Swee, R. G., McLeod, R. A., and Beabout, J. W. Osteoid osteoma: Detection, diagnosis, and localization. *Radiology* 130:117, 1979.

Unni, K. K., et al. Parosteal osteogenic sarcoma. *Cancer* 37:2467, 1976.

7. Endocrine and Reproductive Disease

Janet L. Potter

Disorders of the Thyroid

The normal thyroid is a bilobed gland with a small isthmus connecting the inferior poles of the two lobes. The principal role of the thyroid is to secrete iodinated substances that control tissue metabolism.

HYPERTHYROIDISM. Hyperthyroidism is a syndrome of hypermetabolism and enlargement of the thyroid gland. Excessive amounts of thyroid hormone are produced and released by the gland. Eighty-five percent of cases are caused by Graves' disease, with the remainder caused by multinodular goiter (Plummer's disease), solitary toxic adenoma, or subacute thyroiditis. Radioactive iodine (RAI) uptake at 24 hours is markedly elevated in Graves' disease, and images reveal a diffusely enlarged, "hot" gland (Fig. 7-1). In Plummer's disease, functioning adenoma, or thyroiditis, thyroid images show one or more hot nodules, with little if any background radiation in the gland (Fig. 7-2).

HYPOTHYROIDISM. Hypothyroidism is a clinical syndrome characterized by deficiency of thyroid hormone. More than 95 percent of cases are caused by glandular malfunction, which is commonly secondary to glandular destruction by Hashimoto's thyroiditis, endemic goiter (severe iodine deficiency), external radiation (e.g., in treatment of neoplastic disease of the neck), or previous radioactive iodine therapy for hyperthyroidism.

THYROIDITIS. Thyroiditis is an inflammation of the thyroid gland. The subacute form of the disease may present clinically as hyperthyroidism but the 24-hour RAI uptake is reduced; the hyperthyroid phase is short and is followed by a hypothyroid phase, with eventual return to normal function. Chronic thyroiditis (Hashimoto's and Riedel's diseases) is an autoimmune disease. The gland may be either quite enlarged or normal in size. The radioactive iodine image generally reveals heterogenous uptake or occasionally a solitary nodule that represents the only functioning thyroid tissue remaining (Fig. 7-3).

SOLITARY THYROID NODULES. Solitary thyroid nodules may be either "cold" (i.e., having no uptake of iodine) or "hot" (i.e., taking up iodine at the expense of the rest of the gland). The hot nodule is benign and represents a functioning follicular adenoma. The cold nodule accounts for more than 90 percent of solitary nodules (Fig. 7-4). Approximately 10 percent of cold nodules are cysts, 20 percent are carcinomas, and the remainder are adenomas, local thyroiditis, or early multinodular goiter. Adenomas and carcinomas cannot be reliably distinguished on the basis of ultrasound characteristics (Figs. 7-5, 7-6). Percutaneous aspiration for cytology is required for diagnosis.

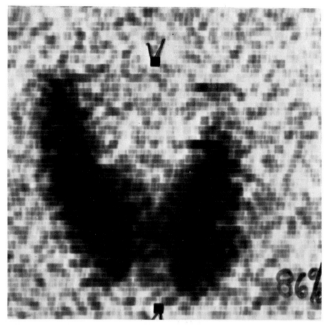

Fig. 7-1. ^{131}I scan of diffusely enlarged thyroid with increased iodine uptake.

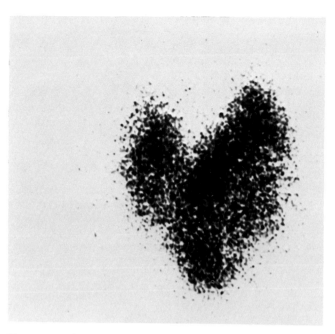

Fig. 7-3. Patchy uptake of ^{131}I is consistent with multinodular goiter.

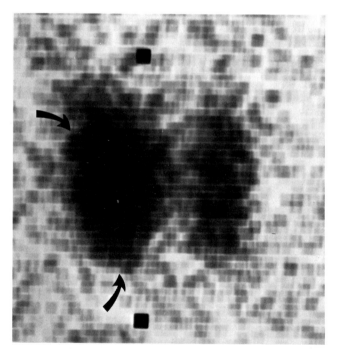

Fig. 7-2. ^{131}I scan of solitary "hot" nodules (*arrows*) in functioning follicular adenoma. Hormonal function of remaining gland is suppressed as evidenced by decreased uptake.

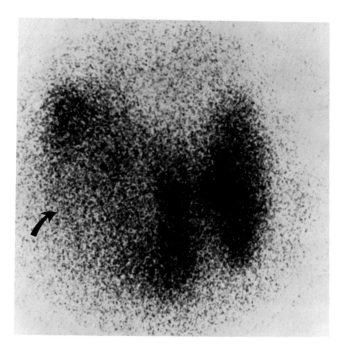

Fig. 7-4. ^{131}I scan of solitary "cold" nodule (*arrow*).

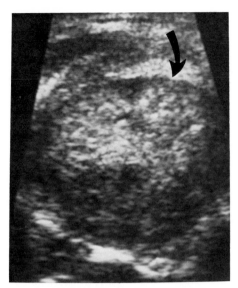

Fig. 7-5. Sonogram of follicular adenoma with halo (*arrow*) and cystic degeneration centrally.

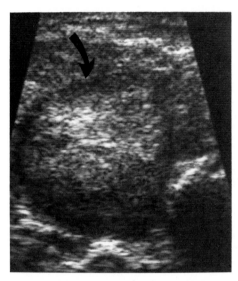

Fig. 7-6. Sonogram of papillary carcinoma also showing peripheral halo (*arrow*).

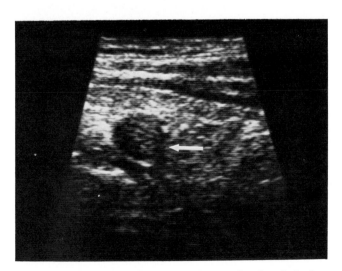

Fig. 7-7. Sonogram of follicular carcinoma that is relatively echopenic (*arrow*).

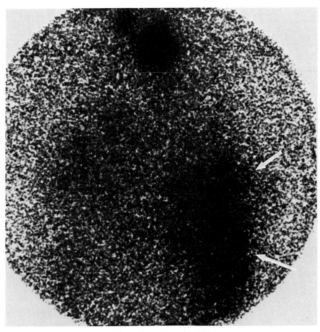

Fig. 7-8. Uptake of ^{131}I by thyroid carcinoma metastases in the right lung (*arrows*) in this posterior projection.

THYROID MALIGNANCIES. Papillary, follicular, and mixed papillary-follicular cell types account for 75 percent of thyroid malignancies. Most of these are relatively low-grade tumors (Fig. 7-7). The papillary type spreads into the cervical lymphatics, whereas dissemination of the follicular type is hematogenous and the metastases may not appear for many years. Fifteen percent of follicular malignancies are anaplastic cancers that occur primarily in patients over age 60 and have a very poor prognosis. Medullary carcinoma accounts for the remaining 10 percent. It is associated with the multiple endocrine neoplasia (MEN) syndromes, but may occur spontaneously. Metastases are blood borne, commonly to the lungs, and can be detected after thyroid ablation by whole-body radioactive iodine scan (Fig. 7-8).

Disorders of the Adrenal Gland

CUSHING'S SYNDROME. Cushing's syndrome is caused by excess ACTH production by the pituitary gland or an ectopic ACTH source, or by excess cortisol secretion by a primary adrenal tumor. Excess ACTH from the pituitary gland accounts for two-thirds of reported cases of this uncommon disorder. Computed tomography is the primary imaging tool for diagnosis of pituitary adenomas. Abdominal CT reveals bilaterally enlarged adrenal glands, which may occasionally be nodular in appearance (Fig. 7-9). Primary adrenal cortisol-secreting tumors may be benign adenomas or malignant carcinomas. Plain films, ultrasound, or CT can demonstrate the tumors, which are frequently large (Fig. 7-10).

PRIMARY ALDOSTERONISM. Primary aldosteronism is caused by adrenal hyperplasia, mineralocorticoid-secret-

212

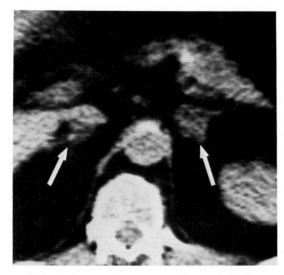

Fig. 7-9. Diffusely enlarged adrenal glands (*arrows*) in Cushing's syndrome secondary to pituitary adenoma.

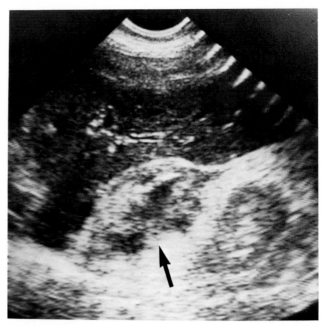

Fig. 7-11. Adrenal carcinoma with central necrosis by ultrasound (*arrow*).

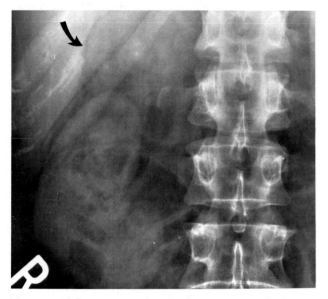

Fig. 7-10. Abdomen x-ray showing large suprarenal adenoma (*arrow*).

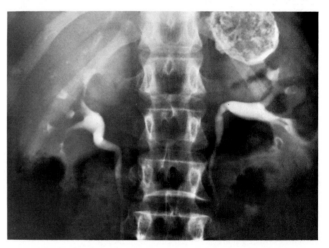

Fig. 7-12. Calcified hematoma of the left adrenal gland.

ing adenomas (Conn's syndrome), and rarely by carcinomas. Adenomas are frequently quite small and must be preoperatively localized by angiography and/or venous sampling for laboratory assay.

ADRENAL CARCINOMAS. About 50 percent of adrenal carcinomas are functional tumors that may cause Cushing's syndrome, feminization or virilization syndromes, and occasionally Conn's syndrome. Computed tomography reveals low-density areas within the mass, and ultrasound shows a complex suprarenal mass (Fig. 7-11). Hepatic metastases are often present at the time of diagnosis.

SOLITARY ADRENAL MASS. Metastases are the most common cause of a solitary adrenal mass. Lung, breast, kidney, ovary, prostate, and melanoma are the most frequent primary tumors that metastasize to the adrenal gland. Chest

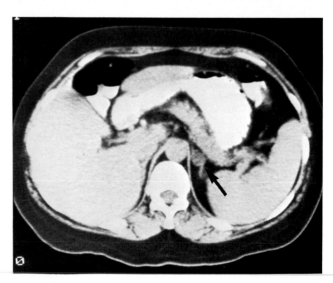

Fig. 7-13. Computed tomography of adrenal adenoma (*arrow*).

CT scans for staging of lung carcinomas should routinely be extended caudad to include the adrenal glands for this reason. There are no CT characteristics that distinguish primary from metastatic adrenal tumors; both may be large and necrotic or contain calcifications.

ADRENAL HEMORRHAGE. Adrenal hemorrhage does occur in the adult, and may present as an incidental finding of suprarenal calcification on abdominal x-ray (Fig. 7-12). Adrenal cysts and nonfunctioning adrenal adenomas may be incidentally identified by CT. The characteristic low-density center and thin periphery confirm the benign nature of the mass (Fig. 7-13).

PHEOCHROMOCYTOMA. The adrenal medulla is part of the sympathetic nervous system. Pheochromocytoma is a catecholamine-producing tumor arising from chromaffin cells in the adrenal medulla or sympathetic ganglia. The catecholamines cause hypertension that is frequently poorly controlled and labile. Approximately 5 percent of pheochromocytomas are malignant, and are often associated with the multiple endocrine neoplasia syndromes. When the clinical and biochemical picture suggests pheochromocytoma, CT is the best imaging modality to localize a tumor. Most extraadrenal pheochromocytomas occur in the abdomen, although sympathetic ganglia in the neck or chest may also give rise to the tumors. Adrenal venography is highly accurate for localized small adrenal lesions.

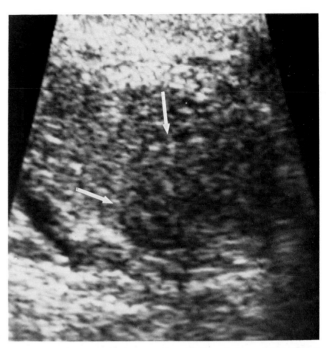

Fig. 7-14. Ultrasound of testis showing focal area of low-level echoes (*arrows*) representing nonpalpable mixed cellular testicular carcinoma.

negative, a CT examination of the abdomen and pelvis is performed.

Disorders of the Testes

TUMORS. Testicular tumors are uncommon but they are frequently malignant. They occur predominantly in young men in their third and fourth decades. Most are of germ cell origin and arise from any of the cellular components of the testes or their embryonal counterparts. Prognosis with a pure seminoma is generally good, but most tumors have mixed elements with poorer prognosis.

Ultrasound is used to diagnose the presence of testicular masses before biopsy, especially if the physical examination is negative, equivocal, or complicated by an associated hydrocele (Fig. 7-14). Ultrasound is a highly sensitive screening tool for testicular masses, but is not very specific. Staging includes abdominal and pelvic CT to evaluate lymphatic spread and chest x-ray for lung metastases. If the CT does not reveal adenopathy, a bipedal lymphangiogram is necessary to evaluate metastatic involvement of normal-sized lymph nodes. The false negative rate of lymphangiography may be fairly high; reported series range from 13 to 35 percent falsely negative lymphangiogram reports. Because most testicular carcinoma patients are young and have minimal body fat, ultrasound is often equivalent to CT in demonstrating abdominal and pelvic adenopathy in such patients, at one-third the cost of CT.

UNDESCENDED TESTICLES. Undescended testicles have a markedly increased malignancy rate. When a testicle cannot be palpated in the scrotal sac or inguinal canal, ultrasound is the initial screening modality because the majority of undescended testicles are located in the inguinal canal between the inner and outer rings. If ultrasound is

Disorders of the Ovaries

PELVIC INFLAMMATORY DISEASE. Ultrasound is the imaging modality of choice in evaluation of pelvic inflammatory disease (PID). Ultrasound usually demonstrates a complex mass with adherent bowel enveloping the fallopian tubes and often extending into the cul-de-sac (Fig. 7-15). The incidence of PID has been increasing over the last decade and has been accompanied by an increased incidence of ectopic pregnancy. Ultrasound often does not image the ectopic gestation itself (Fig. 7-16) but may reveal a pseudogestational sac in the uterus. Failure to demonstrate an intrauterine pregnancy by ultrasound in association with a positive pregnancy test and acute pelvic pain is strongly suggestive of ectopic pregnancy.

ENDOMETRIOSIS. Endometriosis, the presence of foci of endometrium in an extrauterine location, characteristically appears as sonolucent masses on the ovaries, broad ligament, or cul-de-sac.

OVARIAN TUMORS. Ovarian tumors are commonly cystic masses. Dermoids account for approximately 25 percent of ovarian neoplasms and present in younger women. A fat/fluid level on ultrasound, and a characteristic lucent fat density or teeth on abdominal x-rays, are characteristic findings (Figs. 7-17 and 7-18). The serous and mucinous cystadenomas and cystadenocarcinomas are septated cystic adnexal masses (Fig. 7-19). Signs of malignancy include ascites, fixation of bowel loops, and solid areas within the mass. Ovarian carcinomas metastasize to the liver and omentum. Computed tomography is the procedure of

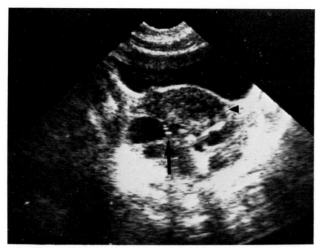

Fig. 7-15. Transverse scan of PID involving both adnexa and the cul-de-sac. Arrowhead indicates uterus. The bright echoes (*arrow*) are caused by air in adherent loops of bowel.

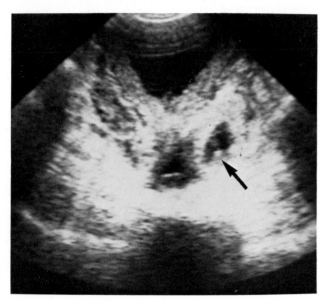

Fig. 7-16. Adnexal gestation sac containing fetal parts (*arrow*).

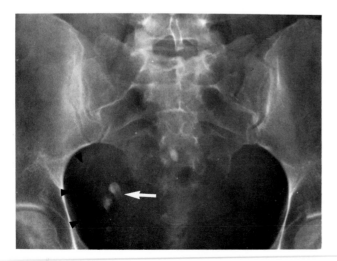

Fig. 7-17. Abdominal x-ray showing lucent mass (*arrowheads*) and teeth (*arrow*) of dermoid cyst.

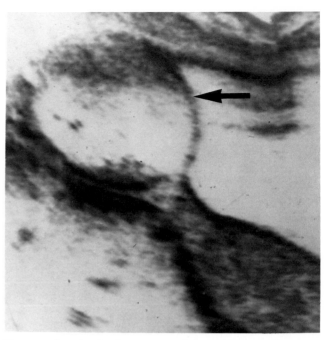

Fig. 7-18. Longitudinal sonogram of dermoid cyst with fat/fluid level (*arrow*).

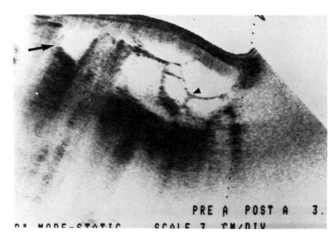

Fig. 7-19. Pelvic cystic mass with septations. Septal thickening (*arrowhead*) and ascites (*arrow*) indicate that this is a cystadenocarcinoma.

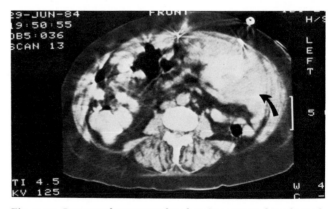

Fig. 7-20. Computed tomography showing omental "cake" of ovarian carcinoma (*arrow*).

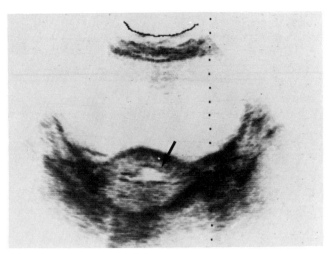

Fig. 7-23. Transverse sonogram of endometrial carcinoma showing typical irregular sonolucent area (*arrow*) in uterine cavity.

acteristic "popcorn" calcifications (Figs. 7-21, 7-22). Ultrasound is frequently employed to determine whether a mass palpated on pelvic examination is a pedunculated fibroid or an adnexal mass. Leiomyosarcoma is uncommon and has no ultrasound features that distinguish it from its benign counterpart. A leiomyoma that increases in size in a postmenopausal woman is most likely malignant.

Endometrial carcinoma is the most common malignancy of the uterus. Ultrasound typically shows an enlarged uterus with irregular sonolucent regions within the endometrium or endometrial cavity (Fig. 7-23).

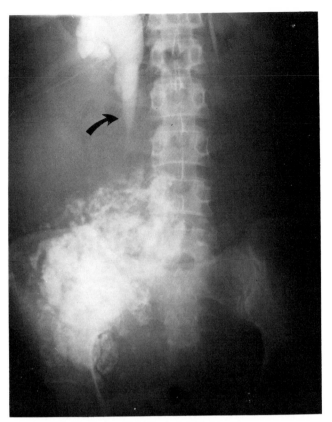

Fig. 7-21. Abdominal x-ray of calcified leiomyoma. The large, pedunculated fibroid caused obstruction of the right ureter (*arrow*).

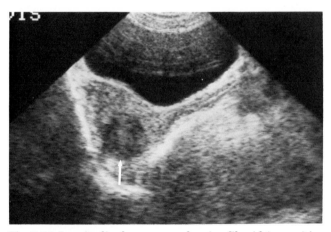

Fig. 7-22. Longitudinal sonogram showing fibroid (*arrow*) in posterior myometrium.

choice to demonstrate spread of ovarian carcinomas to bowel, peritoneum, liver, and retroperitoneal lymph nodes (Fig. 7-20).

Disorders of the Uterus

Leiomyoma of the uterus is best imaged with ultrasound. It may exhibit a variety of sonographic features and often is evident on abdominal x-rays as a pelvic mass with char-

Disorders of the Cervix

Cervical carcinoma is the third most common malignancy in women. Abdominal and pelvic CT is utilized to evaluate pelvic sidewall, parametrial, and lymphatic involvement. Cervical carcinoma frequently involves or compresses the ureters, causing hydronephrosis. Ultrasound readily demonstrates this complication, but CT is required if the level of ureteral obstruction must be demonstrated.

Bibliography

Thyroid
Van Herle, A. J., et al. The thyroid nodule. *Ann. Intern. Med.* 96:221, 1982.

Adrenal
Hussain, S., et al. Differentiation of malignant from benign adrenal masses. *A.J.R.* 144:61, 1985.
Tisnado, J., et al. Computed tomography versus angiography in the localization of pheochromocytoma. *J. Comput. Assist. Tomogr.* 4:853, 1980.

Testis
Batata, M. A., Whitmore, W. F., Jr., and Chu, F. C. H. Cryptorchidism and testicular cancer. *J. Urol.* 124:382, 1980.
Glazer, H. S., et al. Sonographic detection of occult testicular neoplasms. *A.J.R.* 138:673, 1982.
Hainsworth, J. D., and Greco, F. A. Testicular germ cell neoplasms. *Am. J. Med.* 75:817, 1983.

Hricak, H., and Filly, R. A. Sonography of the scrotum. *Invest. Radiol.* 18:112, 1983.

Postkitt, K. J., Copperberg, P. L., and Sullivan, L. D. Sonography and CT in staging nonseminomatous testicular tumors. *A.J.R.* 141:939, 1985.

Wallace, N. Lymphography in the management of testicular tumors. *Clin. Radiol.* 20:435, 1969.

Ovary and uterus

Gross, B. H., et al. Computed tomography of gynecologic diseases. *A.J.R.* 141:765, 1983.

8. Neurologic Disorders

Donald W. Chakeres

Cerebrovascular Disease

There is a wide range of indications for radiographic evaluation of possible cerebrovascular disease, since a wide range of neurologic symptoms can be encountered secondary to ischemia. Frequently the diagnosis of cerebrovascular disease is clear on clinical grounds, but radiographic evaluation is essential both to quantify the extent of disease and establish the underlying cause (e.g., vasculitis, embolus) while excluding other causes so that the proper therapy can follow (Fig. 8-1).

CEREBRAL ISCHEMIA. Computed tomography and MRI are the best screening exams for evidence of cerebral ischemia (Fig. 8-2). In those patients who have transient ischemic attacks (TIA) with no permanent injury to the brain, the exam may fail to demonstrate acute changes. There may be other findings to suggest vascular pathology, such as old infarctions or calcified vertebral, carotid, or superficial temporal arteries. Other screening exams, such as ultrasound of the carotid bifurcations, nuclear medicine flow study (rapid sequence imaging), and intravenous digital subtraction angiography (computer enhanced fluoroscopy) may demonstrate major abnormalities. Standard intraarterial angiography with its greater precision is indicated if surgical intervention or long-term anticoagulation therapy is considered.

Ischemic brain infarctions with permanent injury typically evolve in CT appearance over a matter of months and in a relatively standard fashion. The initial CT exam (done less than 48 hours from onset of symptoms) may be negative despite clinical evidence of major neurologic deficit. After a short interval brain edema occurs, making the infarction appear as a low-density area that conforms to a region of brain supplied by the affected cerebral vessels (Fig. 8-2). Occasionally the dense thrombosed vessel is visible. If the lesion is large, there may be significant mass effect with obliteration of the adjacent cisterns, compression of the adjacent ventricles, and midline shift to the opposite side. The degree of mass effect is usually smaller than a neoplasm involving a similar volume of brain. On CT with contrast injection there may be enhancement at the periphery or center of the infarct secondary to breakdown of the blood-brain barrier; enhancement of the entire infarct is uncommon. Magnetic resonance imaging can show areas of brain edema that are similar in distribution to those shown on CT. At times MRI is more sensitive than CT, but unfortunately MRI findings are nonspecific. Radionuclide brain scans show areas of increased activity on delayed scans that correspond to regions of abnormal blood-brain barrier.

If bleeding occurs within the infarction, the CT image may look like a spontaneous intracerebral hemorrhage and mask the underlying infarction. Differentiation of low-grade tumors from early infarcts may be difficult without sequential scans. With time (weeks to months) the infarction involutes, leaving a residual, nonenhancing, low-density area on CT. Evidence of focal brain atrophy is dem-

218

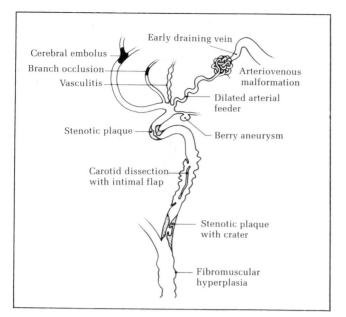

Fig. 8-1. Common pathologic entities associated with vascular disease. This diagram is a lateral view of a common carotid angiogram.

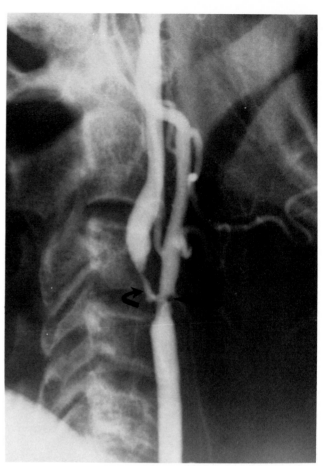

Fig. 8-3. A high-grade stenosis (*curved arrow*) of the origin of the internal carotid artery caused by arteriosclerotic disease is seen on this lateral common carotid angiogram. Note that external carotid artery is also narrowed (*straight arrow*) but to a lesser degree. The caliber of the internal carotid artery at the bifurcation should be similar to that of the common carotid.

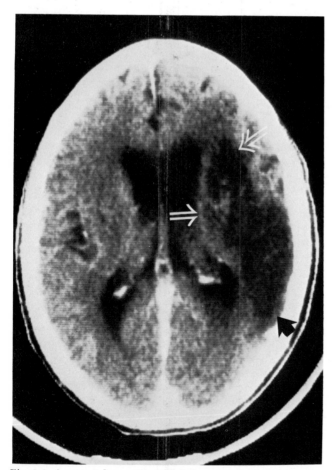

Fig. 8-2. A recent, large, triangular, low-density brain infarction (*arrows*) conforming to the left middle cerebral artery distribution is seen on this axial CT scan. Note mild diffuse mass effect visible by compression of the cisterns and sulci.

onstrated by enlarged adjacent cisternal and ventricular spaces.

Cerebral angiography is the definitive exam for evaluating the cerebral vascular systems; however, intravenous digital studies can demonstrate pathology of the great vessels, dural sinuses, and the major intracranial circulation. Advantages of intravenous digital studies include no arterial puncture, fewer neurologic complications, outpatient care, and high patient acceptance. Disadvantages include less than optimal resolution of small cerebral vessels, inability to study single vessels, dependence on patient cooperation, and good cardiac output. Intraarterial angiography is usually done through an intraarterial catheter. This technique is essential for visualization of small cerebral vessels in great detail and identification of subtle abnormalities, such as vasculitis. The risk of neurologic complications from angiography is higher than for many other diagnostic exams, but the information gained cannot be acquired by any other modality.

Arteriosclerotic Disease. Arteriosclerotic vascular disease most commonly involves the origins of the vertebral, subclavian, and innominate arteries, the carotid bifurcations, and the distal internal carotid. (Ultrasound can be used to visualize the carotid bifurcations.) Stenoses or total occlu-

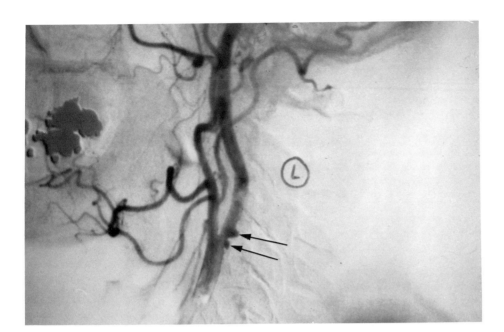

Fig. 8-4. Two small indentations (*arrows*) into a stenotic arteriosclerotic plaque of the internal carotid artery are seen on this lateral selective carotid angiogram. These pockets can be the source of cerebral emboli.

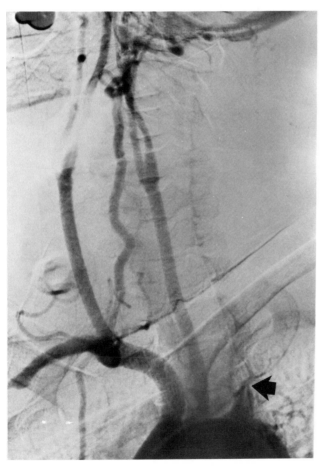

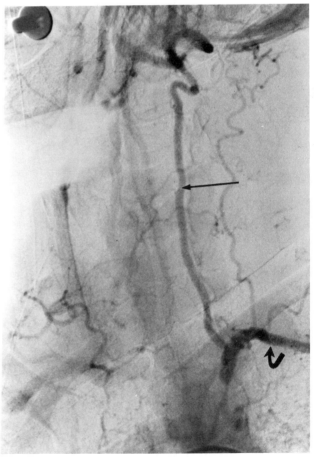

A

B

Fig. 8-5. A. An early arterial film from an oblique arch aortogram demonstrates an occlusion of the proximal left subclavian artery (*arrow*) and no flow within the left vertebral artery. B. On a lateral film of the same angiogram, retrograde flow down the normal left vertebral artery (*straight arrow*) is seen with antegrade flow out the distal subclavian artery (*curved arrow*).

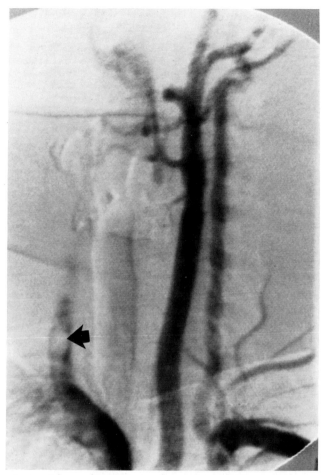

Fig. 8-6. A large embolus (*arrow*) is seen as a filling defect within the lumen of the proximally occluded right carotid artery on this arch aortogram. Note that the right subclavian artery is also occluded. Emboli frequently lodge at vessel bifurcations.

sions are the most common findings (Figs. 8-3, 8-4). Intracranially, arteriosclerotic stenoses or occlusions are seen primarily at vessel bifurcations. Total occlusion of a vessel is recognized by its absence or abrupt termination on the radiograph. Collateral circulation to the brain plays an important role in maintaining tissue viability despite significant vascular occlusions or stenoses. The collateral circulation circumvents the level of obstruction and reconstitutes the blood supply to an ischemic territory. This compensation produces unusual flow patterns. The characteristic angiographic findings of collateral circulation include retrograde flow, small vessel hypertrophy, delayed arterial filling, and tortuosity.

A classic example of collateral circulation producing cerebral ischemia is *subclavian steal syndrome*. This occurs when there is occlusion or high-grade stenosis of a proximal subclavian artery and reverse flow through the ipsilateral vertebral artery to supply the distal subclavian artery (Fig. 8-5A, B), producing a posterior fossa vascular steal and ischemic symptoms.

Cerebral Embolus. Most cerebral emboli originate from the heart (e.g., mural thrombus, atrial myxoma, valvular disease) or from plaques of the carotid bifurcation. Other more unusual emboli include air, bullet fragments, and amniotic fluid. A cerebral embolism can be diagnosed angiographically when a filling defect is visible within a ves-

sel (Fig. 8-6). Emboli usually lodge at bifurcations. Unfortunately, most emboli produce a complete obstruction and differentiation from thrombosis is not possible.

Arteritis-Vasculitis. The angiographic findings of arteritis-vasculitis include tightly spaced focal areas of stenosis and dilatation (arterial beading), small aneurysm formation, vascular occlusions, and extensive collateral circulation development (Fig. 8-7). Differentiation from spasm induced by subarachnoid hemorrhage or severe arteriosclerotic small vessel disease is difficult. The diagnosis of vasculitis is suggested by the clinical history of drug abuse, bacterial endocarditis, elevated sedimentation rate, meningitis, or encephalitis and is confirmed by positive meningeal or temporal artery biopsy.

Carotid Dissection. Carotid dissection, which is more common in females, is seen following trauma, with fibromuscular hyperplasia, or for unknown cause. There may be complete carotid occlusion or only narrowing of the lumen. The characteristic angiographic finding is irregular, undulating narrowing of the internal carotid from the bifurcation to the skull base. A linear filling defect representing the free intimal edge (Fig. 8-8) is occasionally seen.

Fibromuscular Dysplasia. Fibromuscular dysplasia of the carotid arteries is usually seen in females. On angiography the internal carotid artery has a lobulated-beaded contour (Fig. 8-9). High-grade stenosis, dissection, aneurysm, or intracerebral vessel occlusion may be present. Surgical intraluminal dilatation has been used for therapy.

Venous Thrombosis. Patients with cerebral venous thrombosis frequently have a history of severe dehydration, malignancy, recent pregnancy, or hypercoaguable blood. Thrombosis of cortical veins and dural sinuses can be radiographically visualized. The characteristic CT findings include brain edema (low-density areas of the white matter and compression of the ventricles and cisternal spaces) and increased density within the dural sinuses related to clot formation on nonenhanced studies. Following intravenous enhancement there is no change in the density of the dural sinuses, since no contrast reaches them (Fig. 8-10). Angiography and nuclear brain scan can also show lack of flow in the dural sinuses.

INTRACRANIAL HEMORRHAGE. Subarachnoid Hemorrhage. Acute subarachnoid hemorrhage usually presents as a severe acute headache that may be followed by neurologic deficits and coma. Common causes of subarachnoid hemorrhage include aneurysm, arteriovenous malformation, and trauma. Subarachnoid hemorrhage is seen on CT as an area of increased density conforming to a portion of the subarachnoid space. The distribution of the hemorrhage suggests the location and etiology of the bleeding site.

Intraventricular Hemorrhage. Most intraventricular hemorrhages arise from intracerebral or subarachnoid hemorrhages that rupture or reflux into the ventricles. Intraventricular hemorrhage is seen on CT as an area of increased density within the dependent portion of the ventricular system. If only a portion of the ventricle is filled with blood, a blood-fluid level between the blood below and the normal cerebral spinal fluid (CSF) above is visible (Fig. 8-11). Retracted clots may form a cast of the ventricle. Acute hydrocephalus may also occur as blood obstructs normal CSF flow.

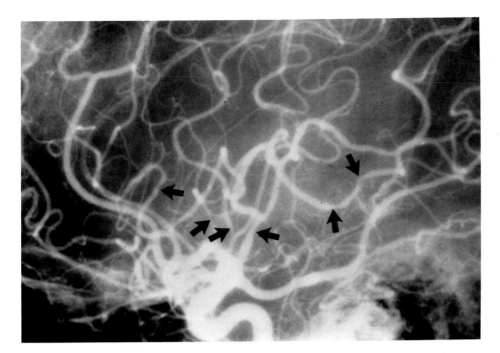

Fig. 8-7. Multiple small intracerebral vessel stenoses (*arrows*) are seen involving the middle cerebral artery on this lateral carotid artery angiogram in a patient with cerebral arteritis. Following inflammation of an artery, occlusions, aneurysms, or unusual cerebral collateral vessels may develop.

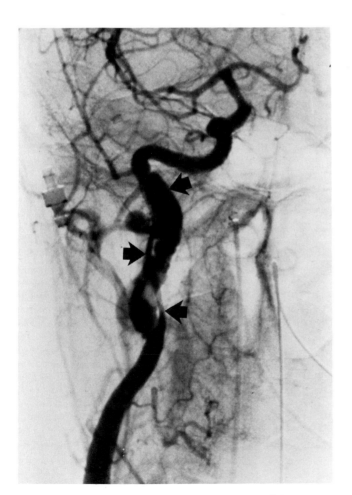

Fig. 8-8. A carotid dissection (*arrows*) is seen on this anterior-posterior angiogram. Note the corrugated appearance of the vessel wall. The linear stripe through the vessel is related to a flap of intima that has been dissected away from the media. Complete occlusion of the cervical carotid can occur.

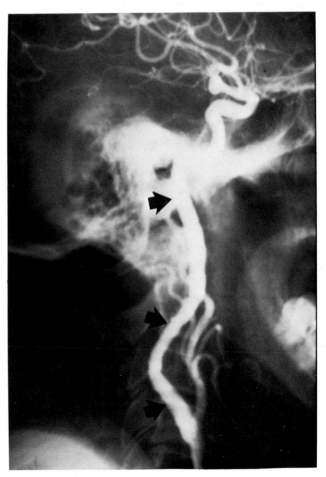

Fig. 8-9. The cervical carotid artery (*arrows*) has a corrugated appearance on this lateral carotid artery angiogram secondary to fibromuscular dysplasia. A similar vascular appearance can be seen involving the renal arteries.

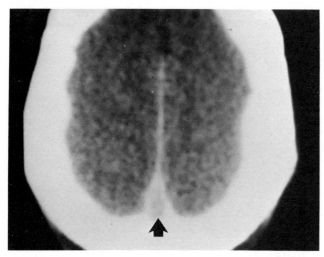

Fig. 8-10. This axial contrast-enhanced CT scan through the vertex of the skull shows a lucent triangle within the superior sagittal venous sinus (*arrow*), which can indicate dural thrombosis, since the sinus should enhance like all of the other vascular structures.

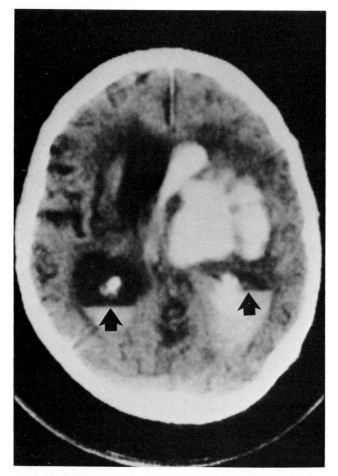

Fig. 8-11. A large hypertensive basal ganglion hemorrhage is seen on this axial non-contrast–enhanced CT scan. Note surrounding edema and mass effect. The hemorrhage (*arrows*) has also ruptured into the lateral ventricles, forming blood-fluid levels in the occipital horns.

Intracerebral Hemorrhage. The cause of an intracerebral hematoma may be a hypertensive bleed, aneurysmal rupture, hemorrhagic infarct, trauma, arteriovenous malformation, coagulopathy, or hemorrhagic tumor. Intracerebral hemorrhage is best evaluated by CT. Almost all intracerebral hemorrhages are dense on initial CT scans, because clotted blood is denser than brain tissue. Although small hemorrhages may not be associated with mass effect, most large hemorrhages do cause compression of the ventricles, obliteration of subarachnoid spaces, herniation, and midline shift. Surrounding brain edema appears as a low-density halo. Hypertensive bleeds usually involve the basal ganglion, cerebellum, brainstem, or periventricular white matter tracts.

Cerebral Aneurysm. Most patients with rupture of a cerebral aneurysm are initially evaluated by CT for a possible intracranial bleed. The distribution of the subarachnoid hemorrhage on CT usually indicates the location of the aneurysm. For example, blood in the inferior portion of the anterior interhemispheric fissure suggests an anterior communicating artery aneurysm. Occasionally, giant (> 1 cm) aneurysms can be seen as circular masses with crescent-shaped peripheral calcifications on CT. The central lumen is enhanced with intravenous contrast.

Once an aneurysm is suspected, intraarterial angiography is essential for defining the number of aneurysms and their size and shape, and helping to assess which one has bled, if aneurysms are multiple (Fig. 8-12). Most aneurysms are seen at vessel bifurcations near the circle of Willis. Mycotic aneurysms characteristically occur more distally, but can mimic idiopathic aneurysms. Lobulated projections from vessels with narrowed necks are most common. Large fusiform aneurysms are more common in elderly patients and present as a mass lesion. The vessels may be displaced if there is an associated intracerebral hemorrhage. Within a week following subarachnoid hemorrhage, diffuse cerebral artery spasm is seen as narrowed areas with slow flow near the aneurysm. Brain infarction may follow.

Arteriovenous Malformation. Patients with arteriovenous malformation (AVM) may be entirely asymptomatic or may present with subarachnoid or intracerebral hemorrhage, focal neurologic symptoms, head bruits, congestive heart failure, or seizures. Arteriovenous malformations have a characteristic CT appearance. Massively enlarged serpentine arteries and veins form a dense mass of clustered abnormal vessels. There may be subarachnoid or intracerebral hemorrhage and small punctate calcifications. Magnetic resonance imaging shows the tortuous vessels as low-intensity loops (Fig. 8-13). Angiography is essential for defining the arterial supply, the nature and location of the vascular malformation, the venous drainage, and possible associated aneurysms. Rapid shunting of blood occurs from the arterial side through the malformation into dilated veins (Fig. 8-14). Some AVMs are poorly seen by any radiographic modality; these are small vessel malformations that do not have rapid flow through them.

Brain Neoplasms

Computed tomography, nuclear medicine brain scan, and MRI all can be used as screening procedures for brain neoplasms. All are very sensitive for detection of lesions, but

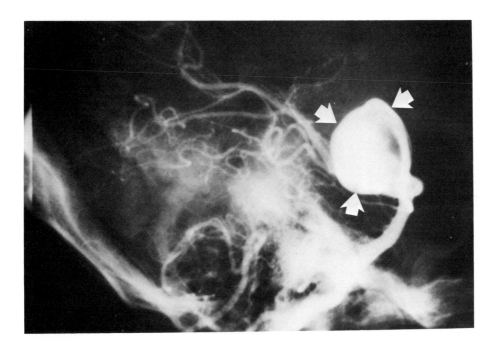

Fig. 8-12. A giant basilar artery aneurysm (*arrows*) is seen on this lateral vertebral angiogram. Aneurysms of this size may present with symptoms related to hemorrhage, mass effect, or hydrocephalus.

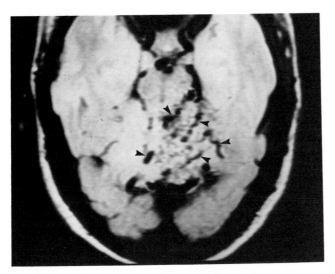

Fig. 8-13. Multiple serpentine low-signal intensity areas related to a cerebral arteriovenous malformation within and adjacent to the cerebellum (*arrowheads*) are seen on this axial MRI. Vessels with high flow usually appear to have no signal on MRI. Occasionally high-signal intensity foci are also seen if there has been an associated hemorrhage.

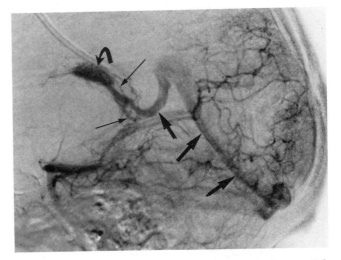

Fig. 8-14. A lateral vertebral angiogram film from the arterial phase demonstrates enlarged arteries (*small arrows*) feeding into a vascular malformation (*curved arrow*), which rapidly drains into the internal cerebral veins and straight sinus (*large arrows*).

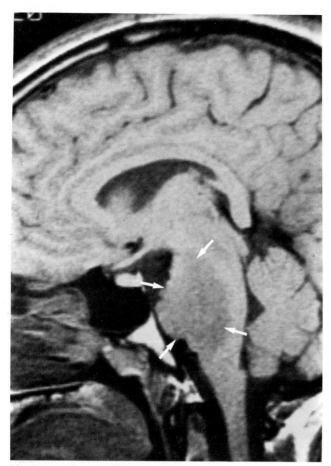

Fig. 8-15. A low-grade pontine glioma (*arrows*) is seen as a low-intensity mass within the brainstem on this sagittal MRI image. Note the irregularity of the exophytic anterior margin and the posterior displacement of the fourth ventricle.

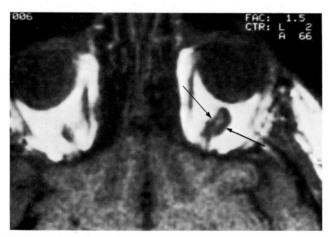

Fig. 8-16. An enlarged tortuous optic nerve secondary to an optic glioma (*arrows*) is seen on this axial MRI image. Differential diagnosis includes meningioma of the optic nerve sheath.

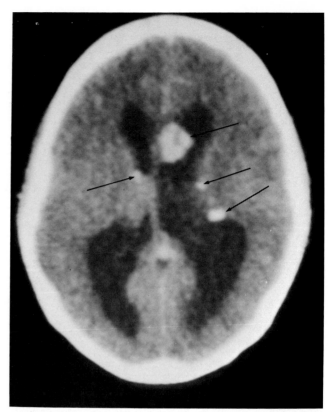

Fig. 8-17. Multiple densely calcified subependymal low-grade astrocytomas (*arrows*) are seen on this axial contrast-enhanced CT scan. The location and calcification of these tumors are characteristic for tuberous sclerosis. Hamartomas of tuberous sclerosis usually involve the cortex and are not periventricular in location.

further studies may be needed for complete characterization. Angiography is indicated to help define the type of tumor, location, arterial supply, vascularity, and dural venous sinus involvement.

GLIOMAS. Gliomas include astrocytomas, oligodendrogliomas, and ependymomas, which are named by their site of origin and their histologic grade. The lower the grade, the less biologically aggressive the tumor. For example, a low-grade glioma arising from the hypothalamus is a grade I hypothalmic glioma. On CT, well-differentiated astrocytomas can be difficult to recognize because of minimal contrast enhancement, little change in brain density, subtle mass effect, and subtle enlargement of brain structures. Metrizamide computed tomography-cisternography may help define small changes in brain surfaces. Bulbous enlargement of the brainstem or optic nerves by gliomas is a classic finding (Figs. 8-15, 8-16). Giant cell astrocytomas are seen most classically as periventricular calcified masses in tuberous sclerosis (Fig. 8-17). Cystic cerebellar gliomas in children present with a small enhancing nodule in the wall of a posterior fossa cyst. A calcification within the temporal lobe without any other finding may be a temporal lobe glioma. Magnetic resonance imaging is more sensitive than CT for the identification of the presence and extent of low-grade gliomas. Magnetic resonance imaging frequently shows changes related to the presence of brain and tumor edema beyond CT findings, particularly for lesions of the posterior fossa. Nuclear medicine scans may show focal areas of increased cerebral accumulation of the

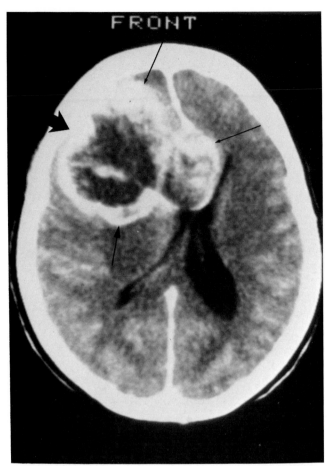

Fig. 8-18. This axial contrast-enhanced CT scan demonstrates a large rim-enhancing frontal high-grade glioma (*arrows*). The mass has an irregular low-density center and is invading the ventricle.

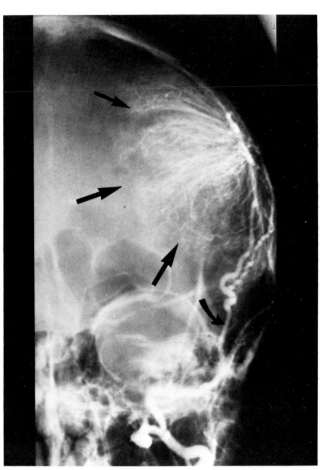

Fig. 8-19. A highly vascular parietal meningioma (*straight arrows*) with radiating stellate tumor vessels within the mass is seen. Note that the arterial blood supply is from a markedly enlarged middle meningeal artery (*curved arrow*).

isotope. Angiography can show displacement of the blood vessels due to the enlarging mass.

On CT aggressively malignant gliomas are more easily recognized than low-grade tumors, since there may be low-density regions within the mass or surrounding white matter tracts, marked irregular contrast enhancement, extensive mass effect, a donut or ring-like appearance, invasion of the ventricles and ependymal surfaces, or extension into the adjacent brain structures following the normal nerve tracts (Fig. 8-18). As an example of the infiltrative invasion through nerve tracts, a glioma can cross from one hemisphere to the opposite via the corpus callosum, forming a butterfly-shaped mass. Differentiation of a glioma from an abscess, lymphoma, metastasis, radiation necrosis, old resolving hematoma, or a large infarct can at times be difficult. Frequently, MRI demonstrates findings similar to those of CT related to mass effect; however, MRI frequently demonstrates extensive changes not visible on CT. Nuclide brain scans show high-activity regions. Angiography may show displacement of cerebral vessels by a mass, a tumor blush, irregular abnormal vasculature within the mass, and veins draining earlier than normal.

MENINGIOMAS. Meningiomas characteristically induce thickening, expansion, and sclerosis (hyperostosis) of the skull. Involvement of the clinoids, or greater wing of the sphenoid or calvarium, may produce characteristic findings on plain radiographs. Less commonly, there is lyt-

ic skull destruction. Enlarged middle meningeal artery impressions on the skull also suggest meningioma, since these vessels frequently supply the tumor (Fig. 8-19).

Most meningiomas are isodense with brain on noncontrast CT, but may be calcified and hyperdense. Contrast enhancement produces a densely enhancing mass related to a dural structure. The lesion may have a flat edge if the dural origin is flat (e.g., the falx or tentorium). Rarely, meningiomas may arise within the ventricles; this is seen particularly in neurofibromatosis. Some meningiomas are associated with little or no mass effect, suggesting very slow benign growth, while others demonstrate severe mass effect. The latter are usually associated with extensive white matter edema. Occasionally, the tumors are partially cystic. Most meningiomas are quite vascular and are easily visible on angiography, which is helpful in defining the type of tumor since the blood supply to these tumors is dual. Enlargement of meningeal arteries supplying the central portion of the tumor is seen. The periphery of the lesion may parasitize cortical cerebral vessels. Magnetic resonance imaging may overlook meningiomas since they appear isodense with brain, but the surrounding edema is visible. Radionuclide brain scans are sensitive to the presence of most meningiomas, unless they are small or near the skull base.

BRAIN METASTASES. Most brain metastases are seen on CT as multiple masses that increase in density following

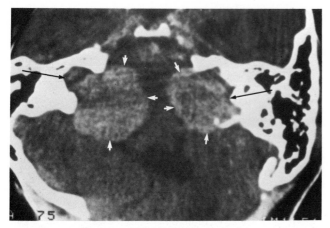

Fig. 8-20. Bilateral acoustic neuromas (*arrows*) are seen on this axial contrast-enhanced CT scan. Circular enhancing masses that indent the fourth ventricle are centered at the enlarged internal auditory canals. This patient also had neurofibromatosis.

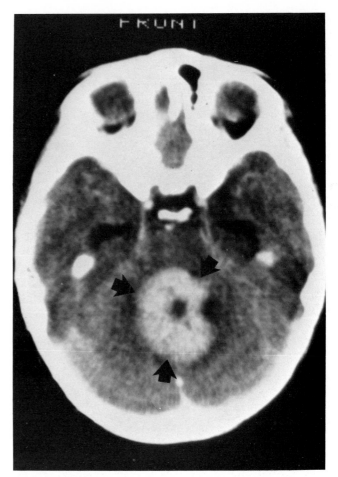

Fig. 8-21. A densely enhancing partially cystic fourth ventricular medulloblastoma (*arrows*) is seen on this axial CT scan. Note the obliteration of the fourth ventricle and dilatation of the temporal horns related to obstructive hydrocephalus.

intravenous contrast infusion. They may be surrounded by extensive white matter edema. Metastases are frequently hemorrhagic, malignant melanoma particularly. Squamous cell carcinomas may be cystic. A single brain metastasis is difficult to differentiate from an abscess or primary neoplasm. Other lesions that may mimic metastases include infarcts, multifocal gliomas, and hemorrhages.

PERIPHERAL NERVE TUMORS. Neurofibromas, neurilemmomas, and schwannomas are related benign tumors that all arise from peripheral nerves. Tumors in the head are named by the nerves from which they arise; for example, acoustic neuromas arise from the eighth cranial nerve and trigeminal neuromas from the fifth cranial nerve. On plain radiographs smooth enlargement of the affected nerve foramen (e.g., the internal auditory canal, foramen ovale) suggests the diagnosis (Fig. 8-20). Computed tomography is necessary to define the soft-tissue component of the tumor, brain edema, hydrocephalus, and mass effect. Most nerve tumors enhance but have little associated mass effect because of slow growth. Acoustic neuromas characteristically enlarge the internal auditory canal asymmetrically. A mushroom-shaped enhancing mass projects into the cerebellar pontine angle on contrast-enhanced CT. Small lesions (< 1 cm in diameter) can be visualized by directing air into the internal auditory canal and then studying it with CT. Trigeminal neuromas extend from the lateral prepontine cistern into the region of Meckel's cave and may extend through the foramen ovale. Hypoglossal and vagal neuromas may also occur. If multiple tumors are present, the diagnosis of neurofibromatosis is suggested.

MEDULLOBLASTOMAS. Most medulloblastomas are seen in children and arise in the anterior vermis of the cerebellum. The tumor appears to fill the fourth ventricle and almost universally produces obstructive hydrocephalus (Fig. 8-21). The tumor may or may not calcify or enhance. Medulloblastomas have a high incidence of metastasis to the surface of the brain, which can be seen on enhanced CT, and to the spinal cord, which can be seen on myelography.

PINEAL REGION TUMORS. Pineal region tumors may be of many different tissue types and include dysgerminoma, pinealblastoma, teratoma, dermoid, and glioma. Some of the tumors have extensive calcifications that can be seen on plain radiographs in the region of the pineal gland. Many of these tumors cause obstructive hydrocephalus by blocking the posterior third ventricle and aqueduct. Most tumors are enhanced on CT and fill the quadrigeminal cistern. Dermoids and teratomas may have fat within them and metastasize to the brain and spinal cord surfaces. Magnetic resonance imaging is helpful in localizing pineal tumors in relation to the aqueduct.

PITUITARY TUMORS. Most pituitary tumors are adenomas, but other tumors, such as carcinomas, dysgerminomas, and metastases, can sometimes arise within the sella tursica. There may be minor changes of the sella, visible on either plain radiographs or complex motion tomography, such as thinning, sloping, or bulging of the floor of the sella; however, these findings are common in normal patients without tumors. These minor findings are not reliable in defining tumor presence. There is also a wide range in the normal volume of the sella. Computed tomography and MRI are much better screening exams, since both the gland and the surrounding structures are visible. Micro-

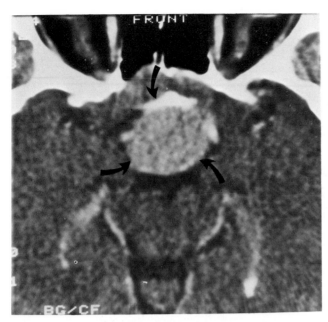

Fig. 8-22. A large circular pituitary adenoma (*arrows*) is seen expanding the sella on this axial CT. The mass has eroded the posterior clinoids and fills the suprasellar cistern.

adenomas (< one cm in diameter) remain within the sella and may be seen as small, low-density areas within the gland on CT. The definitive diagnosis is more accurately made by clinical and laboratory criteria.

Macroadenomas (> 1 cm in diameter) expand or destroy the sella walls, producing a circular configuration of the sella, eroding the clinoids, and extending superiorly into the suprasellar cistern, inferiorly into the sphenoid sinus, or laterally into the cavernous sinus (Figs. 8-22, 8-23). Most enhance, and some are cystic. Suprasellar extension is important since compression of the optic chiasm or hypothalamus may be present. Angiography shows lateral displacement of the cavernous portion of the carotid arteries and elevation of the anterior cerebral arteries. Magnetic resonance imaging is an excellent modality for study of pituitary tumors, since the relation of the tumor to adjacent structures can be imaged by direct coronal or sagittal slices without the need for contrast (Fig. 8-24).

EMPTY SELLA SYNDROME. Empty sella syndrome is seen when the subarachnoid space fills either a portion or all of the pituitary fossa. Most cases are incidentally discovered and usually have no clinical significance. Empty sella can be seen following surgical or radiation therapy of sella tumors, in pseudotumor cerebri, and in conjunction with pituitary tumors. On plain radiographs the sella may be enlarged and egg-shaped rather than circular. Plain film distinction from a tumor may not be possible. Computed tomography or MRI show the sella filled either partially or completely with cerebral spinal fluid. Visualization of the pituitary stalk descending from the hypothalamus to the sella floor helps exclude a cystic sellar mass. Metrizamide cisternography unequivocally confirms empty sella syndrome, since contrast fills the sella. An empty sella and pituitary tumor can exist simultaneously.

CRANIOPHARYNGIOMAS. Craniopharyngiomas can occur at any age, but are most frequently seen in children or middle-age adults. Since many craniopharyngiomas calcify,

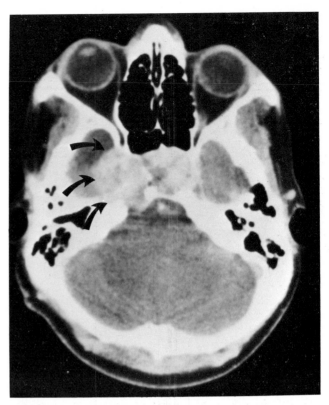

Fig. 8-23. A massive pituitary adenoma (*arrows*) is seen extending out of the sella into the right temporal fossa. Note the circular expansion of the sella.

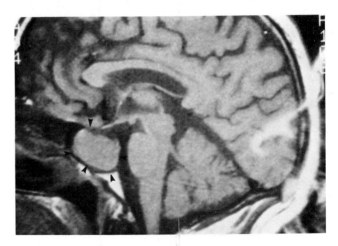

Fig. 8-24. This sagittal MRI demonstrates an enlarged sella (*arrowheads*) secondary to a prolactin-producing tumor. MRI has the advantage of being able to best demonstrate the relationship of the tumor to the optic apparatus.

the tumor can be seen as suprasellar calcifications on plain radiographs. The clinoids may be deformed, but the sella usually is not significantly enlarged. On CT more subtle calcification may be evident (Fig. 8-25). The tumors may be solid or cystic. Some craniopharyngiomas attain large volumes, with the tumor invaginating deeply into the brain (e.g., frontal lobes, thalamus).

CHORDOMAS. Chordomas arise from cell remnants of the notochord and most commonly appear along the clivus,

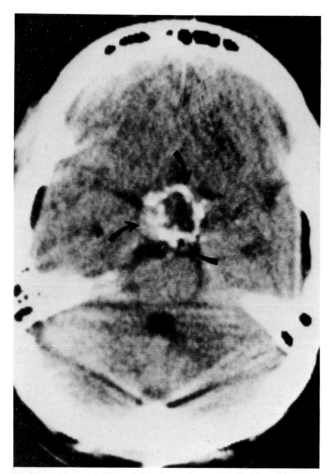

Fig. 8-25. A partially calcified cystic craniopharyngioma (*arrows*) is seen on this axial CT scan. The tumor fills much of the suprasellar cistern.

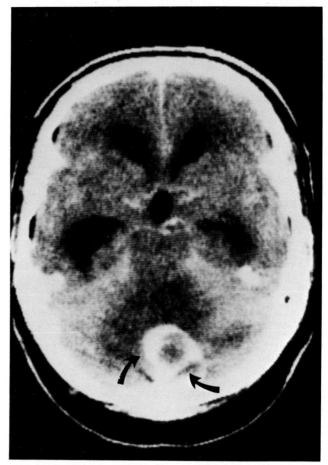

Fig. 8-26. A densely enhancing, partially cystic hemangioblastoma of the cerebellum (*arrows*) with surrounding edema is seen on this axial CT scan. A number of patients with von Hippel-Lindau syndrome also have multiple hemangioblastomas of the brain, spinal cord, and retina.

upper cervical region, and sacrum. Plain films may show destructive changes of the involved bone. Computed tomography better delineates the bony changes, while both CT and MRI can define the soft-tissue component of the tumor. The mass can extend anteriorly into the nasopharynx and posteriorly into the brainstem. On angiography of clivus chordomas the basilar artery and brainstem are displaced posteriorly.

CHOROID PLEXUS PAPILLOMAS. Choroid plexus papillomas can produce communicating or obstructive hydrocephalus by occluding the ventricle. Most tumors are seen on CT as densely enhancing pedunculated masses within a dilated ventricular system. They can arise from any portion of the choroid plexus but are most commonly seen in the trigone of the lateral ventricle, the third ventricle, and the lateral recess of the fourth ventricle. Angiography is of value, since enlarged choroidal vessels supply these vascular tumors.

HEMANGIOBLASTOMAS. Hemangioblastomas usually involve the cerebellum, but also can be seen within the spinal cord. There is a high association between von Hippel-Lindau syndrome and cerebellar hemangioblastomas. These tumors are seen on CT as densely enhancing cerebellar masses (Fig. 8-26). A large adjacent cyst with obstructive hydrocephalus may also be present. Angiography shows a dense, highly vascular mass.

COLLOID CYSTS. Colloid cysts are seen only at the foramen of Monro. They usually present with symptoms related to chronic obstructive hydrocephalus. CT findings in colloid cysts are quite characteristic. A circular mass is centered in the midline at the foramen of Monro and projects into the lateral and third ventricles, with secondary ventricular enlargement. The mass may be lucent or calcified. Colloid cysts may or may not enhance. Angiography is of little value except to exclude aneurysm.

EPIDERMOID, TERATOMA, DERMOID, AND LIPOMAS. Epidermoid tumors are related to retained epithelial rests within the brain or skull base. They are benign, slow-growing tumors filled with desquamated cells, and may be calcified, similar to brain in density, or fatty. They are commonly seen in the cerebellar pontine angle and petrous apex regions, but can occur in almost any location.

Dermoids, teratomas, and lipomas frequently contain fat, which is easily recognized by CT (Fig. 8-27). Many are benign incidental findings involving the corpus callosum. More aggressive tumors, such as pineal teratomas, can seed throughout the subarachnoid space.

SUBARACHNOID CYST. Subarachnoid cysts (Fig. 8-28) usually involve the middle fossa but can occur anywhere.

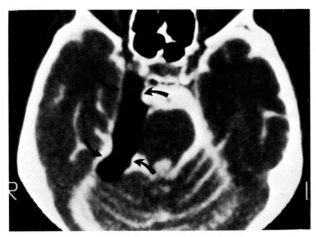

Fig. 8-27. An epidermoid containing fat (*arrows*) is seen extending from the region of Meckel's cave out into the ambient cistern on this metrizamide cisternogram axial CT scan. These soft tumors frequently invaginate into multiple small crevices about the brain.

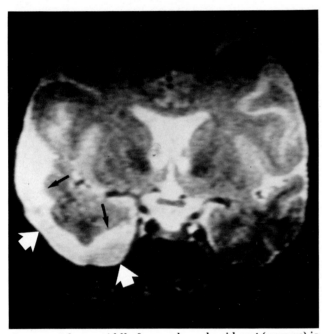

Fig. 8-28. A large middle fossa subarachnoid cyst (*arrows*) is seen expanding the bony margins of the skull base on this coronal MRI. Note that the intensity of the cyst is identical to that of the other normal subarachnoid spaces.

Suprasellar subarachnoid cysts can produce precocious puberty. They are most commonly seen as incidental findings in normal patients, but can cause mass effect and brain compression. On CT and MRI they appear as cystic spaces within or adjacent to the brain. Midline shift, hydrocephalus, or distortion of underlying structures may be present. The skull may be expanded, indicating that the lesion is a developmental change. Magnetic resonance imaging and intrathecal contrast CT studies can help confirm that the cyst is filled with spinal fluid. Occasionally, the cysts are difficult to differentiate from cystic tumors.

PSEUDOTUMOR CEREBRI. Pseudotumor cerebri is most commonly seen in young obese females. They present with headaches and papilledema suggesting brain tumors, but

their course is benign. Computed tomography or MRI does not demonstrate a mass or hydrocephalus; instead, the ventricles are small due to generalized brain edema. Some patients may also demonstrate an empty sella. Exclusion of dural sinus thrombosis or some other cause for generalized brain edema (e.g., toxins, infection) must be made before the diagnosis of idiopathic pseudotumor cerebri is made.

Hydrocephalus

Hydrocephalus is abnormal enlargement of the ventricular system of the brain. Radiographic evaluation is indicated to identify the cause and degree of hyrocephalus, to evaluate the possibility of increased intracranial pressure, and to followup intervention (i.e., ventricular shunt placement). Computed tomography and MRI are the initial exams of choice in adults; ultrasound can be used with infants. If more invasive evaluation, such as a lumbar puncture, is necessary, caution is needed in those patients with suspected increased intracranial pressure to avoid possible precipitation of brain herniation. Placement of a ventricular shunt for pressure measurement and drainage may be indicated before lumbar puncture in patients with apparent hydrocephalus and intracranial pressure.

It is important to understand that the morphologic information on the images can be used to infer intracranial and ventricular pressure, but actual measurement is needed for accurate assessment. For example, a patient may have large ventricles and normal pressure secondary to brain atrophy, with CT findings that are very similar to those of another patient with elevated intracranial pressure and obstructive hydrocephalus. Patients with small ventricles may have elevated intracranial pressure secondary to brain edema. Ventriculography or cisternography with air, metrizamide, or radioisotopes can give insight into the physiology of the cerebral spinal fluid (CSF) circulation (Fig. 8-29).

Fig. 8-29. An anterior view of the skull from a normal radionuclide cisternogram is demonstrated. The isotope that was injected into the lumbar subarachnoid space twenty-four hours earlier has now ascended to fill the upper cervical canal (*black arrows*), basal cisterns (*open white arrow*), and partially extends over the convexities (*arrowheads*).

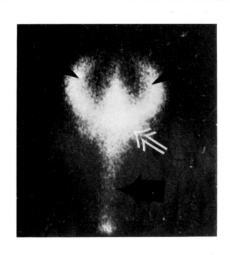

Table 8-1. Obstructive Hydrocephalus

Dilated Ventricular Structures	Level of Obstruction	Common Etiologies
Isolated frontal, temporal, or occipital horns	Within the lateral ventricle	Intraventricular pathology, such as a congenital web; intraventricular tumor, such as a choroid plexus papilloma or an extrinsic compression by brain mass lesions
Single lateral ventricle	One foramen of Monro	Congenital stenosis, primary brain mass, such as a subependymal giant cell astrocytoma of tuberous sclerosis
Both lateral ventricles	Both foramens of Monro	Anterior third ventricular mass, such as colloid cyst, lymphoma, or glioma
Third and both lateral ventricles	Aqueduct or posterior third ventricle	Aqueductal stenosis, posterior third ventricular tumor, such as brainstem glioma, pineal tumor, or cerebellar mass
Third, fourth, and both lateral ventricles	Outlets of fourth ventricle, basal cisternal block, block over the convexities, no obstruction	Communicating hydrocephalous, subarachnoid hemorrhage, meningitis, or generalized brain atrophy

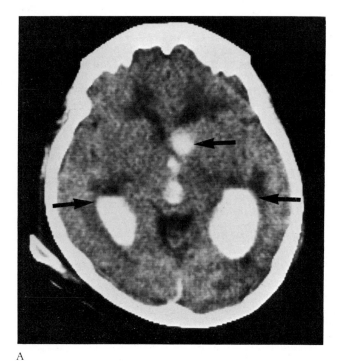

A

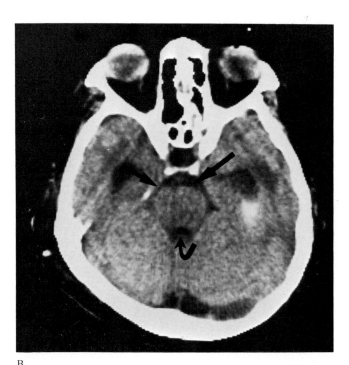

B

Fig. 8-30. A. Intraventricular metrizamide (*arrows*) is seen on this axial CT scan. Note the dilatation of the lateral and third ventricles secondary to a ventricular obstruction below. **B.** A section made through the fourth ventricle (*curved arrow*) fails to demonstrate normal free flow of contrast into the more inferior ventricular and cisternal spaces (*straight arrows*). This study confirms the presence of an aqueductal obstruction.

OBSTRUCTIVE HYDROCEPHALUS. Obstructive hydrocephalus occurs when there is an anatomic block to the normal circulation of CSF within the ventricular system (Table 8-1). Common etiologies of obstructive hydrocephalus include tumors, congenital anomalies (e.g., aqueductal stenosis, Arnold-Chiari malformation, Dandy-Walker syndrome), clot, and ventriculitis. Obstructive hydrocephalus is best documented by the use of a subarachnoid contrast agent (Fig. 8-30). An obstruction to free movement of the contrast agent throughout the complete ventricular and cisternal system is seen. Computed tomography, ultrasound, and MRI can predict the level of obstruction (Fig. 8-31). All of the ventricular structures proximal to the block dilate (Table 8-1). For example, if only one lateral ventricle is enlarged, with contralateral midline shift, then the block is at the foramen of Monro. When the lateral and third ventricles are symmetrically dilated, the level of obstruction is at the aqueduct or posterior third ventricle. If all of the outlets of the fourth ventricle are obstructed then the ventricles are universally dilated. Another CT finding that suggests obstructive hydrocephalus is bulbous enlargement of the ventricular contours (particularly the temporal horns) greater than would be expected for the patient's age. On CT, leakage of CSF through the ventricular walls is seen as low-density areas in the periventricular, frontal, and occipital regions of the white matter (Fig. 8-32). As the ventricles expand, the sulci over the hemispheres are compressed and seem to disappear.

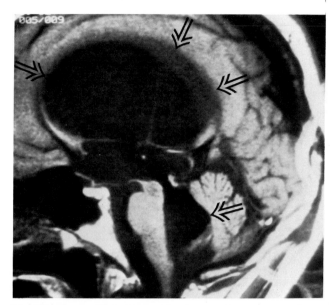

Fig. 8-31. Large dilated ventricles (*arrows*) are seen on this sagittal MRI image of the midline brain. This patient demonstrates bulbous expansion of all of the ventricular structures secondary to congenital obstruction.

COMMUNICATING HYDROCEPHALUS. Communicating hydrocephalus occurs when there is enlargement of the ventricles without an identifiable anatomic obstruction within the ventricular system. The most common causes are prior subarachnoid hemorrhage, infection, normal pressure hydrocephalus, or choroid plexus papilloma. In communicating hydrocephalus there is free flow of a ventricular contrast agent (e.g., air, metrizamide, radioactive isotope) throughout the ventricles, suggesting an abnormality outside the ventricles as the site of underlying pathology. Free movement of the agent through the foramen of the ventricles implies either a basilar cisternal block, an overproduction of CSF, or a problem in reabsorption of CSF in the Pacchionian granulations over the hemispheres. Nuclear cisternography can show both the absence of normal flow of CSF over the convexities and the level of block. Computed tomography shows universal bulbous enlargement of the ventricles, including the fourth ventricle (Fig. 8-33). There may be leakage of CSF through the white matter tract of the frontal or occipital lobes, producing fan-shaped low densities.

OVERPRODUCTION OF CSF. Overproduction of cerebrospinal fluid is an uncommon cause of hydrocephalus. The source is usually a choroid plexus papilloma. On CT the papilloma is an intraventricular pedunculated tumor that arises from a choroid plexus. Choroid plexus papillomas can arise from any portion of the choroid plexus, but most commonly occur in children in the trigone of the lateral ventricles.

NORMAL PRESSURE HYDROCEPHALUS. Normal pressure hydrocephalus occurs in elderly patients and is characterized by gait difficulties, incontinence, and dementia. The diagnosis is made predominantly on clinical grounds. The radiographic exam can exclude other causes, but there are no radiographic pathognomonic findings. Most patients have brain atrophy consistent with their age, so there are no good CT criteria for the diagnosis. Radionuclide cisternography may show reflux of the isotope into the lat-

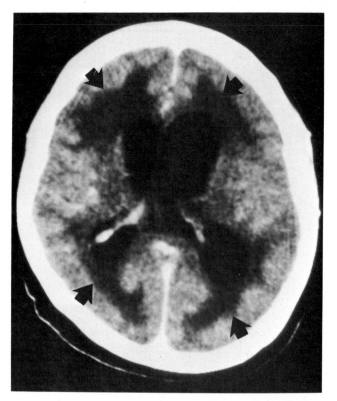

Fig. 8-32. Large low-density areas are seen surrounding dilated lateral ventricles (*arrows*) on this axial CT scan of the brain. These areas are related to leakage of cerebrospinal fluid through the ventricular walls (transependymal reabsorption) in patients with hydrocephalus.

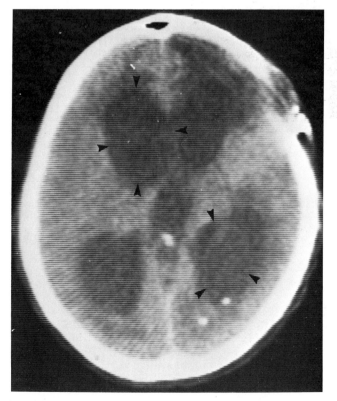

Fig. 8-33. CT scan demonstrates massive ventricular enlargement (*arrowheads*) following the development of communicating hydrocephalus secondary to trauma.

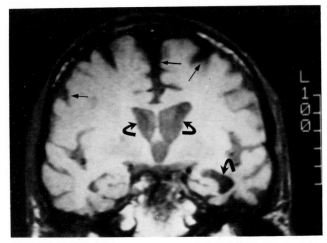

Fig. 8-34. Coronal MRI of a patient with senile dementia demonstrates marked enlargement of the ventricular (*curved arrows*) and cisternal spaces (*arrows*) about the brain secondary to atrophy rather than obstruction.

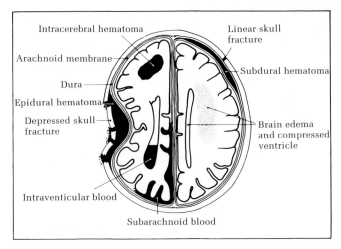

Fig. 8-35. The multiple locations for the accumulation of hemorrhage secondary to cerebral trauma are shown. Their characteristic appearances are also shown.

eral ventricles following a lumbar injection. Unfortunately, despite findings that suggest normal pressure hydrocephalus, there is no good radiographic exam that predicts significant improvement following ventricular shunt.

ATROPHIC HYDROCEPHALUS. Ventricular enlargement is commonly seen in any disorder associated with generalized brain atrophy (hydrocephalus exvacuo) (Fig. 8-34). As the brain shrinks, the adjacent ventricular and cisternal spaces compensatorily enlarge. Differentiation of acute communicating or obstructive hydrocephalus from atrophy is frequently difficult in elderly patients. The findings on CT or MRI that suggest atrophic hydrocephalus include no mass effect, no CSF leakage into the white matter tracts, and simultaneous enlargement of ventricles and sulci due to loss of brain mass.

Cerebral Trauma

Radiographic evaluation following cerebral trauma characterizes the nature and extent of the injury (brain contusion vs. subdural hematoma, for example) so that appropriate therapy can follow (Fig. 8-35). There is a wide range of indications for radiographic evaluation, including loss of consciousness, skull fracture, head bruit, otorrhea, focal neurologic findings, and altered mental status. Even in the absence of any significant clinical findings, a major abnormality, such as subdural hematoma, may be present.

NONDEPRESSED SKULL FRACTURE. Recognition of nondepressed linear skull fractures is of disputed clinical significance. There is poor correlation between significant brain injury and skull fracture; therefore, the presence or absence of skull fracture should not be the primary clinical finding used to direct the patient's care. Computed tomography is the appropriate exam for evaluation of possible brain injury.

The characteristic plain radiographic finding of nondepressed skull fracture is a linear lucency unassociated

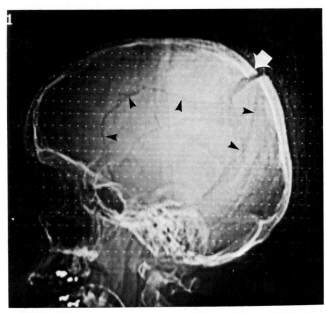

Fig. 8-36. Multiple linear fractures of the skull (*arrowheads*) are seen on this lateral skull image. Note the slight overlapping of the fragment related to depression (*white arrow*).

with a normal structure, such as a suture or vascular impression (i.e., middle meningeal artery) (Fig. 8-36). A fracture does not follow normal anatomic structures unless it is in the form of diastasis of an affected suture. In general, routine skull radiographs are more sensitive than CT for identifying calvarial fractures. Fractures may not be visible if they involve the skull base. In this specialized case, opacification of the sphenoid sinus or mastoid may be circumstantial evidence for a fracture crossing the skull base. Computed tomography may be very useful for evaluating the skull base.

DEPRESSED SKULL FRACTURES. The findings on plain radiographs suggesting depressed fracture include linear increased density related to two layers of calvarium superimposed on one another, and evidence by tangential films that a bony fragment is displaced below the contour of the adjacent normal skull. Depressed skull fractures may be

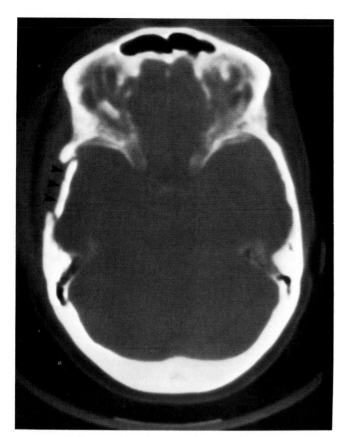

Fig. 8-37. A depressed squamous temporal bone fracture (*arrowheads*) is seen on this axial CT image. Note the overlying soft-tissue swelling.

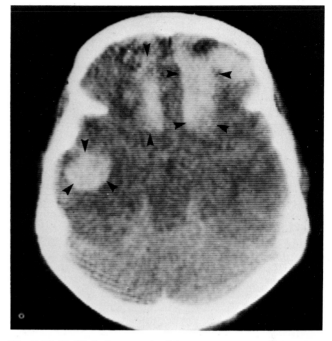

Fig. 8-38. Multiple intracerebral hemorrhages (*arrowheads*) with surrounding edema secondary to brain contusions are seen on this axial CT. Most contusions involve the temporal and frontal lobe poles.

associated with underlying brain injury; therefore, CT is an important study on every patient with depressed fracture (Fig. 8-37). A step-off of the cortical margins of the depressed fragment is visible. Associated brain contusion or blood collection may be visible on CT.

LEPTOMENINGEAL CYST. Occasionally following a linear skull fracture the meninges herniate through the fracture, producing a growing fracture that expands over weeks and can be associated with a palpable scalp soft-tissue mass. This entity may radiographically mimic a benign bone tumor of the skull and occurs most frequently in children.

BRAIN EDEMA AND CONTUSION. Over a period of hours to days after trauma brain edema occurs, causing an isodense expansion of the affected part of the brain on CT. This mass effect obliterates the cisternal spaces, compresses the ventricles, and causes midline shift to the contralateral side if asymmetric. Brain edema alone may account for a very large mass effect without associated hematoma. Focal intraparenchymal hemorrhages are commonly seen as high-density areas within the frontal, temporal, and occipital lobes. These lobes are the ones most frequently contused against the falx and skull base, though any segment of brain can be involved. Follow-up CT in 24 to 48 hours is indicated since delayed hemorrhage into areas of injured brain is common (Fig. 8-38). Those patients who develop infarct-like lesions on CT should undergo vascular evaluation, since carotid or vertebral dissection or traumatic cervical aneurysm may have occurred. In general, angiography adds little to the evaluation of routine head trauma. Radionuclide brain scans are not helpful. Most severely injured patients are not candidates for MRI.

ACUTE SUBDURAL HEMATOMA. Most acute subdural hematomas are seen on CT as high-density, crescent-shaped densities that overlie and compress the adjacent cerebral hemispheres (Fig. 8-39). When a hemispheric subdural hematoma is large, the brain is displaced, with herniation below the falx. The ventricles are shifted to the opposite side and bowing of the falx may be present. If bilateral symmetrical subdural hematomas are present there may be no midline shift, but compression of the ventricles toward the midline will be evident. Collections may also form adjacent to the tentorium or falx; these are seen as high-density stripes, usually with little mass effect. Cerebral angiography demonstrates displacement of the cortical arteries and veins away from the inner table of the skull. Displacement of the anterior cerebral artery and internal cerebral veins across the midline may also be present if the subdural hematoma is unilateral.

Acute hemorrhages are poorly seen on MRI. Brain edema and areas of contusion are more easily identified.

CHRONIC SUBDURAL HEMATOMA. Chronic subdural hematomas may be traumatic in origin but can also be secondary to coagulopathy, anticoagulation, or prior ventricular shunt placement, or can be spontaneous. Chronic subdural hematomas have shape and appearance similar to those of acute subdural hematomas, but the former usually have less associated brain edema. Compression of the sulci and ventricles with brain displacement is seen. When symmetrically bilateral, the ventricles are not shifted from the midline but are displaced medially to form parallel slits (Fig. 8-40). Hemorrhage within the subdural space undergoes a gradual reabsorption process. The blood is metabolized and over a period of weeks begins to resemble spinal fluid. These changes are reflected by CT

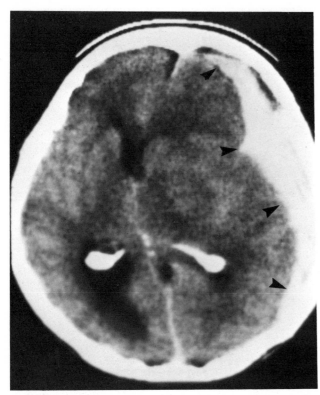

Fig. 8-39. An acute subdural hematoma (*arrowheads*) is seen as a high-density crescent conforming to the contour of the skull on this axial CT. There is associated brain edema and shift of the ventricles to the opposite side.

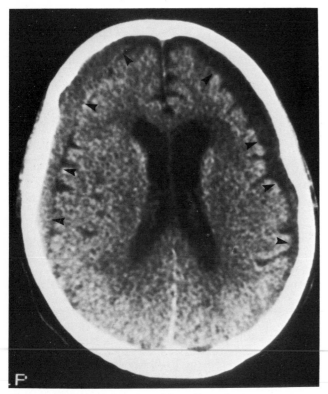

Fig. 8-40. Bilateral chronic subdural hematomas (*arrowheads*) are seen on this axial CT as low-density crescents over the hemispheres. The crescent on the right has a small amount of acute hemorrhage within it, raising its density slightly.

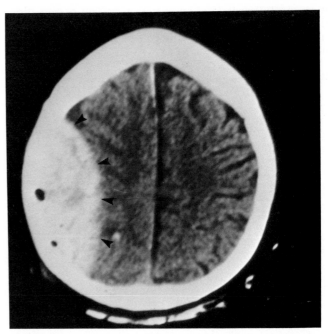

Fig. 8-41. An acute epidural hematoma (*arrowheads*) is seen as a lenticular high-density on this axial CT. There is compression of the adjacent brain and obliteration of the sulci.

scanning. An acute subdural hematoma is initially seen as a dense, crescent-shaped lesion paralleling the inner table of the skull. This same collection gradually decreases in apparent density until it is similar to normal brain on CT. At this time contrast enhancement may be necessary to show an enhancing membrane between the brain and the fluid collection. Late chronic subdural hematomas can be similar to cerebrospinal fluid in density, and differentiation from brain atrophy may be difficult if there is minimal mass effect. Occasionally, acute hemorrhage is seen in chronic subdural hematomas. Radionuclide brain scans can show avascular crescents over the cerebral hemispheres on early images (related to the avascular fluid collections) and areas of increased activity on delayed studies. Cerebral angiography is occasionally of value to confirm the presence of fluid in the subdural space.

Magnetic resonance imaging can more accurately assess the extent and presence of chronic subdural hematomas than can CT. The hematomas stand out as high-intensity crescents over the hemispheres, even though they cannot be differentiated from cerebrospinal fluid on CT. The mass effect is similar to that seen on CT.

EPIDURAL HEMATOMA. Epidural hematomas form a characteristic lenticularly shaped area of increased density underlying the inner table of the skull (Fig. 8-41). Many epidural hematomas are associated with a skull fracture (e.g., of the squamous portion of the temporal bone) and a resulting tear of a dural vessel (e.g., of the middle meningeal artery). In contrast to subdural hematomas, which parallel the skull and subarachnoid spaces, epidural hematomas form a convex margin facing the brain, with more abrupt edges. Essentially all epidural hematomas are dense on CT, since they are acute. When large, the hematoma compresses the adjacent brain, causing brain herniation. The findings on cerebral angiography that suggest an epidural hematoma are displacement of the meningeal vessels away from the skull, formation of an arteriovenous fistula of the meningeal vessels, and an extracerebral fluid collection displacing the underlying brain. Since most epidural hematomas are associated with an arterial bleeding source and a progressively expanding mass, patients do not survive without acute surgical intervention. This accounts for the absence of chronic epidural hematomas.

Demyelinating and Degenerative Diseases

MULTIPLE SCLEROSIS. Multiple sclerosis is an idiopathic disorder causing focal regions of demyelination and is associated with exacerbation and remission of clinical findings. Radiographic evaluation is indicated initially to help confirm the diagnosis or exclude other treatable entities that may mimic the symptoms of multiple sclerosis. In most cases there are few CT findings early in the course of the disease. Late in the disease generalized brain atrophy occurs, with diffuse low-density areas within the white matter. During an active phase of the disease, small focal regions of low-density surrounded by contrast enhancement are most classically seen involving the white matter. Occasionally the lesions are greater than 2 cm in diameter and simulate masses. Any white matter track can be involved, including the optic nerves, which may enlarge transiently in patients with optic neuritis. The CT findings and the clinical symptoms are often transient. Magnetic resonance imaging has been found to be much more sensitive in identifying plaques within the white matter tracks (Fig. 8-42). These plaques are usually seen as regions of high intensity on T_2 weighted images and of low intensity on T_1 weighted images. Visualization of even subtle lesions within the brainstem and spinal cord have been described with MRI. Radionuclide brain scans are of little value.

CENTRAL PONTINE MYELINOLYSIS. Central pontine myelinolysis is a demyelinating disorder seen in alcoholics. Necrosis and demyelination of the fibers of the pons can be seen as a low-density area in the brainstem on both CT and MRI. Patients are frequently disabled by the interruption of the brainstem fibers.

DISMYELINATING DISEASES. Dismyelinating diseases are disorders of the white matter related to abnormal myelin development rather than demyelination of normal myelin, as seen in multiple sclerosis and other acquired diseases. Dismyelinating diseases include the leukodystrophies, Krabbe's disease, and Canavan's disease. The majority of these disorders are hereditary and progressive. The characteristic CT findings include focal low-density areas in the distribution of white matter that may or may not enhance during periods of active degeneration. With time, these involved areas frequently atrophy. In contrast to multiple sclerosis, the extent of dismyelinating disease is usually greater, the onset earlier, and the progression more rapid.

ALZHEIMER'S DISEASE. Alzheimer's disease is a common degenerative process of the brain seen primarily in elderly patients. Some patients may present clinically with dementia before there are significant CT changes. Com-

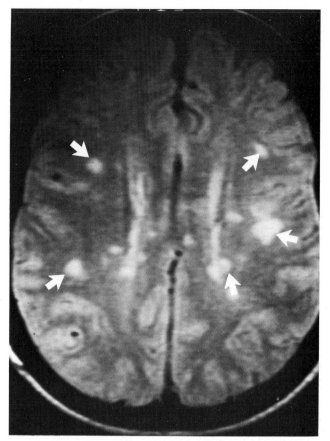

Fig. 8-42. Multiple areas of high-signal intensity (*arrows*) are seen on this axial spin echo MRI image of the white matter tracks on a patient with multiple sclerosis.

puted tomography shows enlarged ventricles and cisternal spaces secondary to brain atrophy. The ventricles may be so large that it is difficult to differentiate Alzheimer's disease from some type of obstructive or communicating hydrocephalus. Detailed volumetric analysis has shown increased ventricular size in those patients with Alzheimer's disease compared to normal controls. There are normal involutional changes of the brain in the elderly that are similar in appearance, but different in degree. Interpretation of CT scans, therefore, needs to be performed in light of the patient's age. Unfortunately, confident diagnosis of Alzheimer's disease in elderly patients based on CT interpretation is poor. Prediction of brain function based on CT appearance for patients generally is also poor.

SPINOPONTINECEREBELLAR DEGENERATION. These are a group of disorders associated with varying degrees of progressive myelopathy, as well as brainstem and cerebellar dysfunction. There may be a family history of similar disease, and some patients have retinitis pigmentosa. Computed tomography and MRI demonstrate atrophy of the affected structures. The volume of the brainstem and cerebellum is decreased (Fig. 8-43). There is compensatory enlargement of the cisterns, including the ambient, prepontine, cerebellopontine, and cisterna magna. The folia of the cerebellum may be quite prominent. Similar changes can be acquired from alcoholic or other toxic injuries to the brainstem.

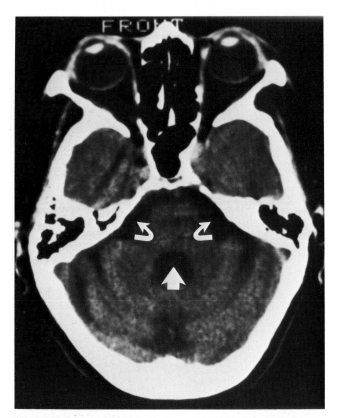

Fig. 8-43. Enlarged cisternal spaces about the cerebellum (*curved arrows*) and a large fourth ventricle (*straight arrow*) are seen on this axial CT scan of a young patient with spinocerebellar degeneration. The degree of atrophy is out of proportion to the patient's age.

HUNTINGTON'S CHOREA. Huntington's chorea is a hereditary autosomal dominant disease that is associated with chorea, dementia, and rigidity and usually presents at middle age. The CT findings described with this disorder include generalized brain atrophy with enlarged ventricles and cisternal spaces. The most characteristic finding on CT is focal exaggerated atrophy of the caudate nuclei and basal ganglia, creating rectangular frontal horns of the lateral ventricle.

PARKINSON'S DISEASE. Parkinson's disease can have a delayed onset after encephalitis, but most cases are idiopathic. There are no consistent radiographic findings. Since most of these patients are elderly, generalized brain atrophy is present. Computed tomography is of value to rule out other treatable causes.

HEPATOLENTICULAR DEGENERATION. Hepatolenticular degeneration, or Wilson's disease, is a hereditary disease associated with abnormal accumulation of copper due to an error in copper metabolism. Many patients may have nervous dysfunction from both degeneration of the basal ganglion and hepatic encephalopathy. Computed tomography is not used as the definitive diagnostic exam. Occasionally, low-density regions of brain necrosis involving the putamen and globus pallidus can be seen.

Brain Infection

In those patients with known central nervous system infection (positive cultures from brain or CSF), radiographic evaluation is important to exclude possible septic complications (abscess, dural sinus thrombosis) and to discover the source of the infection (sinusitis, mastoiditis, or cardiac valve disease).

CEREBRAL ABSCESS AND CEREBRITIS. Early cerebritis presents as low-density areas that may not enhance on CT scan. The appearance may mimic that of a brain infarct or other nonspecific finding. Following a short interval (days), a better developed circular lesion with a low-density center is seen on CT. It enhances at its margins following intravenous contrast, classically appearing as a donut- or ring-shaped lesion (Fig. 8-44). Focal, surrounding white matter edema and mass effect are usually present. Differentiation from a neoplasm at this time on radiographic grounds alone is impossible. Multiple cerebral abscesses suggest a cardiac source or an immunodeficiency accounting for the dissemination. In those patients who are immunosuppressed (by leukemia, AIDS, or chemotherapy), the classic appearance of an enhancing ring- or donut-shaped lesion may be absent secondary to the altered host response. Poorly enhancing focal low-density areas without mass effect are encountered.

Radionuclide brain scanning demonstrates alterations in the blood-brain barrier that are related to infections. Abscesses and cerebritis are seen as regions of increased activity. Occasionally nuclear medicine studies may be positive before changes on CT scans appear. Magnetic resonance imaging can also show brain edema and mass effects prior to CT.

Angiography is indicated in patients with brain abscesses when surgery is planned; no neurosurgeon wants to be surprised by an unexpected mycotic aneurysm. The majority of brain abscesses are avascular masses that displace and distort the cerebral vessels. With severe infection, an associated vasculitis may occur. Vasculitis results in areas of focal vessel narrowing and dilatation, producing the appearance of a string of beads. Complete intracerebral vessel occlusions most commonly occur with opportunistic infections, such as those caused by *Nocardia* or *Aspergillus*. In patients with subacute bacterial endocarditis, the septic emboli may produce mycotic cerebral aneurysms that may rupture and present as cerebral hemorrhages. Dural sinus thrombosis and cortical vein thrombosis can occur in conjunction with severe infections. Such thromboses are more common with an adjacent septic focus, such as osteomyelitis, sinusitis, mastoiditis, and orbital cellulitis. Thrombosed dural sinuses appear dense on CT, due to clotted blood. On CT with intravenous contrast the lumen of the dural sinus appears lucent, due to the lack of blood flow.

MULTIFOCAL LEUKOENCEPHALOPATHY. Multifocal leukoencephalopathy is seen as scattered low-density areas involving primarily the white matter tracts. It is seen usually in patients with suppressed immune responses, due to disorders such as leukemia, lymphoma, or carcinomas, or in patients treated with chemotherapy and steroids. This disorder may be related to a viral etiology.

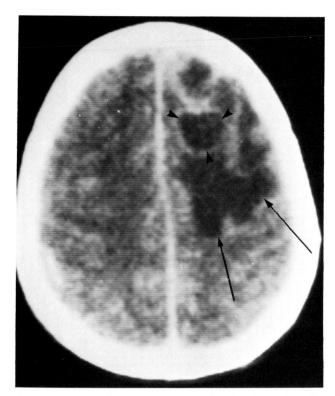

Fig. 8-44. A brain abscess is seen as a circular ring-enhancing mass (*arrowheads*) with surrounding edema (*arrows*) on this axial CT.

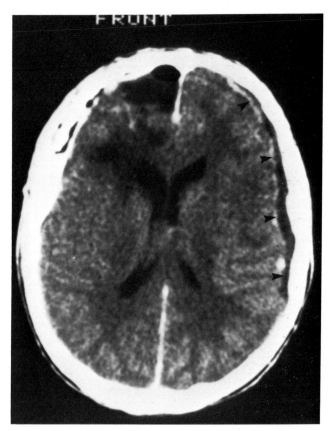

Fig. 8-45. Following drainage of a frontal abscess a CT scan demonstrates a small crescent-shaped low-density subdural empyema collection (*arrowheads*) with an enhancing border overlying the left hemisphere.

MENINGITIS. Despite dramatic clinical symptoms, acute meningitis usually has few significant findings on CT. Enhancement of the subarachnoid spaces and pial membranes following contrast infusion may be seen, particularly at the skull base. In those patients who develop generalized brain edema, obliteration of the ventricular and cisternal spaces may occur, with transtentorial or tonsilar herniation. Acute or chronic hydrocephalus may follow meningitis.

VENTRICULITIS. Ventriculitis is seen in patients with severe purulent meningitis or with abscesses that rupture into the ventricle, as a postsurgical complication (i.e., infected ventricular shunt), and occasionally with aseptic inflammation secondary to rupture of tumors (craniopharyngioma) into the ventricles. Marked contrast enhancement of the ventricular walls and hydrocephalus are characteristic CT findings.

SUBDURAL EMPYEMA. Subdural empyemas usually occur with brain abscesses, open skull fractures, purulent meningitis, or as postoperative complications. They appear on CT as low-density, crescent-shaped fluid collections over the convexity of the brain conforming to the subdural space, and are similar in appearance to chronic subdural hematomas (Fig. 8-45). There may be obliteration of the cerebral sulci and marked mass effect, with compression of the ventricles and shift of the brain to the contralateral side. Computed tomography with contrast demonstrates a densely enhancing membrane at the interface of the brain and subdural fluid collection. Nuclide

brain scan shows increased activity over the affected hemisphere.

SUBDURAL HYGROMA. Subdural hygromas are spinal fluid-like collections in the subdural space that are frequently seen in children after bacterial meningitis. On CT they resemble chronic traumatic subdural hematomas with low-density crescent-shaped fluid collections over the hemispheres. Magnetic resonance imaging may help differentiate these collections from empyemas.

EPIDURAL EMPYEMA. Epidural empyemas are usually seen adjacent to a focus of osteomyelitis of the skull. Primary infections can arise from open skull fractures, postsurgical complications, mastoiditis, or sinusitis. They appear on CT as lens-shaped fluid collections conforming to the epidural space. They resemble acute epidural hematomas in shape, but are of low-density. The epidural abscess margin frequently enhances on CT with contrast infusion, much like the ring around a cerebral abscess. An abnormality of the adjacent skull may be evident, usually as a lytic lesion. Dural sinus displacement or thrombosis frequently occurs in this clinical setting.

ENCEPHALITIS. Encephalitis often has a paucity of radiographic findings. If there is generalized brain edema, CT

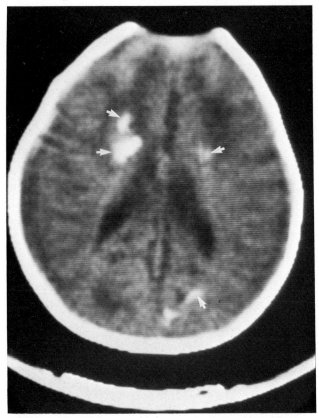

Fig. 8-46. Periventricular calcifications (*arrows*) and large lateral ventricles are seen on this CT of a child with microcephaly secondary to intrauterine infection of toxoplasmosis.

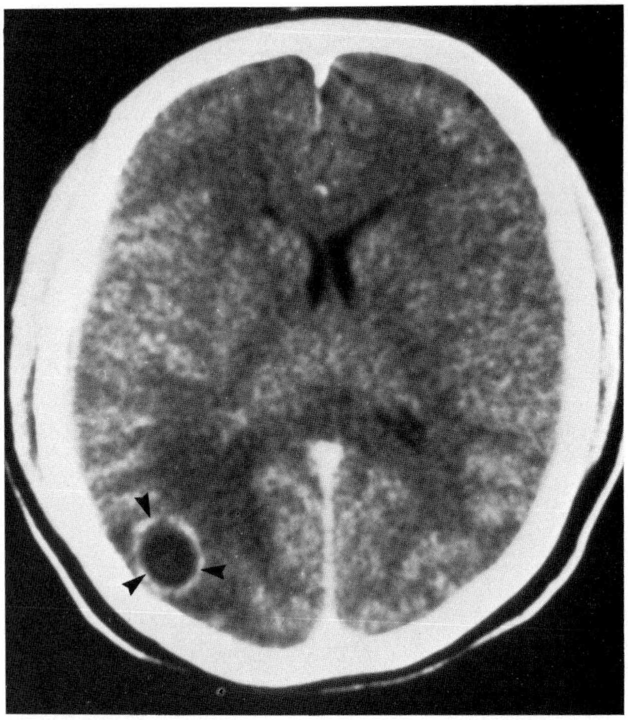

Fig. 8-47. A circular thin ring-enhancing cysticercotic cyst (*arrowheads*) is seen on this axial CT image. Most cysts have a CSF density center. Occasionally eccentric punctate calcification is also present within the mass or elsewhere in the brain.

demonstrates obliteration of the subarachnoid spaces about the brain, compression of the ventricles and possible brain herniation. Herpes encephalitis involves primarily the temporal and frontal lobes. In most cases the disease is bilateral, though asymmetric. Magnetic resonance imaging is frequently more sensitive than CT in subtle cases. Patients are often symptomatic for a few days before the CT scan demonstrates the findings of focal temporal lobe edema. Low-density expansile masses that are slightly enhanced at their margins in the temporal lobes are most commonly seen on CT with contrast infusion. Nuclear medicine brain scan studies may demonstrate areas of increased activity within the temporal fossa related to the hyperemia and inflammation prior to CT changes.

TOXOPLASMOSIS. Toxoplasmosis is usually the result of a congenital intrauterine infection. Severely affected patients frequently present in infancy with microcephaly, seizures, or failure to thrive. The most characteristic finding is multiple periventricular calcifications (Fig. 8-46). There may also be hydrocephalus, regions of brain destruction, and calcifications in the globes. Similar findings can be seen in many congenital central nervous system infections, such as herpes, cytomegalic inclusion disease, and rubella.

CYSTICERCOSIS. Cysticercosis is a parasitic infection endemic to many underdeveloped countries. There is a wide range of radiographic findings associated with this para-

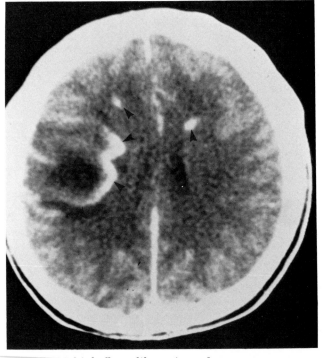

Fig. 8-48. Multiple flame-like regions of contrast enhancement (*arrowheads*) are seen within the white matter tracts of this young male with AIDS. These types of lesions are common in patients with AIDS. The exact etiology of cerebral lesions usually cannot be determined radiographically. They can be secondary to opportunistic infection or neoplasm.

sitic infection. Plain skull x-rays and CT demonstrate multiple small ovoid calcifications, the size and shape of rice grains, scattered throughout the brain (Fig. 8-47). Extremity radiographs also demonstrate similar calcifications within the muscles. Small circular cysts with eccentric punctate calcifications are characteristic on CT.

ACQUIRED IMMUNE DEFICIENCY SYNDROME. Acquired immune deficiency syndrome (AIDS) is associated with a wide range of radiographic brain findings that are usually nonspecific. Flame-like areas of abnormal brain (Fig. 8-48) involving the white matter tracts are commonly seen on both MRI and CT. There may be mass effect and contrast enhancement. Multiple ring lesions or a single large brain mass can be seen. Late in the disease brain atrophy is common. The etiology of these abnormalities can be secondary to infection (e.g., cytomegalic inclusion disease or with toxoplasmosis and other opportunistic organisms) or tumors (e.g., lymphoma, Kaposi's sarcoma). Even with brain biopsy the exact cause may be difficult to ascertain.

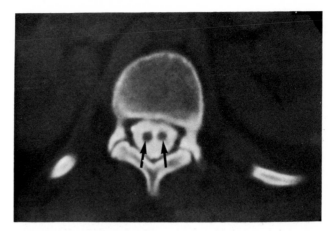

Fig. 8-50. A split thoracic spinal cord (*arrows*) is seen on this axial CT image following a myelogram. Note that there is no division of the spinal canal by either a bony or a soft-tissue plane.

Spinal Cord Pathology

Indications for radiographic evaluation of myelopathy include paralysis, spasticity, sensory change, incontinence, and spine pain (Fig. 8-49). Plain radiographs of the spine are used as a screening procedure to recognize major bony abnormalities. Myelography and CT are essential for a detailed exam of the dural contents. Magnetic resonance imaging and radionuclide bone scans can generate unique clinical information and are essential for diagnosis of certain entities.

INTRAMEDULLARY PATHOLOGY. Intramedullary lesions originate within the spinal cord. These lesions include neoplasms, degenerative disorders, congenital abnormalities, and hemorrhages. Intramedullary abnormalities usually deform the outer surface or central architecture (central canal) of the spinal cord. The normal smooth oval

Fig. 8-49. This schematic diagram illustrates the location of intra-, extra-, and intradural extramedullary lesions involving the spine. The location of the lesion is important to establish an accurate differential diagnosis.

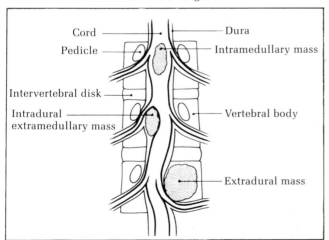

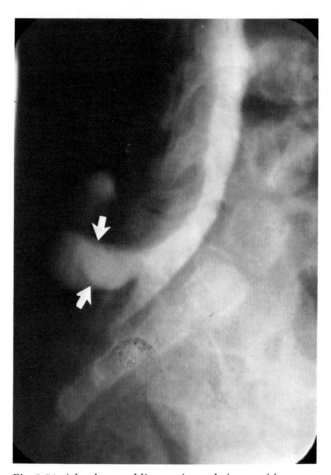

Fig. 8-51. A lumbosacral lipomeningocele (*arrows*) is seen on this lateral radiograph from a lumbar myelogram. The subarachnoid space protrudes into the soft-tissue spaces posteriorly through a defect in the sacrum.

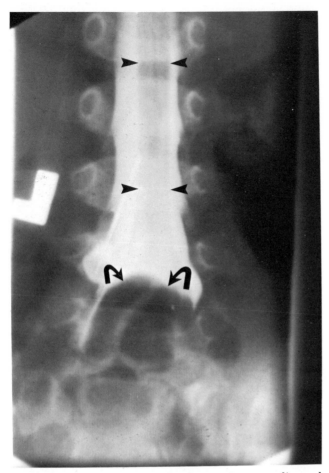

Fig. 8-52. This anteroposterior lumbar myelogram radiograph demonstrates the spinal cord (*arrowheads*) descending to the low lumbar level. The cord widens out to blend into an intradural lipomatous malformation (*curved arrows*) that expands the dural sac and spinal canal.

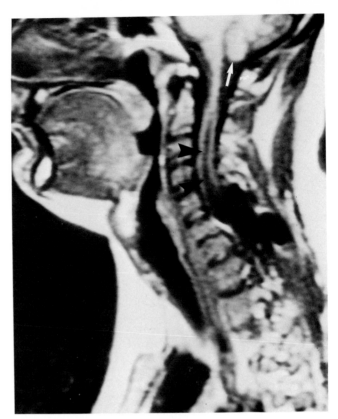

Fig. 8-53. A syrinx (*arrowheads*) is well-demonstrated on this sagittal MRI image of the cervical canal. Note the low-intensity cavity within the central portion of the enlarged spinal cord, similar to spinal fluid in intensity. This patient also has low cerebellar tonsils (*white arrow*) related to Arnold-Chiari malformation type I, which is common with a syrinx.

outer contour of the spinal cord may be expanded or irregular if a mass is present. The cord may be shrunken and flat if atrophic.

Diastematomyelia and Diplomyelia. Diastematomyelia is seen when there is division of the spinal cord into two segments, with or without a bony or cartilaginous spur separating the segments (Fig. 8-50). Diplomyelia is much less common and is a complete duplication of the spinal cord and nerve roots. In both cases plain films frequently show multiple congenital anomalies of the spine, including dysraphism, block vertebrae, hemivertebra, midline spinal canal bony spurs, neuroenteric cysts, and meningoceles. Computed tomography, myelography, and MRI show division of the cord into two parts. There may be narrowing, expansion, or division of the subarachnoid space and bone canal.

Tethered Cord. Patients with tethered cords usually present with caudal root and cord symptoms. Most tethered lumbar spinal cords become symptomatic in childhood and are related to Arnold-Chiari type II malformation, spinal dysraphism, a lumbosacral meningocele, and sacral lipoma (Fig. 8-51). Tethered cords can be occult and might not present with symptoms until adulthood. Magnetic resonance imaging shows that the spinal cord descends well below the normal level of the second lumbar vertebra. In

most patients an ectatic dural sac and a posterior fatty mass (lipoma) continuous with the spinal cord at the level of the dysraphism can be seen. Myelography and CT also show the posteriorly placed low cord (Fig. 8-52). Horizontal or vertical orientation of the roots, which abnormally ascend to exit the neural foramina rather than descend in the normal configuration, may be visible.

Spinal Cord Cysts. Patients with spinal cord cysts usually present with myelopathy, pain, or neuropathic joints. Hydromyelia occurs when there is abnormal enlargement of the central canal. *Syrinx* is another term for spinal cord cyst, but it implies that the cyst is separate from the central canal. Radiologic distinction is not always possible between these disorders and other fluid collections. Abnormal fluid spaces within the spinal cord are often idiopathic, but can be seen in association with tumors, trauma, hydrocephalus, low cerebellar tonsils (Arnold-Chiari type I malformation), and arachnoiditis (Fig. 8-53). Magnetic resonance imaging is the most convenient and accurate means of evaluation, but a combination of CT and myelography can also be used.

Spinal Cord Neoplasms. The same primary tumors of glial origin that involve the brain also affect the spinal cord (e.g., glioma, ependymoma, hemangioblastoma). Most patients present with a long, progressive history of myelopathy. Gliomas usually show a smooth, fusiform expansion of the affected spinal cord (Fig. 8-54). Since some of these

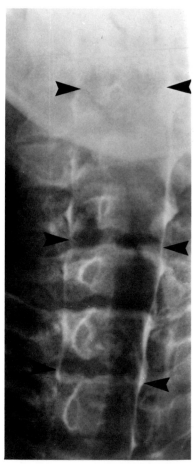

Fig. 8-54. An enlarged cervical spinal cord (*arrowheads*) secondary to an intramedullary glioma is seen on this anteroposterior metrizamide myelogram. Note that the spinal cord expands and fills the spinal canal with only a thin rim of subarachnoid space about the cord.

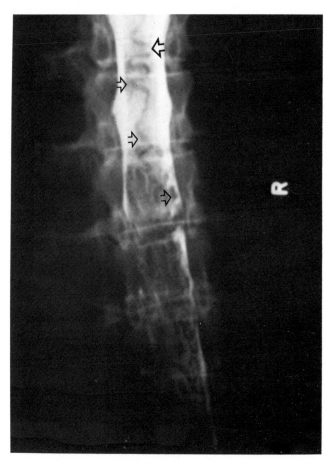

Fig. 8-55. Multiple dilated vessels are seen over the surface of the thoracic spinal cord on this anteroposterior myelogram. Most of these vessels (*arrows*) are draining veins from an arteriovenous malformation. The cord can be enlarged related to an intramedullary hemorrhage. Large vessels can also be seen with spinal cord tumors.

tumors are very slow-growing, enlargement of the bony spinal canal may be visible on plain radiography. Myelography in conjunction with CT shows circular, or less commonly, eccentric enlargement of the affected spinal cord, which fills the available subarachnoid space. Myelography usually shows fusiform enlargement of the cord with narrowed adjacent subarachnoid spaces. There may be total spinal block, with the tapering portions of the more normal cord visible above and below. The spinal cord alone may be enlarged, or the tumor may extend across the foramen magnum into the brainstem. Computed tomography images delayed several hours after intrathecal injection of water-soluble contrast are needed to define possible associated cysts. Magnetic resonance imaging has the advantage of locating the mass and possible associated cord cysts or syrinx without the need of intrathecal contrast. Intraoperative ultrasound is very helpful for tumor localization.

Ependymomas can involve the central canal of the spinal cord and appear very similar to spinal cord gliomas. Some ependymomas are exophitic, producing a polyp-like mass that may mimic an extramedullary extradural tumor. The most common location of ependymomas is the conus medullaris, where an intramedullary tumor that expands to fill the lumbar canal is visible using MRI or computed tomography-myelography. Spinal canal bony enlargement can be seen in severe chronic cases.

Occasionally, metastases may lodge in the spinal cord at any level. They rarely have distinguishing features. He-

mangioblastomas can be seen as densely enhancing intramedullary masses on CT with intravenous contrast injection.

Spinal Arteriovenous Malformation. Spinal arteriovenous malformations (AVM) may present with subarachnoid hemorrhage, back pain, or myelopathy. Most are first recognized on myelography by the presence of large, tortuous vessels over the surface of the spinal cord (Fig. 8-55). The cord might be enlarged if there has been an intraspinal hemorrhage. Magnetic resonance imaging may also show serpentine channels about the cord. Angiography best delineates enlarged spinal arteries filling a dense cluster of abnormal vessels (Fig. 8-56). Rapid flow into dilated veins confirms the diagnosis.

Transverse Myelitis. Transverse myelitis presents as sudden para- or quadraplegia. Transverse myelitis can be seen with multiple sclerosis, spinal artery occlusion, spinal cord hemorrhage, or from unidentifiable causes. Edema producing smooth, focal, fusiform enlargement of the cord may be transiently seen with computed tomography-myelography. Magnetic resonance imaging shows the focal edematous changes. Differentiation from other intramedullary masses on a single exam is not possible. Follow-up exams show that the process is not one of progressive cord enlargement, as would be seen with a tumor.

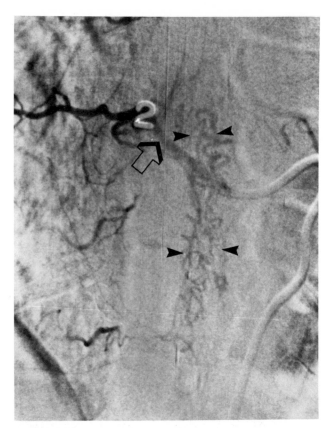

Fig. 8-56. This anteroposterior film from a selective lumbar (*arrow*) angiogram demonstrates enlarged spinal vessels (*arrowheads*) centered in the spinal canal. These vessels supply an arteriovenous malformation. The appearance of the spinal lesions are similar to those in the brain, with enlarged arteries and early-draining veins.

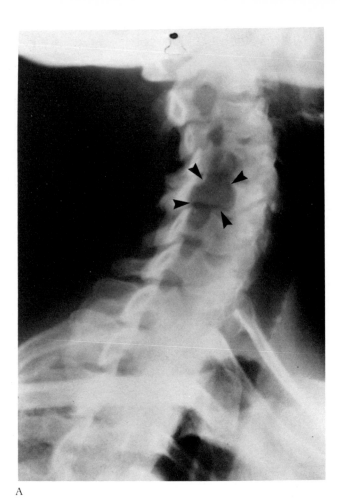

A

B

Fig. 8-57. A. Oblique cervical spine radiograph of an enlarged neural foramen (*arrowheads*). Neurofibroma has eroded both adjacent pedicles as well as the vertebral body. B. Oblique film from a cervical myelogram shows an extradural impression (*straight arrows*) and an intradural mass (*curved arrows*). This mass is seen because the dumbbell-shaped neurofibroma extends through the dural sac to exit the foramen.

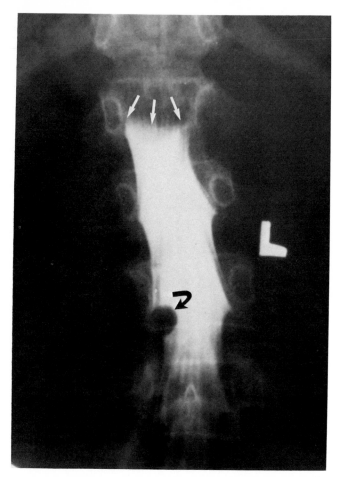

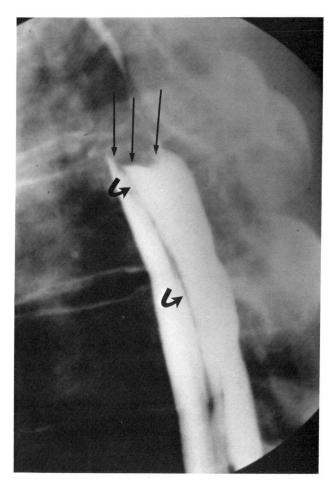

Fig. 8-58. Multiple intradural neurofibromas are seen on this lumbar myelogram with the patient positioned head down. A small circular mass (*curved arrow*) is seen arising from a nerve root. A large convex mass (*straight arrows*) totally obstructs the spinal canal at the upper lumbar area. The mass was found to be a malignant neurofibroma in a patient with neurofibromatosis.

Fig. 8-59. A thoracic meningioma (*straight arrows*) is seen on this lateral myelogram radiograph of a middle aged woman. The patient was positioned head down; there is nearly complete obstruction secondary to the tumor. The dentate ligament of the spinal cord (*curved arrows*) is also displaced anteriorly by the mass.

INTRADURAL EXTRAMEDULLARY PATHOLOGY. Intradural extramedullary lesions arise within the subarachnoid space between the spinal cord and dura but are not of cord origin. A subarachnoid mass shifts the cord to the contralateral side, with obliteration of the subarachnoid space at the level of the mass. Above or below the mass the subarachnoid space is paradoxically enlarged. There is no narrowing of the dural sac paralleling the bony spinal canal.

Peripheral Nerve Tumors. Peripheral nerve tumors can be neurofibromas, neurilemmomas, schwannomas, or malignant neurofibrosarcomas. Radiographic distinction between the different types is usually not possible. Since these tumors grow along the course of the peripheral nerves, one lesion can be both intra- and extradural. The extradural distal portion of the tumor circumferentially expands the margins of the neural foramen by erosion, and is apparent on plain radiographs (Fig. 8-57A, B). Neural foramen enlargement is the most characteristic finding of this type of tumor. The intradural component displaces the spinal cord and adjacent nerve roots to the contralateral side. Magnetic resonance imaging, CT, and myelography are all essential to evaluating the complete extent of the tumor.

Multiple nerve tumors are seen in neurofibromatosis (von Recklinghausen's disease) (Fig. 8-58). The neurofibromas may be of varying size and cause multiple spinal blocks. They also fill the dural sac, causing massive irregular enlargement of the spinal canal, with involvement of the vertebral bodies and posterior elements. Enlargement of the spinal canal with scalloping of the posterior margins of the vertebral bodies and severe scoliosis can also occur in the absence of a neurofibroma. Malignant neurofibrosarcomas of the peripheral nerves are frequently very large (> 5 cm), infiltrate the adjacent fascial planes, recur after surgery, and may metastasize.

Meningioma. Many patients with meningiomas have minimal symptoms for many years. Slowly progressive myelopathy is the most common presentation. Meningiomas can arise wherever there is pia mater, but they have a propensity to involve certain regions. Spinal meningiomas are most common in middle-aged women and are usually located in the thoracic region (Fig. 8-59). Less common sites include the cervical and foramen magnum regions. Meningiomas are very rare in the lumbar spine. Occasionally the tumors may be densely calcified, appearing as calcified intraspinal masses on plain radiographs. There are no other associated bone findings. A single, smooth or lobu-

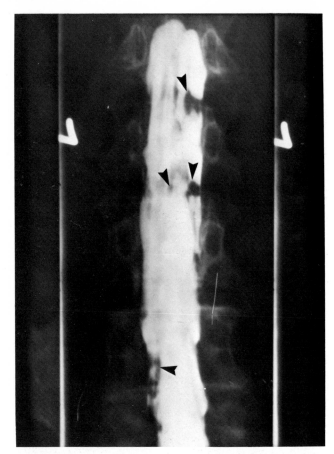

Fig. 8-60. Multiple filling defects (*arrowheads*) secondary to drop metastases are seen on this anterior posterior lumbar myelogram. Differentiation from multiple neurofibromas or inflammatory nodules may be difficult.

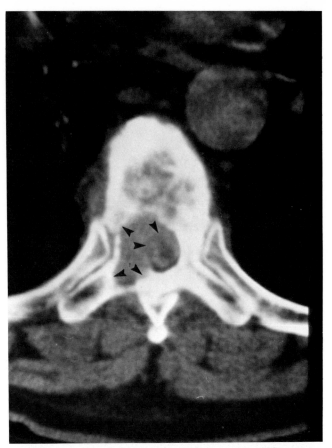

Fig. 8-61. An axial CT image demonstrates a destructive mass (*arrowheads*) that involves the pedicle, lamina, and epidural space. The spinal cord and subarachnoid space are displaced to the left. These findings suggest that the mass arose within the bone and extended into the spinal canal.

lated, extramedullary, and intradural mass is seen on CT, myelography, or MRI. There may be extensive displacement of the spinal cord and root to the contralateral side.

Drop Metastases. Subarachnoid seeding of metastatic tumor frequently presents as a multiple radiculopathy in a patient with known tumor. Drop metastases to the spinal subarachnoid space develop most commonly with lung and breast carcinomas, cerebellar medulloblastomas, and pineal teratomas. Most patients with spinal carcinomatosis by CSF cytology do not have positive CT or myelographic changes since the tumor foci are microscopic. Those tumors that are large enough to be seen radiographically produce multiple filling defects within the subarachnoid space (Fig. 8-60). Unless there are bone metastases, plain films are not positive. Myelography is essential for diagnosis. The tumors may thicken the nerve roots in a nodular fashion (mimicking neurofibromas), or form plaque-like lesions on the dura or spinal cord. Rarely is there complete spinal block.

EPIDURAL SPINAL PATHOLOGY. Epidural abnormalities arise within the spinal canal but outside the dural sac. Epidural pathology displaces the dura centrally away from the bony canal, producing narrowing of the underlying subarachnoid space. There is displacement of the dura, spinal cord, and nerve roots away from the epidural mass.

Epidural Metastases. Sudden or gradual onset of quadra- or paraplegia is very commonly seen with epidural meta-

static tumor. It may be the first manifestation of an otherwise occult tumor. Epidural metastases are much more common than drop subarachnoid metastases and may originate from tumor foci in the epidural veins or the bony vertebrae. If the initial metastasis is within the adjacent bone, then destruction or sclerosis of the pedicle and vertebral body may be visible on plain radiographs. Radionuclide bone scans are more sensitive than plain radiographs in recognizing the presence of tumor within the vertebrae but cannot indicate whether there is encroachment on the spinal canal. Myelography, CT, or MRI is frequently needed to show compression or obstruction of the subarachnoid space with secondary cord compression (Fig. 8-61).

Epidural Abscess. Epidural abscesses can be seen in patients with symptoms of myelopathy or radiculopathy who have a history of fever, immune suppression, recent spinal surgery, or back pain. Most abscesses present as epidural masses causing a block on myelography. Plain films are not helpful in general, but a gallium nuclear scan may help confirm a focus of infection (Fig. 8-62). Occasionally, associated osteomyelitis of the vertebral body, septic discitis, or a retroperitoneal abscess is visible on CT. Differentiation from tumor is difficult.

Osseous Epidural Pathology. Any osseous expansile process of the bones forming the spinal canal can produce an epi-

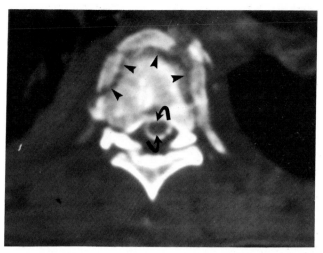

Fig. 8-63. This axial CT image obtained after a myelogram through the upper lumbar region demonstrates a comminuted fracture (*arrowheads*) of the vertebral body. The spinal cord (*curved arrows*) is surrounded by a thin rim of contrast within the subarachnoid space. There is mild distortion of the dural sac but no frank cord compression.

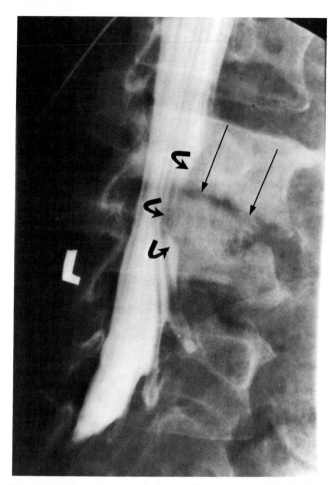

Fig. 8-62. Sclerosis, irregularity, and narrowing of the lumbar interspace (*straight arrows*) is seen on this oblique lumbar myelogram. The dural sac is also compressed by a broad epidural mass (*curved arrows*) secondary to an epidural septic fluid collection.

dural spinal obstruction or stenosis. Paget's disease, fibrous dysplasia, giant cell tumors, metastases, osteoblastomas, and chondrosarcomas can all compress the dural contents. Plain radiographs demonstrate bony expansion and sclerosis or destruction of the affected vertebrae. Estimation of the narrowing of the spinal canal is best made by CT. Magnetic resonance imaging and myelography define the effect on the subarachnoid space, nerve roots, and spinal cord.

SPINAL CORD TRAUMA. There is a wide range of possible spinal cord findings produced by trauma ranging from minor contusions to transections. Plain radiographs can demonstrate spinal fractures and dislocations. One of the most important assessments is whether the spinal canal is narrowed by the affected adjacent bony structures. If narrowing is present an estimation of the degree of spinal cord compression is possible (Fig. 8-63). A severe cord injury can occur in the absence of plain film findings. Computed tomography and myelography are essential for detailed evaluation of the spinal cord (Fig. 8-64). Spinal contusions may be associated with only mild enlargement of the cord or slight to moderate stenosis of the spinal canal by fragments displaced toward the dural sac. With more severe trauma there may be spinal block, evidence of extravasation of myelographic contrast into the soft tissues related to a dural tear, expansion of the cord by hemorrhage and

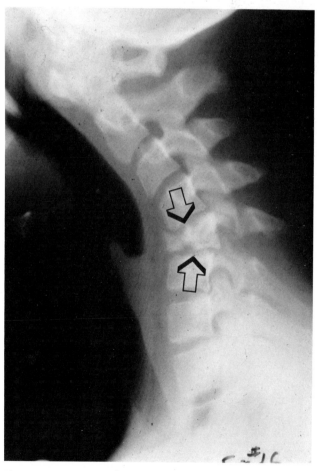

Fig. 8-64. A severe midcervical spine compression fracture (*arrows*) is seen on this lateral cervical radiograph. Note the reverse of the normal lordotic curve and expansion of the vertebral body. The spinal canal is only slightly narrowed.

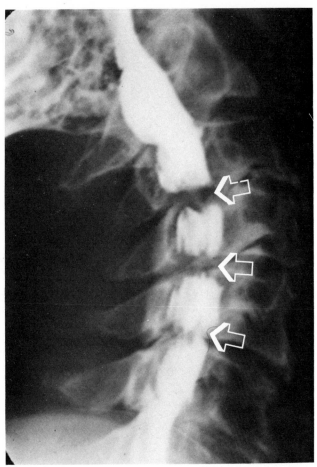

Fig. 8-65. Multiple degenerative stenoses (*arrows*) are seen at nearly every interspace of the cervical spine on this lateral radiograph from a myelogram. The spinal cord is compressed by bony spurs and enlarged ligaments.

edema, and penetration of contrast into the cord suggesting transection or laceration.

Spondylosis

Spondylosis is a term used to describe the variety of spinal changes seen with spinal degenerative joint disease. Patients present with neurologic symptoms when combined bony and soft-tissue changes impinge on the spinal cord or nerve roots. Plain radiographs and CT show bony changes, but computed tomography-myelography or MRI are necessary to evaluate the contents of the dural sac. Nuclear medicine bone scans frequently demonstrate areas of increased activity related to degenerative changes, but are nonspecific and of little clinical value.

Bony changes visible on plain radiographs or CT include narrowing of the disk interspaces and facet spaces, irregularity and sclerosis of the joint surfaces, ligamentous hypertrophy or calcification, and hypertrophic bony overgrowth at the edges of the joints (osteophytes). These bony changes are identical to any other joint affected by similar degenerative changes. Osteophytes from the posterior rim of the vertebral bodies can indent the anterior margin of the dural sac. On myelography or MRI ridge-like indentations of the subarachnoid space at each interspace can be

seen (Fig. 8-65). Very large osteophytes can create a complete block in the subarachnoid space.

Hypertrophy of the facets can be seen in conjunction with narrowing of the facet joints. Gas may actually be visible within the joint spaces. This is called *vacuum joint phenomenon* and is a sign of joint degeneration. If the hypertrophic degenerative changes cause the facet to enlarge laterally and posteriorly there may be no associated spinal stenosis. However, if the facet forms osteophytes anteriorly the posterior lateral spinal canal is encroached upon. Enlargement of the facets and vertebral end plates produces hemispheric impressions on the spinal canal at the level of the interspaces. Usually, the spinal canal is circular or oval in shape, with a wide subarachnoid space about the cord. The hypertrophic changes produce a triangular canal with small dimensions. In general, narrowing of the canal below 16 mm in the anterior-posterior dimension produces significant narrowing of the dural sac. If the bony canal is one cm or less in anterior-posterior dimension, complete or near-complete block is present.

Either a posterior vertebral end plate osteophyte or a large superior facet can narrow the neural foramen. On plain radiographs, oblique views of the cervical spine or lateral views of the remaining spine show bony spurs projecting into the neural foramen. Computed tomography is the most accurate exam for evaluating neural foraminal stenosis, since the anterior to posterior dimension of the foramen and the nerve roots can be seen simultaneously.

DEGENERATIVE DISK DISEASE. Degeneration of the intervertebral disks is a normal aging process. With increasing age the disks lose their water content and elasticity. This can be associated with loss of disk height, protrusion of disk material into the spinal canal, and secondary degenerative bony changes of the vertebral end plates and facets.

Bulging Annulus. The earliest radiographic finding of degenerative disk disease is loss of the water content of the lower lumbar disks, which can be visualized by MRI. This finding frequently precedes any clinical symptoms and is very common. With further degeneration, the disk circumferentially expands to protrude beyond the limits of the vertebral end plates. Narrowing of the interspace may be evident on plain radiographs. On CT the bulging contour of the disk forms a symmetric, circumferential halo around the end plates of the adjacent vertebral bodies. The anterior margin of the dural sac may be slightly indented, but in general the nerve roots are unaffected. This is a common finding on CT in asymptomatic patients and is not associated with radiculopathy in general. Myelography shows symmetric compression of the dural sac at the interspace level. In general, the root sleeves fill symmetrically and the roots are not thickened.

Disk Herniation. A disk herniation occurs when there is a tear in the annulus of the disk with protrusion of its contents into the epidural space. On plain radiographs narrowing of the interspace may be evident but need not be associated with a protrusion. Therefore, plain film findings of spondylosis are suggestive but not diagnostic; CT is a more sensitive and definitive exam. The lower lumbar disks are most commonly involved. Mid- and lower cervical protrusions are the next levels most commonly involved. Thoracic disk herniation is rare. Disk protrusions at different levels have a similar appearance.

A soft-tissue density extending asymmetrically beyond the posterior edge of the vertebral end plate is most char-

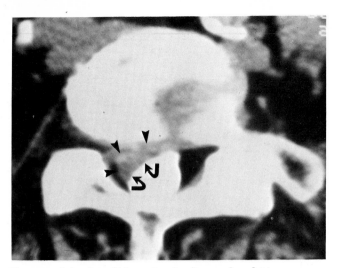

Fig. 8-66. A lumbar disk protrusion (*arrowheads*) is seen on this axial CT lumbar spine section made following a myelogram. The dural sac is compressed (*curved arrows*) and the nerve root sheath fails to fill with subarachnoid contrast.

acteristic on CT (Fig. 8-66). If the protrusion is central (midline) in location, the dural sac may be compressed symmetrically, with narrowing of the subarachnoid space at the level of the interspace. A soft-tissue density similar to the disk is seen filling the epidural space anterior to the dura. Occasionally gas or calcium may be seen within an extruded disk. If the protrusion is more lateral it unilaterally compresses the dural sac and nerve root. A far lateral disk protrusion may involve only the neural foramen and root without compromise of the dural sac. Computed tomography in conjunction with myelography may be of more value for evaluating the extent of involvement than either study separately.

Myelography or MRI best depict the dural contents. Most disk protrusions cause a smooth impression of the adjacent dural sac at the level of the affected interspace. The root sleeve may be obliterated or may fill asymmetrically. The affected nerve root within the dural sac may be thickened and displaced over the protruding disk. Large disk protrusions can produce complete spinal block by displacing the sac posteriorly. Even a small disk protrusion can cause severe subarachnoid compromise in a patient with preexisting spinal stenosis from another cause (e.g., degenerative hypertrophic joint disease).

Bibliography

Cerebrovascular disease
Ford, K. K., and Sarwar, M. Computed tomography of dural sinus thrombosis. *A.J.N.R.* 2:539, 1981.
Houser, O. W., et al. Spontaneous cervical cephalic arterial dissection and its residuum: Angiographic spectrum. *A.J.N.R.* 5:27, 1984.
Newton, T. H., and Potts, D. G., (eds.). *Radiology of the Skull and Brain: Angiography,* Vol. 2, Book 4. St. Louis: Mosby, 1984.
Osborne, A. *Introduction to Cerebral Angiography.* Philadelphia: Harper & Row, 1980.

Brain neoplasm
Brandt-Zawadski, M., et al. Primary intracranial tumor imaging:
A comparison of magnetic resonance and CT. *Radiology* 150:435, 1984.
Hawkes, R. C., et al. Application of NMR imaging to the evaluation of pituitary and juxtasellar tumors. *A.J.N.R.* 4:221, 1983.
Latchaw, L. *Computed Tomography of the Head, Neck, and Spine.* Chicago: Year Book, 1985.

Hydrocephalus
Gado, M., et al. Aging, dementia, and brain atrophy: A longitudinal computed tomographic study. *A.J.N.R.* 4:699, 1983.
Naidich, T. P., Schott, L. H., and Baron, R. L. Computed tomography in the evaluation of hydrocephalus. *Radiol. Clin. North Am.* 20:143, 1982.
Naidich, T. P., et al. Computed tomographic signs of Chiari II malformation: I. Skull and dural partitions. *Radiology* 134:65, 1980.

Cerebral trauma
Moon, K. L., et al. Nuclear magnetic resonance imaging of CT-isodense subdural hematomas. *A.J.N.R.* 5:319, 1984.
Zimmerman, R. A., and Bilaniuk, L. T. Computed tomographic staging of traumatic epidural bleeding. *Radiology* 144:809, 1982.

Demyelinating and degenerative diseases
Jackson, J. A., et al. Magnetic resonance imaging in multiple sclerosis: Results in 32 cases. *A.J.N.R.* 6:171, 1985.

Brain infection
Enzmann, D. R., Brandt-Zawadski, M. N., and Britt, R. H. CT of central nervous system infections in immunocompromised patients. *A.J.R.* 135:263, 1980.

Spinal cord pathology
Harwood-Nash, D. C., and Fitz, C. R. (eds.). *Neuroradiology in Infants and Children.* St. Louis: Mosby, 1976.
Newton, T. H., and Potts., D. G. (eds.). *Modern Neuroradiology, Advanced Imaging Techniques,* Vol. 2. San Anselmo, CA: Clavadel, 1983.
Shapiro, R. *Myelography* (3rd ed.). Chicago: Year Book, 1975.

Spondylosis
Resnick, D. Degenerative diseases of the vertebral column. *Radiology* 156:3, 1985.

9. Medical Complications of Pregnancy

Janet L. Potter

Medical disorders that occur during pregnancy present special problems to the clinician. Diagnosis is often complicated by the normal biochemical and physiologic changes of gestation. Radiation risk to the fetus is an important concern when imaging is required to assist in diagnosis.

Imaging with ultrasound is the primary and often the only modality required for diagnosis of many pregnancy-associated diseases. When x-rays are unavoidable, the fetus can be shielded externally from direct but not from scatter radiation. When imaging with radioactive agents is required, nuclides with very short half-lives are used to minimize dosage. Because of the risk of inducing fetal cretinism, radioactive iodine studies are contraindicated in pregnancy. Computed tomography scanning of the maternal head for neurologic complications carried essentially no risk to the developing fetus.

Renal Complications

From early pregnancy the maternal renal collecting system is mildly dilated, more so on the right side than the left (Fig. 9-1). The urinary tract returns to its normal size within two weeks to three months post partum. When a pregnant patient presents with signs and symptoms of ureteral calculus, ultrasound can confirm obstruction but often fails to visualize the stone. Mild degrees of hydronephrosis, especially right-sided, cannot be distinguished from pseudoobstruction of pregnancy. Fortunately, because the collecting system is dilated in pregnancy, persistent obstruction is rare and an intravenous pyelogram (IVP) or retrograde study can usually be avoided. Acute pyelonephritis occurs in 1 to 2 percent of pregnancies. Subsequent development of renal or perirenal abscess is rare and can be diagnosed with a high degree of accuracy by ultrasound (Fig. 9-2).

RENAL FAILURE. Acute renal failure is uncommon in pregnancy. Failure may be on the basis of acute cortical necrosis, acute tubular necrosis, or renal vein thrombosis and is usually associated with obstetric disasters such as eclampsia, abruptio placentae, or amniotic fluid embolus. Occasionally a seemingly uncomplicated pregnancy presents with renal failure. The cause is usually deterioration of previously undiagnosed chronic renal insufficiency. In all of these situations ultrasound is used to rule out hydronephrosis and often provides additional useful information. Markedly enlarged and swollen kidneys suggest renal vein thrombosis (Fig. 9-3), which requires selective venography for confirmation. Small kidneys are indicative of chronic renal failure.

Fig. 9-1. IVP showing
pseudoobstruction of pregnancy,
more pronounced on the right side.

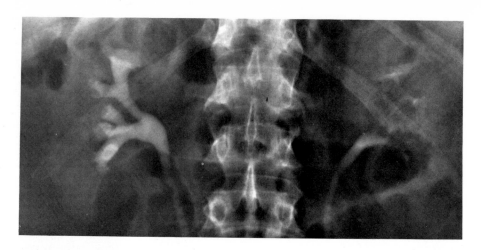

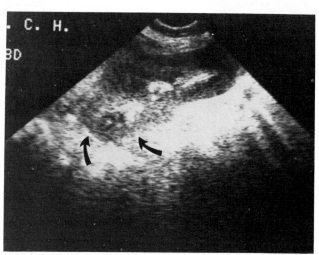

Fig. 9-2. Ultrasound showing enlarged left kidney upper pole (*arrows*) consistent with uncomplicated acute pyelonephritis. The perinephric space is normal in appearance.

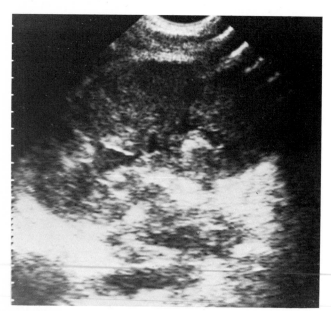

Fig. 9-3. Ultrasound showing swollen echogenic kidney consistent with renal vein thrombosis in preeclamptic patient with acute renal failure.

Liver, Biliary System, and Pancreas Complications

GALLSTONES. Gallstones are diagnosed by ultrasound with greater than 95 percent accuracy. In certain population groups gallstones occur in younger women and may precipitate acute cholecystitis or biliary pancreatitis. Because treatment is usually conservative during pregnancy, radionuclide hepatobiliary scanning is often deferred.

CHOLESTASIS. Cholestasis of pregnancy appears after 24 weeks' gestation. It is a self-limited disorder, marked by jaundice and pruritis, that resolves quickly post partum. Viral hepatitis and acute fatty liver of pregnancy present as abdominal pain and jaundice. Ultrasound confirms that jaundice is not due to biliary obstruction.

LIVER COMPLICATIONS. Common liver complications of toxemia include localized periportal hemorrhage, subcapsular hemorrhage, and occasionally hepatic rupture with intraperitoneal hematoma. These complications usually occur in the third trimester, during labor, or in the immediate postpartum period. Hepatic hematoma and/or rupture have also been reported in uncomplicated pregnancies associated with trauma, seizures, or excessive vomiting. The patient complains of sudden onset of right upper quadrant pain and has a drop in hematocrit. Diagnosis of subcapsular hematoma and hepatic rupture can be made by ultrasound. Frequently CT is employed to evaluate the size and extent of subcapsular and intraperitoneal blood (Fig. 9-4).

Computed tomography usually displays anatomic relationships to better advantage, but the cost of ultrasound is one-third that of CT, and the more limited ultrasound examination is frequently sufficient for diagnosis and follow-up.

ACUTE PANCREATITIS. Acute pancreatitis is not common in pregnancy. Fifty percent of cases are caused by passage of a gallstone and the remainder are idiopathic. The disease usually presents in the third trimester or puerperium. It is a serious complication that carries a maternal mortality rate of up to 20 percent. Ultrasound can evaluate for a biliary etiology and demonstrate necrotic areas, phlegmon, and pseudocyst formation (Fig. 9-5). In the postpartum period, CT is employed for complications of pancreatitis be-

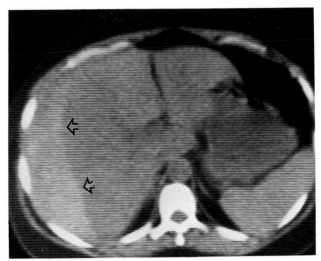

Fig. 9-4. CT showing curvilinear subcapsular collection (*arrows*) with high CT coefficient consistent with blood in eclamptic patient post partum.

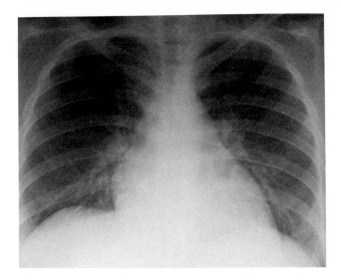

Fig. 9-6. Markedly enlarged globular heart in cardiomyopathy of pregnancy.

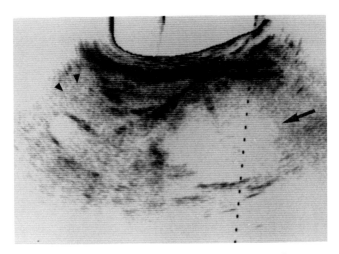

Fig. 9-5. Longitudinal ultrasound of pancreatic pseudocyst (*arrow*); arrowheads indicate the liver.

cause of its improved diagnostic accuracy in identifying pseudocysts, abscesses, and phlegmon.

Thromboembolism

Risk of deep venous thrombosis is increased after cesarean section and in the older and multiparous patient. Clinical evaluation of deep venous thrombosis is often difficult in pregnancy. Signs of superficial venous thrombosis, unilateral symptoms, or a history of previous thrombophlebitis in pregnancy increases clinical suspicion. A lower extremity venogram with fetal shielding is necessary before instituting heparin therapy. A radionuclide fibrinogen study is contraindicated because the nuclide is iodine.

Suspected pulmonary embolus is diagnosed by a radionuclide ventilation-perfusion scan. A perfusion defect with normal ventilation and a clear chest x-ray confirm the diagnosis.

Septic pelvic thrombophlebitis occurs approximately 8 to 10 days after cesarean section and presents as chills and

fever. It is a diagnosis of exclusion and is suspected when symptoms are unabated after four days of antibiotic therapy. Computed tomography has been successful in demonstrating clots in pelvic veins in a few reported cases. Venography by catheter through the inferior vena cava and selection of ovarian veins has a higher success rate than CT, but is an invasive procedure. Septic pulmonary embolus is a potential complication.

Cardiac Complications

Chest x-ray and echocardiography are the primary imaging tools for cardiac problems first presenting in pregnancy. Endocarditis can develop during pregnancy, but there is no increased risk of the disease in pregnant women. Diagnosis is made by demonstrating valvular vegetations by echocardiography.

Cardiomyopathy of pregnancy is an uncommon complication presenting in the postpartum period as congestive heart failure. The disorder is more common in toxemia and twin pregnancies, and among black and multiparous women. Chest x-ray reveals a diffusely enlarged heart, and echocardiography shows dilated chambers, sometimes visualizing thrombi along the flaccid walls (Fig. 9-6). Only half of patients recover normal cardiac configuration and function post partum.

Respiratory System Complications

The most serious respiratory system complication is shock lung (adult respiratory distress syndrome [ARDS]), which can occur after aspiration, hypovolemic shock, amniotic fluid embolus, septic abortion, or in association with disseminated intravascular coagulopathy (DIC). Chest x-rays are required to follow development of this serious condition.

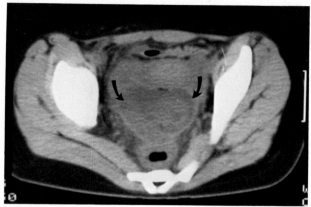

Fig. 9-7. CT shows postpartum uterus and pelvic abscess (*arrows*).

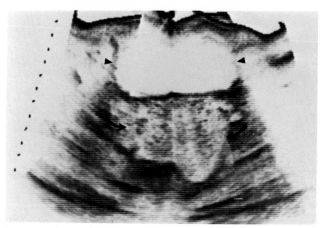

Fig. 9-8. Transverse ultrasound scan of uterus filled with a complex mass characteristic of a molar pregnancy (*arrows*). Bladder is echo-free (*arrowheads*).

Neurologic Complications

Seizures unassociated with eclampsia may occur during labor or puerperium. Pseudotumor cerebri, a syndrome of increased intracranial pressure of unknown etiology, is not common and usually improves post partum. Patients complain of headache. Papilledema is present and bitemporal visual field loss may develop suddenly. Brain CT reveals normal or small ventricles and no tumor or mass effect.

The most serious neurologic complications are associated with toxemia of pregnancy. Intracerebral hemorrhage usually occurs in the immediate pre- or postpartum period. The mortality rate is high. Hemorrhage is often a solitary collection of blood in the white matter, basal ganglia, or brainstem. Small petechial hemorrhages or multiple nonhemorraghic areas may be seen postmortem. Central venous thrombosis may occur and also carries a poor prognosis.

PITUITARY INFARCTION. Pituitary infarction is an uncommon complication that ultimately produces panpituitary insufficiency, or Sheehan's syndrome. It is associated with postpartum hemorrhage. The insufficiency is gradual in onset. It may present as an inability to lactate postpartum or make a delayed appearance as irregular or absent menstrual cycles. The role of CT is to rule out pituitary tumor, which can also destroy the gland and produce hypopituitarism.

Postpartum Infection

Puerperal sepsis is an acute endometritis that can progress to pelvic cellulitis and peritonitis. It develops three days or more post partum. Both ultrasound and CT are used to define pelvic abscess (Fig. 9-7) and plan a surgical approach.

Neoplasms in Pregnancy

Malignancy in the pregnant woman is uncommon. With the exception of choriocarcinoma, no cancers are unique to the pregnant woman. The cancer itself, whether it is breast, cervix, lymphoma or melanoma, threatens the life of the mother. Treatment for the cancer is hazardous to the fetus. In the first trimester elective abortion is often recommended so that needed therapy can be started. It is at this time that the fetus is most vulnerable to teratogenic effects of radiation and chemotherapeutic agents.

TROPHOBLASTIC DISEASE. Choriocarcinoma is a malignancy of the fetal trophoblastic epithelium. It is the most malignant form of a spectrum of trophoblastic disorders; hydatidiform mole is benign and invasive mole is intermediate. Hydatidiform mole is suspected when the uterus enlarges more rapidly than expected for a singlet pregnancy or the woman develops toxemia in the first trimester. Bleeding and excessive vomiting also may be presenting symptoms. Diagnosis of trophoblastic disease is suggested by ultrasound demonstration of a complex intrauterine mass. (Fig. 9-8). Computed tomography of the abdomen and pelvis and chest x-ray are required for staging. Choriocarcinoma tumor fragments may embolize diffusely to the lungs, producing severe respiratory compromise, but more typically present with multiple asymptomatic parenchymal nodules. Hematogenous metastases also involve the liver, bone, and brain in advanced disease.

Bibliography

Hibbard, L. T. Spontaneous rupture of the liver in pregnancy. *Am. J. Obstet. Gynecol.* 126:334, 1976.

Raja Rao, A. K., Zucker, M. and Sacks, D. Right ovarian vein thrombosis with extension to the inferior vena cava. *Br. J. Radiol.* 53:160, 1980.

Ramsay, L. E. Impact of venography on the diagnosis and management of deep vein thrombosis. *Br. Med. J.* 286:698, 1983.

Steven, M. M. Pregnancy and liver disease. *Gut* 22:592, 1981.

Index

Abdominal aortic aneurysm, 7
Abdominal plain film, 1–9
  of calcifications, 7
  of fluids, 7–8, 9
  of gas patterns, 1–7
Abruptio placentae, 249
Acetabulum
  ankylosing spondylitis and, 158
  Paget's disease of, 179
  pyogenic septic arthritis of, 189
  rheumatoid arthritis and, 154
Achalasia, 11, 12
Acquired immune deficiency syndrome
    (AIDS), 100–101
  brain findings in, 239
  monilial esophagitis and, 10
Acroosteolysis, 160
Acroosteosclerosis, 185
Adenomyomatosis, 36
Adrenal gland
  adenoma of, 212
  calcified adenoma of, 212
  carcinoma of, 212
  disorders of, 211–213
  hemorrhage of, 212, 213
  solitary mass, 212–213
Adrenocorticotropic hormone, in
    Cushing's syndrome, 211
Adult polycystic kidney disease, 127–
    128, 129
  liver cysts in, 30
Adult respiratory distress syndrome, 92,
    100, 102
  in pregnancy, 251
Adynamic ileus, 1–2
AIDS. See Acquired immune deficiency
    syndrome (AIDS)
Air bronchogram, 67, 68
Airway disease, upper, 79–81
Alcohol abuse, cirrhosis and, 30
Alcoholic pancreatitis, 9
Aldosteronism, primary, 211–212
Alimentary canal. See Gastrointestinal
    tract
Alkaptonuria, 166, 167
Allergic bronchopulmonary
    aspergillosis, 90
Alpha₁ antitrypsin deficiency, 82
Alpha thalassemia, 181
Alveolar proteinosis, 102
Alzheimer's disease, 235
Amebiasis, 22
Amniotic fluid embolism, 249, 251
Analgesic nephropathy, 123
Anemia, 181–182
Aneursymal bone cyst, 198–199
Angiitis, 137
  granulomatous, 96, 97
Angiography
  in angiomyolipoma, 131
  in cerebral embolism, 220
  in decreased renal failure, 136
  in hypernephroma, 135
Angiomyolipoma, 131
Ankle
  gouty arthritis of, 162
  hemophiliac arthropathy of, 183
  Reiter's syndrome of, 161
  staphylococcal osteomyelitis of, 188
Ankylosing hyperostosis, of spine, 171
Ankylosing spondylitis, 157–159

Ankylosis, intraarticular bony, 161–162
Ann Arbor Staging Classification, of
    lymphomas, 147
Annular pancreas, 39
Annulus fibrosis, 157
Anthracosilicosis, 84
Aortic aneurysm, 63–64
  abdominal, 7
  descending, 109
Aortic arch, 219
Aortic insufficiency, congestive heart
    failure and, 54–55
Aortic valve aneurysm, 63
Aortography, 55
Apophyseal joint osteoarthritis, 171, 172
Appendicitis, 27
Appendicolith, 7, 9
Appendix, disorders of, 27
Arnold-Chiari malformation, 240
Arteriography, in renal infarction, 138
Arteriosclerotic disease, cerebral, 218–
    220
Arteriovenous malformation
  intracranial hemorrhage and, 222, 223
  vs. solitary pulmonary nodule, 76, 77
  of spine, 241
Arteritis, cerebral, 220, 221
Arthritis, 151–172
  ankylosing spondylitis and, 157–159
  calcium pyrophosphate dihydrate
      crystal deposition disease, 162–
      165
  crystal-induced, 162–167
  degenerative joint disease of spine,
      168–171
  gouty, 162
    thalassemia and, 182
  hemochromatosis and, 165
  hepatolenticular degeneration and,
      165–166
  hydroxyapatite crystal deposition
      disease, 165
  juvenile chronic, 154–157
  neuroarthropathy, 171–172
  ochronosis, 167
  osteoarthritis, 167–168
    erosive, 168
  psoriatic, 159–160
  pyogenic septic, 189–190
  Reiter's syndrome and, 160–162
  rheumatoid, 151–154
  septic
    pyogenic, 189–190
    sickle cell disease and, 180
  seronegative spondyloarthropathies,
      157–162
  spondyloarthritis, with inflammatory
      bowel disease, 159
  Wilson's disease and, 165–167
Asbestos, -related malignant
    mesothelioma, 111
Asbestosis, 85–86
Ascending cholangitis, 36
Ascites, 7–8, 9, 30
Ask-Upmark kidney, 117
Aspergillosis, 90
Aspiration
  foreign body, 70, 79
  radiographic contrast materials, 92–93
Aspiration pneumonia, 91–93
Asthma, 82, 83

Asthma—Continued
  donuts in, 84
Astrocytoma, 224–225
Atelectasis
  foreign body aspiration and, 79
  Legionnaire's disease and, 100
  subsegmental, 72
Atherosclerotic heart disease, 63–64
Atlantoaxial ligament, rheumatoid
    arthritis and, 154
Atlantoaxial subluxation, rheumatoid
    arthritis and, 154
Atrium, myxoma of, 64
Autonephrectomy, 120
Avascular necrosis, 185–187

Bacterial infection, pneumonia, 69
Barium enema
  in Crohn's disease, 27–28
  double contrast, 22
  single contrast, 22, 23
  in ulcerative colitis, 28–29
Barlow's syndrome, 55–56
Barrett's esophagus, 10
Beckwith-Wiedemann syndrome, 132
Berylliosis, 86
Beta thalassemia, 181
Bezoar, 18
Big bang theory, of vesicoureteral reflux,
    117
Bile duct
  cholangiocarcinoma of, 36
  diseases of, 34–36
Biliary pancreatitis, in pregnancy, 250
Biopsy, in breast cancer, 141, 143
Bipedal lymphangiogram
  in lymphoma, 147
  in prostate carcinoma, 148
Bjork-Shiley prosthetic valve, 58, 59
Blastema, Wilms' tumor derived from,
    132
Blastomycosis, 90
Blebs, 34, 83
"Blue bloater," 81
Bone disease, 151–206
  arthritis, 151–172. See also under
      Arthritis
  bone tumors, 195–206
  disorders of unknown origin, 183–185
  hemoglobinopathies and anemias,
      179–182
  infarction of, 181
    osteonecrosis in, 186
  infections, 187–195
  medullary infarctions, 181
  metabolic, 172–179
  neoplasms, 195–206
    aneursymal bone cyst, 198–199
    benign, 197–200
    breast metastases, 144
    chondroblastoma, 198
    chondrosarcoma, 203
    enchondroma, 199, 200
    eosinophilic granuloma, 199–200
    Ewing's sarcoma, 203, 204
    fibrous cortical defect, 197–198
    giant cell tumor, 200, 201
    malignant, 200–206
    malignant fibrous histiocytoma,
        204–206
    metastatic carcinoma, 205, 206

Bone disease, neoplasms—*Continued*
  myeloma, 204
  nonossifying fibroma, 197–198
  osteochondroma, 199
  osteogenic sarcoma, 200–203
  osteoid osteoma, 198
  prostate metastases, 149–150
  radiographic approach to, 195–197
  reticulum cell sarcoma, 204
  sites of origin, 196
  solitary bone cyst, 198, 199
  osteonecrosis, 185–187
Boutonniere deformity, in rheumatoid
    arthritis, 154
Bowel
  large. *See* Large bowel
  lymphoma of, 145–146
  small. *See* Small bowel
Bowleg deformity, 175
Brain
  astrocytoma, 224–225
  chordoma, 227–228
  choroid plexus papilloma, 228
  collateral circulation of, 220
  colloid cyst, 228
  contusion, 233
  craniopharyngioma, 227, 228
  edema, 233
  ependymoma, 224–225
  epidermoid tumor, 228
  focal atrophy of, 217–218
  glioma, 224–225
  hemangioblastoma, 228
  lipoma, 228
  medulloblastoma, 226
  meningioma, 225
  neoplasms of, 222–229
    metastases, 225–226
  oligodendroglioma, 224–225
  pineal region tumors, 226
  pseudotumor cerebri, 229
  subarachnoid cyst, 229
  teratoma, 228
Brainstem, 235
Breast
  cancer of, 139–144
    calcifications, 140, 141
    diaphanography in, 143
    lobular, 142
    lung metastases, 75
    mammography in, 140–143
    microcalcification in, 141, 142
    osseous metastasis, 206
    prognosis, 140
    risk factors, 139–140
    staging and followup, 144
    "tail," 140
    thermography in, 143–144
    ultrasound in, 143
  cyst, 140
  degenerating fibroadenoma of, 141
  nonpalpable lesions of, 141
    hook wire in, 141, 142
  palpable lesions of, 140
Breast Cancer Detection Demonstration
    Projects, 141
Brodie's abscess, 189, 190
Bronchial adenoma, 75
Bronchiectasis, 90–91
  hypertrophic osteoarthropathy and,
    184
Bronchitis, chronic, 82
Bronchogenic carcinoma, 72–76
  hypertrophic osteoarthropathy and,
    184
  radiation exposure and, 95

Bronchogenic cyst, 108
Bronchography, in bronchiectasis, 91
Brown tumors, hyperthyroidism and,
    176, 177
Budd-Chiari malformation, liver in, 34
Bullae, 83, 84
Burkitt's lymphoma, 144

Café au lait spots, 183
Calcific tendinitis, 165, 166
Calcium oxalate stones, 124
Calcium phosphate stones, 124
Calcium pyrophosphate dihydrate
    crystal deposition disease (CPPD),
    162–165
Calculous disease, 34, 123–125
Calvé's disease, 200
Campylobacter infection, 22
Canavan's disease, 235
Cancer. *See specific type and location*
Caplan's syndrome, 85
Cardiomyopathy
  congestive heart failure and, 56–58
  of pregnancy, 251
Cardiovascular disease, 45–65
  aortic diseases, 63–64
  calcifications, 58–61
  computed tomography in, 48–51
  congestive heart failure, 51–58
  echocardiography in, 45–48, 49
  imaging tools, 45–51
  magnetic resonance imaging in, 51
  pericardial disease, 58–61
  peripheral atherosclerosis, 64
  peripheral venous thrombosis, 64, 65
  in pregnancy, 251
  prosthetic valves, 58, 59
  pulmonary embolism and, 61–63
  pulmonary hypertensive heart disease,
    61–63
  radionuclide imaging in, 51
  thoracic radiographs in, 45, 46–47
  tumors, 64–65
Carotid artery
  bifurcation, 218–220
  dissection, 220, 221
  fibromuscular dysplasia of, 220
Catecholamines, neuroblastoma and,
    134
Cecum, volvulus, 2, 4
Celiac sprue, 22
Central pontine myelinolysis, 235
Central venous thrombosis, in
    pregnancy, 252
Cerebral abscess, 236, 237
Cerebral aneurysm, 222, 223
Cerebral angiography, 218
Cerebral embolism, 220
Cerebral infarction, 217, 218
Cerebral ischemia, 217–220
Cerebral trauma, 232–235
Cerebritis, 236
Cerebrospinal fluid, in intraventricular
    hemorrhage, 220
Cerebrovascular accident, acute
    aspiration and, 92
Cerebrovascular disease, 217–223
  arteriosclerotic disease, 218–220
  arteriovenous malformation, 222, 223
  arteritis, 220, 221
  carotid dissection, 220, 221
  cerebral aneurysm, 222, 223
  cerebral embolism, 220
  cerebral infarction, 217, 218
  cerebral ischemia, 217–220
  intracerebral hemorrhage, 222

Cerebrovascular disease—*Continued*
  intracranial hemorrhage, 220–223
  intraventricular hemorrhage, 220, 222
  pathologic entities, 218
  vasculitis, 220, 221
  venous thrombosis, 220, 222
Cervical spine
  apophyseal joint osteoarthritis of, 171
  juvenile chronic arthritis of, 156
  rheumatoid arthritis of, 154
  "stair-step" deformity of, 154
Cervix, carcinoma of, 215
Cesarean section, venous thrombosis
    and, 251
Charcot's joint, 171–173
Chemotherapeutic agents
  induced lung disease, 94–95
  teratogenicity, 252
Chest x-ray
  in adult respiratory distress syndrome,
    251
  in cardiovascular disease, 45, 46–47
  in lymphoma, 147
Children
  asthma in, 82, 83
  Brodie's abscess in, 189, 190
  rickets in, 175–177
  sickle cell disease in, 179
  vesicoureteral reflux in, 117
  Wilms' tumor in, 131–133
Chlamydia infection, pneumonia from,
    100
Cholangiocarcinoma, 36
Cholangitis
  ascending, 36
  sclerosing, 35
Cholecystitis, 34–35
Cholecystosis, hyperplastic, 36
Choledochal cysts, 36
Cholelithiasis, 34
Cholestasis, of pregnancy, 250
Cholesterolosis, 36
Chondroblastoma, 198
Chondrocalcinosis
  CPPD and, 162, 163–165
  gouty arthritis and, 162
  hyperparathyroidism and, 177
  thalassemia and, 182
Chondrosarcoma, 203
Chordoma, 227–228
Choriocarcinoma, 252
Choroid plexus papilloma, 228
Chronic obstructive pulmonary disease
    (COPD), 81–83
  alpha₁ antitrypsin deficiency, 82
  asthma, 82, 83
  chronic bronchitis, 82
  complications of, 83
  cor pulmonale, 83
  emphysema, 81–82
Cirrhosis, 30
Claudication, atherosclerotic stenosis
    and, 64
Coal worker's pneumoconiosis, 83–85
Coccidioidomycosis, 89–90
Codman's triangle, 197
Colitis
  infectious, 24
  pseudomembranous, 22, 24
  ulcerative, 2, 28–29, 157
Collagen vascular disease, 96
Collecting system, renal
  duplication, 115
  in pregnancy, 249–250
  staghorn calculi of, 124
Colloid cyst, 228

Colon
  adenocarcinoma of, 25
  angiodysplasia, 40
  carcinoma of, 3
  diseases of, 22–27
  gas in, 2
  infection of, 22–24
  lipoma of, 25
  lymphoma of, 25, 146
  obstruction of, 3, 24–26
  polyps, 24
  villous adenomas of, 25
Colonoscopy, 24
Computed tomography
  in adrenal adenoma, 212
  in angiomyolipoma, 131
  in arteriovenous malformation, 222
  in basal ganglion hemorrhage, 222
  in cardiovascular disease, 48–51
  in cerebral aneurysm, 222
  in cerebral ischemia, 217, 218
  in cirrhosis, 30
  in dural thrombosis, 222
  in empyema, 111
  gated, 48
  in genitourinary tuberculosis, 120
  in giant cell tumor of bone, 201
  in hypernephroma, 134, 135–136
  in intracranial hemorrhage, 222
  in lung cancer, 74–75
  in lymphoma, 147
  in neuroblastoma, 133
  in pericardial disease, 61
  in pneumoconiosis, 86
  in polycystic kidney disease, 127–128
  in prostate carcinoma, 148
  in pyelonephritis, 118
  in pyogenic infectious spondylitis,
     190, 191
  in shock lung, 102
  in simple renal cysts, 126
  in spinal cord pathologies, 239
  in subarachnoid hemorrhage, 220
  in toxemia of pregnancy, 250
  in trophoblastic disease, 252
  in Wilms' tumor, 132–133
  in xanthogranulomatous
     pyelonephritis, 119, 120
Congenital heart disease, hypertrophic
     osteoarthropathy and, 184
Congestive heart failure, 51–58
  left ventricular contour in, 53, 54–55
  mitral contour in, 55–56
  vascularity evaluation in, 51–54
Conjunctivitis, Reiter's syndrome and,
     160
Connective tissue disease,
     tracheobronchomegaly and, 80
Consolidation, in pulmonary disease, 67
Cooley's anemia, 181–182
COPD. See Chronic obstructive
     pulmonary disease (COPD)
Cor pulmonale, 83
Coronary artery, calfication of, 58
Coronary artery disease, 60
Corrosive esophagitis, 10
Corrosive gastritis, 18
Cortisol-secreting tumors, 209
CPPD. See Calcium pyrophosphate
     dihydrate crystal deposition
     disease (CPPD)
Craniopharyngioma, 227, 228
Crohn's disease, 27–28, 157
  calculi in, 124
Crohn's ileitis, 28
Crossed renal ectopia, 117

Cryptosporidium, 20
Crystal-induced arthropathies, 162–167
  alkaptonuria, 166, 167
  calcium pyrophosphate dihydrate
     crystal deposition disease, 162–
     165
  gouty arthritis, 162
  hemochromatosis, 165, 166
  hepatolenticular degeneration, 165–
     167
  hydroxyapatite crystal deposition
     disease, 165, 166
  ochronosis, 166, 167
  Wilson's disease, 165–167
Crystalline stones, 124
Cushing's syndrome, 211, 212
  pituitary adenoma and, 212
Cystic fibrosis, bronchiectasis and, 91
Cysticercosis, 238–239
Cystourethrography, voiding, 130
Cytomegalovirus infection, of bone, 195

Dactylitis, sickle cell disease and, 180
DeBakey dissecting aortic aneurysm, 63
Degenerative disease
  disk, 246–247
  joint. See Degenerative joint disease
  neurologic, 235–239
  spinal, 168–171, 246–247
Degenerative enthesopathy, vs.
     enthesitis, 159
Degenerative joint disease, 167–171
  apophyseal joint osteoarthritis, 171,
     172
  diffuse idiopathic skeletal
     hyperostosis, 171
  erosive osteoarthritis, 168, 169
  intervertebral osteochondrosis, 171
  osteoarthritis, 167–168
  of spine, 168–171
  spondylosis deformans, 168–171
Demyelinating disease, 235–239
Dermatomyositis, hydroxyapatite
     crystals in, 165
Dermoid cyst, ovarian, 214
Diaphanography, in breast cancer, 143
Diaphragm, extraluminal air, 2
Diastematomyelia, 239, 240
Diffuse idiopathic skeletal hyperostosis,
     170, 171
Digital clubbing, hypertrophic
     osteoarthropathy and, 184
Digital examination, in prostate
     carcinoma, 147
Digital subtraction angiography, in
     exertional dyspnea, 61
Diplomyelia, 240
Diskitis, pyogenic, 191
Dismyelinating disease, 235
Disseminated intravascular coagulation,
     in pregnancy, 251
Diverticula, of esophagus, 14
Diverticulitis, large bowel, 25–26
Diverticulosis, 20
  large bowel, 25–26
Drug therapy
  induced esophagitis, 10
  induced respiratory injury, 94–95
Duodenal ulcer, 16
  bleeding, 41
Duodenitis, 14
Duodenum, diseases of, 14–19
Dysphagia, 8
Dyspnea, exertional, 62

Echinococcal cysts, of liver, 30

Echocardiography, 45–48, 49
  in hypertensive heart disease, 63
  M-mode, 48
  in rheumatic heart disease, 55
  two-dimensional, 48, 49
Eclampsia, 249
Ectopic pregnancy, 213
Edema
  laryngeal, 80
  pulmonary. See Pulmonary edema
Egg shell calcification, in silicosis, 83–
     84, 85, 93
Ehlers-Danlos syndrome, hydroxyapatite
     crystals in, 165
Elbow
  CPPD of, 163
  gouty arthritis of, 162
  hemophiliac arthropathy of, 183
  rheumatoid arthritis, of, 154
Electrocardiogram, 45
Emphysema, 81–82
  hypertrophic osteoarthropathy and,
     184
Empty sella syndrome, 227
Empyema
  vs. abscess, 111
  epidural, 237
  subdural, 237
Encephalitis, 237–238
Enchondroma, 199, 200
Endocardium, calcification of, 58
Endocrine disease, 209–215
Endometrial carcinoma, 213
Endometriosis, 213
Endoscopy, in cirrhosis, 30
Endotoxins, pyelonephritis and, 117
Endotracheal intubation, 79, 80
  tracheal stenosis and, 80
End-stage lung disease, 98
Enteroclysis, 19
Enthesitis, 158
  ankylosing spondylitis and, 158–159
  psoriatic arthritis and, 160, 161
  Reiter's syndrome and, 161
Eosinophilic granuloma, 199–200
Eosinophilic pneumonia, 93
Ependymoma, 224–225, 240–241
Epidemic dysentery, Reiter's syndrome
     and, 161
Epidermoid tumor, 228
Epidural abscess, 244, 245
Epidural empyema, 237
Epidural hematoma, 234–235
Epiglottis, 80
Epiglottitis, 79
Epiphyseal end plate
  fusion, in thalassemia, 182
  overgrowth, hemophilia and, 182
Epiphysis
  osteonecrosis of, 185–186
  slipped, 177
Erlenmeyer flash deformity, thalassemia
     and, 182
Erosive osteoarthritis, 168, 169
Esophageal diseases, 8–14
  diffuse spasm, 11
  diverticula, 14
  hiatal hernia, 12–13
  infection, 10–11
  inflammation, 8–10
  leiomyoma, 11
  Mallory-Weiss tear, 14
  motor disorders, 11, 12
  neoplasms, 11–12, 13
  parasternal hernia, 13–14
  rupture, 14

Esophageal diseases—*Continued*
  stricture, 10
  webs, 14
Esophagitis
  corrosive, 10
  drug-induced, 10
  herpes, 11, 12
  monilial, 10–11, 12
  peptic, 8–10
  radiation, 10
Ewing's sarcoma, 203, 204
Excretory urography
  in decreased renal function, 136
  in renal failure, 136
  in renal infarction, 137
Extremities, neuroarthropathy of, 171–172

Facial bones, fibrous dysplasia of, 183, 184
Familial polyposis, 20, 25
Fatty liver, 34
Feet
  gouty arthritis of, 162
  Reiter's syndrome of, 161
Femur
  fibrous dysplasia of, 183
  hypertrophic osteoarthropathy of, 184
  metastatic carcinoma of, 205
  prostatic carcinoma metastases to, 149
  pyogenic septic arthritis of, 189
  shepherd's crook deformity of, 179
Fibromuscular dysplasia, of carotid artery, 220
Fibrous cortical defect, 197–198
Fibrous dysplasia, 183–184
Fibrous histiocytoma, malignant, 204–206
Fibula
  fibrous dysplasia of, 183
  hypertrophic osteoarthropathy of, 184
Finger, primary idiopathic osteoarthritis of, 167
Floating fragment sign, in solitary bone cyst, 198
Fluoroscopy, in tracheal stenosis, 80
Foot, leprosy of, 192
Foreign body aspiration, 78, 79
  atelectasis and, 70
Forrestier's disease, 171
Fracture
  ankylosing spondylitis and, 158
  osteoporosis and, 173
  Paget's disease and, 179
  spontaneous, 183
Fungal infection
  of bone and joint, 195
  of esophagus, 10
  of respiratory system, 87–90

Galactography, 141
Gallbladder disease, 34–36
Gallium citrate imaging, in sarcoidosis, 94
Gallstone ileus, 36
Gallstones
  plain films of, 7
  in pregnancy, 250
Gardner's syndrome, 20, 24
Gas patterns, 1–7
  abscess, 5, 6
  bowel obstruction, 2, 3–4
  extraperitoneal air, 6
  hepatobiliary air, 6, 7
  ileus, 1–2
  intramural air, 5–7

Gas patterns—*Continued*
  pneumoperitoneum, 2–5, 6
  toxic megacolon, 2, 5
Gastric ulcer, 14–16
Gastrinoma, 19
Gastritis, 14
  chronic atrophic, 17
  corrosive, 18
  erosive, 15
  hypertrophic, 18
Gastrointestinal bleeding, 7, 42
Gastrointestinal disease, 1–42
  abdominal plain film in, 1–8
  abscess, 5
  bleeding, 7, 42
Gastrointestinal tract, Hodgkin's lymphoma and, 144
Genitourinary disease, 115–138
  benign tumors, 131
  calculous disease, 123–125
  congenital abnormalities, 115–117
  decreased renal function, 136
  duplication, 115
  hydronephrosis, 120
  intrarenal arterial aneurysms, 136–137
  malignant tumors, 131–136
  nephrocalcinosis, 123, 125
  nephrolithiasis, 123–125
  obstructive disease, 120–122
  papillary necrosis, 122–123
  pyelonephritis, 117–119
  reflux uropathy, 117
  renal cysts, 125–130
  renal infarction, 137–138
  renal transplantation, 138
  tuberculosis, 120
  ureteropelvic obstruction, 120–122
  vesicoureteral reflux, 117
  xanthogranulomatous pyelonephrosis, 119
Genu varum, 175
Gestational sac, 214
Giant cell tumor, 200, 201
  Paget's disease and, 179
Glioma, 224–225, 240–241
Glomerulonephritis, acute, 136
Glomerulus, hyalinization, 123
Goiter, multinodular, 209, 210
Gout, uric acid stones and, 124
Gouty arthritis, 162
  articular destruction in, 164
  soft tissue masses in, 164
  thalassemia and, 182
Granulomatous angiitis, 96, 97
Granulomatous colitis, 29
Graves' disease, hyperthyroidism and, 209

HADD. *See* Hydroxyapatite crystal deposition disease (HADD)
Haemophilus influenzae, in airway obstruction, 79–80
Hamartoma, vs. solitary pulmonary nodule, 76, 77
Hammon-Rich syndrome, 96
Hampton's line, 14
Hand
  CPPD of, 163, 165
  gouty arthritis of, 162
  hemochromatosis of, 166
  juvenile chronic arthritis of, 155, 156
  leprosy of, 192
  Ollier's disease and, 200
  rheumatoid arthritis of, 151, 152
Hand-foot syndrome, 180
Hand-Schüller-Christian disease, 98, 200

Hansen's disease. *See* Leprosy
Hashimoto's thyroiditis, 209
Heart
  anatomy of, 45
  calcifications, 58–61
  magnetic resonance imaging of, 52
  prosthetic valves, 58, 59
  rhabdomyoma of, 64–65
  tumors of, 64–65
Heartburn, 8
Heel, psoriatic arthritis of, 161
Hemangioblastoma, 228, 240–241
Hematogenous infection, pyelonephritis, 117
Hemidiaphragm, pleural effusion and, 109
Hemochromatosis, 165, 166
  of liver, 33–34
  secondary, thalassemia and, 182
Hemoglobinopathies, 179–182
  anemia, 181–182
  hemophilia, 182
  iron-deficient anemia, 182
  sickle cell disease, 179–181
  thalassemia, 181–182
Hemolytic anemia, 182
Hemophilia, 182
Hemosiderosis, idiopathic pulmonary, 98–99
Hepatobiliary air, 6, 7
Hepatolenticular degeneration, 165–167, 236
Hepatoma, 32
Hernia, 12–14
Herpes infection, of esophagus, 10–11, 12
Hiatal hernia, 12–13
Hilar adenopathy
  in adult respiratory distress syndrome, 102
  in berylliosis, 86
  in pneumoconiosis, 83
  in sarcoidosis, 93
Hip
  ankylosing spondylitis of, 158
  CPPD of, 163, 165
  juvenile chronic arthritis of, 156
  osteoarthritis of, 167, 168
  osteonecrosis of, 186
  osteoporosis of, 174
    in juvenile chronic arthritis, 156
  in Paget's disease, 179
  pyogenic septic arthritis of, 189
  rheumatoid arthritis of, 151, 153
Histiocytoma, malignant fibrous, 204–206
Histiocytosis, 98
Histoplasmosis, 89, 90
Hodgkin's lymphoma, 105, 106, 144
  staging of, 147
Horseshoe kidney, 115–117
Huntington's chorea, 236
Hydatidiform mole, 252
Hydrocarbon aspiration, 92
Hydrocephalus, 229–232
  atrophic, 232
  cerebrospinal fluid overproduction and, 231
  communicating, 231
  normal pressure, 231–232
  obstructive, 230
Hydronephrosis, 120
  in pregnancy, 249
  Wilms' tumor and, 133
Hydroxyapatite crystal deposition disease (HADD), 165, 166

Hypernephroma, 134–136, 205
  angiomyolipoma and, 131
  hypovascular, 119
Hyperparathyroidism, 176, 177
  hydroxyapatite crystals in, 165
Hypersensitivity pneumonitis, 86–87
Hypertension
  chest x-ray in, 63
  portal, 30
  pulmonary, 51, 61–63
Hypertensive heart disease, 54, 61–63
Hyperthyroidism, 209, 210
Hypertrophic osteoarthropathy, 184–185
Hyperuricemia, sickle cell disease and,
      180
Hypokinesis, in aortic insufficiency, 55
Hypoparathyroidism, 177
  hydroxyapatite crystals in, 165
Hypophosphatasia, 177
Hypothyroidism, 209, 210

Idiopathic inflammatory bowel disease,
      27–29
Idiopathic pulmonary hemosiderosis,
      98–99
Ileitis
  backwash, 29
  Crohn's, 28
Ileocecal valve, 28–29
Ileum, 19
  carcinoid tumor of, 21
Ileus, 1–2
  gallstone, 36
Immotile cilia syndrome, 91
Immunosuppression, septic arthritis
      and, 190
Infantile polycystic disease, 127–128
Infarction
  cerebral, 217
  myocardial, 53
  pituitary, 252
  renal, 137–138
Infection
  bone and joint, 187–195
    fungal, 195
    leprosy, 193
    pyogenic hematogenous
        osteomyelitis, 187–189
    pyogenic infectious spondylitis,
        190–192
    pyogenic septic arthritis, 189–190
    skeletal tuberculosis, 192
    syphilis, 193–195
    viral, 195
  in cardiomyopathies, 56
  of colon, 22–24
  of esophagus, 10–11
  extrapulmonary, in lymphoma, 147
  postpartum, 252
  of small bowel, 19–20
Infectious enteritis, seronegative
      spondyloarthropathies and, 157
Infectious spondylitis, 190–192
Inflammatory bowel disease
  hypertrophic osteoarthropathy and,
      184
  idiopathic, 27–29
  spondyloarthritis and, 159
Interstitial lung disease, 69–70, 96–98
  honeycombing pattern in, 70
  Kerley B lines in, 69, 70
  miliary pattern, 70
Interstitial pneumonia, 96
Intervertebral disk
  bulging annulus, 246
  degenerative disease, 246–247

Intervertebral disk—Continued
  herniation, 246
  ossification of, 157
  psoriatic arthritis and, 160
  pyogenic infection of, 191
  pyogenic infectious spondylitis of,
      191
  vacuum phenomenon, 171
Intervertebral osteochondrosis, 171
Intestinal bypass surgery, seronegative
      spondyloarthropathies and, 157
Intestine. See Bowel
Intracerebral hemorrhage, 222
Intracranial hemorrhage, 220–223
Intramural air, 5–7
Intrarenal reflux, acute pyelonephritis
      and, 117
Intraventricular hemorrhage, 220, 222
  cerebral, 220, 222
Involucrum, in osteomyelitis, 188
Iodine 131 scan
  in hyperthyroidism, 209, 210
  in mediastinal adenopathy, 105
  in thyroid carcinoma, 211
Iron-deficient anemia, 182
Ischemic heart disease, 51, 54
Ischial ramus, spiculating bony
      proliferation at, 159
Islet cell tumor, 19
Ivory phalanx, 160

Jaundice, 34
  in pregnancy, 250
Jejunum, 19
  non-Hodgkin's lymphoma of, 20
Joint disease
  apophyseal osteoarthritis, 171, 172
  arthritis, 151–172. See also Arthritis
  arthritis multilans, 160, 161
  disorders of unknown origin, 183–185
  effusions of, 182
    in pyogenic hematogenous
        osteomyeltis, 187
  hemochromatosis, 166
  hemoglobinopathies and anemias,
      179–182
  infections, 187–195. See also
      Infection, bone and joint
  joint mice, 168
  loose bodies, 168
  metabolic bone diseases, 172–179
  osteonecrosis, 185–187
  "pencil-in-cup" deformity, 160
  space narrowing
    in CPPD, 163
    in erosive osteoarthritis, 168
    in juvenile chronic arthritis, 155–
        157
    in osteoarthritis, 167, 168, 169
    in rheumatoid arthritis, 151–154
    in tuberculosis, 189
Juvenile chronic arthritis, 154–157
  vs. hemophilia, 182

Kaposi's sarcoma, 100, 101
Kerley A lines
  in interstitial lung disease, 69
  in pulmonary edema, 101
Kerley B lines
  in congestive heart failure, 51
  in interstitial lung disease, 69
  in pulmonary edema, 101
  in rheumatic heart disease, 55
Kidney
  abscess, vs. focal pyelonephritis, 118
  adenocarcinoma of, 134–136

Kidney—Continued
  adenoma of, 131
  angiomyolipoma of, 131
  Ask-Upmark, 117
  benign tumors of, 131
  "bouquet of flowers" cysts, 130, 131
  calculous disease of, 123–125
  collecting system duplication, 115
  congenital abnormalities of, 115–117
  congenital hypoplasia of, 117
  crossed renal ectopia, 117
  cysts, 125–130
  decreased function, 136
  enlarged, 115
  hamartoma of, 131
  horseshoe, 115–117
  hydronephrosis, 120
  hypernephroma of, 134–136
  infarction, 137–138
  intrarenal arterial aneurysms, 136–137
  ischemia, 123
  lymphoma of, 146
  malignant tumors of, 131–136
  medullary calcification, in
      nephrocalcinosis, 125
  medullary sponge, 130–131
  metanephric blastema, 115
  multicystic disease of, 128–131
  neuroblastoma of, 133–134
  papillary necrosis of, 122–123
  parenchymal calcification, 119, 120
  pelvic, 117
  polycystic disease of, 127–128, 129
  in pregnancy, 249–250
  prostate carcinoma and, 149
  renal cell carcinoma, 134–136
  squamous cell carcinoma of, 136
  transitional cell carcinoma of, 136
  transplantation, 138
  Wilms' tumor of, 131–133
Klebsiella infection, pneumonia and, 69
Knee
  CPPD of, 163
  giant cell tumor of, 200
  gouty arthritis of, 162
  growth deformity, 156
  hemophilia and, 182, 183
  osteoarthritis of, 167, 168
  pyrophosphate arthropathy of, 163
  Reiter's syndrome of, 161
  rheumatoid arthritis of, 151, 153
  septic arthritis of, 189, 190
Krabbe's disease, 235
Kupffer cells, 32

Large bowel
  dilatation of, 2
  infection of, 22–24
  obstruction of, 24–26
Larynx, edema, 80
Laurence-Moon-Biedl syndrome,
      polycystic kidney disease and,
      128, 129
Left to right shunt, 51
Left ventricle, aneurysm, 54
Left ventricular stress, 53
Legionnaire's disease, 100
Leiomyoma, of uterus, 215
Leiomyosarcoma, of uterus, 213
Leprosy, 193
Leptomeningeal cyst, 233
Letterer-Siwe disease, 98, 200
Leukoencephalopathy, multifocal, 236
Ligament of Treitz, 19
Lingula, consolidation of, 68
Linitis plastica, 17

Lipoma, 228
Liver
  abscess of, 30, 31
  adenoma of, 31–32
  benign neoplasms of, 31–32
  Budd-Chiari syndrome of, 34
  cavernous hemangioma of, 31, 32
  cirrhosis of, 30
  cysts, 30
  diseases of, 29–34
  fatty infiltration of, 34
  focal nodular hyperplasia of, 31, 32
  hematoma of, 250
  hemochromatosis of, 33–34
  lymphoma of, 146
  malignant neoplasms of, 32–33
    metastases, 32–33
  masses, 30–33
  ovarian metastases to, 213
  portal hypertension, 30
Loeffler's syndrome, 93
Loop of Henle, necrosis, 123
Lumbar spine
  apophyseal joint osteoarthritis of, 171,
    172
  diffuse idiopathic skeletal
    hyperostosis of, 171
  infectious spondylitis of, 191
  Paget's disease of, 180
  psoriatic spondyloarthritis of, 160
Lumbosacral spine
  ankylosing spondylitis of, 157, 158
  lipomeningocele, 239
Lung
  abscess, vs. empyema, 111
  coin lesion of, 76
  collapse. See Atelectasis
  end-stage disease of, 98
  Hodgkin's lymphoma and, 144, 145
  lower lobe
    atelectasis of, 71
    consolidation of, 68
  marble lesion of, 76
  middle lobe, atelectasis of, 71
  neoplasms of, 72–76
    adenocarcinoma, 72–73
    alveolar cell carcinoma, 73–74
    bronchial adenomas, 75
    bronchoalveolar carcinoma, 73–74
    bronchogenic carcinoma, 72–75
    epidermoid carcinoma, 72
    large cell undifferentiated
      carcinoma, 72
    metastases to, 75–76
    oat cell carcinoma, 72
    small cell undifferentiated
      carcinoma, 72
    squamous carcinoma, 72, 73
    staging, 74–75
  solitary nodule
    causes of, 76
    differential diagnosis of, 76–79
  upper lobe
    atelectasis of, 72
    blastomycosis of, 90
    emphysema of, 82
Lupus erythematosus, 98
  peripheral vascular disease in, 65
Lymphoma, 144–147
  Ann Arbor Staging Classification, 147
  Burkitt's, 144
  histiocytic, 144, 145
  mixed, 144
  radiographic follow-up in, 147
  radiographic manifestations of, 144–
    146

Lymphoma—Continued
  staging, 146–147
  of stomach, 17
Lymphomatoid granulomatosis, 96

Maffucci's syndrome, 199
Magnesium ammonium phosphate
    stones, 124
Magnetic resonance imaging
  in cardiovascular disease, 51, 52
  in cerebral ischemia, 217, 218
  in degenerative disk disease, 247
  in hepatic metastases, 33
  in osteonecrosis, 185, 186
  in pericardial disease, 61
  in prostate carcinoma, 148–149
  in spinal cord pathologies, 239
  in transverse myelitis, 241
Malabsorption syndromes, 21, 22
  lymphoma and, 144, 145
Malignant fibrous histiocytoma, 204–
    206
Malignant mesothelioma, pleural masses
    in, 111
Mallory-Weiss tear, 14
Mammography, 140–143
  film-screen, 140
  indications for, 141
  radiation exposure in, 143
  xero-, 140
Marfan's syndrome, aortic aneurysm
    and, 63
McCune-Albright syndrome, 183
Meckel's diverticulum, 20–21, 22
Mediastinal masses, 104–109
  adenopathy, 105, 106
  anterior, 104–105
  cystic, 106, 108
  Hodgkin's lymphoma and, 144
  lymph nodes, 105–108
  middle, 105–108
  paraspinal bulging, 109
  posterior, 108–109
  substernal thyroid, 105
  teratoma, 105
  thymoma, 104–105
  vascular structures, 107, 108
Mediterranean anemia, 181–182
Medullary sponge kidney, 130–131
Medulloblastoma, 226
Meningioma, 225
Meningiosarcoma, 243–244
Meningitis, 237
Meningocele, 98
Meniscus, pleural effusion and, 109, 110
Mesentery, diseases of, 40–41
Mesoblastic nephroma, 132
Mesothelioma
  malignant, 111
  of peritoneum, 40
Metabolic bone diseases, 172–179
  hyperparathyroidism and, 176, 177
  hypoparathyroidism and, 177
  hypophosphatasia and, 177
  osteomalacia, 173–175
  osteoporosis, 172–173
  Paget's disease, 178–179
  pseudohypoparathyroidism and, 177
  pseudopseudohypoparathyroidism
    and, 177
  rickets, 175–177
Metacarpophalangeal joint, CPPD of,
    163, 165
Metatarsal, pseudohypoparathyroidism
    of, 178

Metatarsophalangeal joint, in gouty
    arthritis, 162, 164
Milk-alkali syndrome, hydroxyapatite
    crystals in, 165
Mineralocorticoids, Conn's syndrome
    and, 212
Mitral valve
  atrial myxoma and, 64
  calcification of, 58
  prolapse, 55–56
  prosthetic, 58, 59
Monilial infection, of esophagus, 10–11
Monoarticular juvenile chronic arthritis,
    155
Motor disorders, of esophagus, 11, 12
Mounier-Kuhn syndrome, 80–81
Mucocele, 27
Multicystic kidney disease, 120, 128–
    130
Multifocal leukoencephalopathy, 236
Multiple endocrine neoplasia, 211
Multiple sclerosis, 235
Mycobacterium leprae, 193
Myelitis, transverse, 241
Myelography
  in degenerative disk disease, 247
  in spinal pathologies, 239
Myeloma, 204
Myocardial infarction, radionuclide
    scintigraphy in, 53
Myoclonic seizure, neuroblastoma and,
    134
Myometrium, fibroid tumor of, 215

Needle biopsy
  in liver cysts, 30
  in simple renal cysts, 126–127
Nephritis, acute bacterial, 118
Nephrocalcinosis, 123, 125, 126
Nephrography, of simple cyst, 126
Nephrolithiasis, 123–125
Nephroma, mesoblastic, 132
Nephropathy, analgesic, 123
Neurilemmoma, 243
Neuroarthropathy, 171–172, 173
Neuroblastoma, 133–134
Neurofibroma, 243
Neurofibromatosis, 96–98
Neurofibrosarcoma, 243
Neurologic disorders, 217–247
  brain neoplasms, 222–229
  cerebral trauma, 232–235
  cerebrovascular disease, 217–222
  degenerative disease, 235–239
  demyelinating disease, 235–239
  hydrocephalus, 229–232
  in pregnancy, 252
  spinal cord pathology, 239–246
  spondylosis, 246–247
Noncardiogenic pulmonary edema, 101–
    102
Non-Hodgkin's lymphoma, 144
  of stomach, 17
Nonossifying fibroma, 197–198
Nuclear scintigraphy, in renal
    transplantation, 138

Ochronosis, 166, 167
Odontoid process, fracture of, 154
Oligodendroglioma, 224–225
Ollier's disease, 195
  chondrosarcoma and, 203
  enchondroma and, 199
Omentum
  ovarian metastases to, 213
  tumors of, 40, 41

Oncology, 139–150. *See also specific type of disease and location*
Oral contraceptives, hepatic focal nodular hyperplasia and, 32
Organ of Zuckerkandl, neuroblastoma of, 133
Osler-Rendu-Weber syndrome, 42
Osseous neoplasm. See Bone disease, neoplasms
Osteoarthritis, 166–168
  apophyseal joint, 171, 172
Osteochondroma, 199
Osteochondrosis, intervertebral, 171
Osteoclastoma, hyperparathyroidism and, 176, 177
Osteogenic sarcoma, 200–203
Osteoid osteoma, 198
Osteomalacia, 173–175
Osteomyelitis
  bacterial, 187–189
  Brodie's abscess and, 189, 190
  leprous, 193
  pyogenic hematogenous, 187–189
  sickle cell disease and, 180
  staphylococcal, 188
  vertebral, 191
Osteonecrosis, 185–187
  hyperparathyroidism and, 177
Osteopenia, sickle cell disease and, 179
Osteophyte
  hook-like, in hemochromatosis, 165, 166
  osteoarthritis and, 168
Osteoporosis, 172–173
  disorders associated with, 173
  gouty arthritis and, 162
  psoriatic arthritis and, 160
  rheumatoid arthritis and, 151, 152
  sickle cell disease and, 180
Osteoporosis circumscripta, 178
Osteosarcoma, 200
Osteosclerosis
  hypoparathyroidism and, 177
  Paget's disease and, 178
  sarcoidosis and, 185
Ovary, tumors of, 213–215
Oxygen toxicity, 95

Pachydermoperiostosis, 184
Paget's disease, 178–179
  pseudofractures of, 174
Pancoast's tumor, 73–74
Pancolitis, acute, 24
Pancreas
  annular, 39
  carcinoma of, 38–39
  diseases of, 36–39
  endocrine tumors of, 39
  exocrine tumors of, 39
  inflammation of, 37–38
  lymphoma of, 146
  neoplasms of, 39
  pseudocyst, 38, 39, 251
  trauma to, 39
Pancreatitis
  acute, 37
    in pregnancy, 250–251
  chronic, 37, 38
    calcification in, 7, 9
  complications of, 37
Pansinusitis, 91
Paraesophageal hernia, 13–14
Paralytic ileus, 1–2
Paraplegia, 241, 244
Parasternal hernia, 13–14

Parathyroid hormone, osteoclast activation and, 177
Parkinson's disease, 236
Patent ductus arteriosus, 51
Patulous ileocecal valve, 28–29
Pauciarticular juvenile chronic arthritis, 155
Pelvic inflammatory disease, 213, 214
Pelvis
  cellulitis of, 252
  eosinophilic granuloma of, 199
  hyperparathyroidism and, 177
  infectious spondylitis of, 190
  metastatic carcinoma of, 205
  prostatic carcinoma metastases, 149–150
  thrombophlebitis of, 251
Peptic ulcer disease, 14–16
  lymphoma and, 144
Percutaneous aspiration cytology
  in pyogenic infectious spondylitis, 191
  in thyroid nodules, 209
Percutaneous transhepatic cholangiogram, 39
Periarteritis, 136–137
Pericardial disease, 58–61
Pericardial effusion, 58, 61
Pericarditis, acute, 58
Periostitis
  hemochromatosis and, 165
  in leprosy, 193
Peripheral atherosclerosis, 64
Peripheral nerve tumors, 226, 242, 243
Peripheral vascular disease, 64
Peripheral venous thrombosis, 64, 65
Peristalsis, 11, 12
Peritendinitis calcarae, 165, 166
Peritoneum, diseases of, 39–40
Peritonitis, 40
Peutz-Jeghers syndrome, 17, 20, 21
Phalanges, psoriatic arthritis of, 160
Pheochromocytoma, 213
Phlegmon, pancreatic, 38
Phytobezoar, 18
Pia mater, meningiosarcoma of, 243
Pineal region tumors, 226
"Pink puffer," 81
Pituitary gland
  adenoma of, 211
  infarction, in pregnancy, 252
  tumors, 226–227
Placental transfer, in congenital syphilis, 193
Plain film radiograph, in pulmonary embolism, 103
Pleural disease, 109–111
  asbestosis, 85–86
  effusions, 86, 109–111
    in collagen vascular disease, 96
    vs. solitary pulmonary embolism, 76–77
  masses, 110, 111
  mesothelioma, hypertrophic osteodystrophy and, 184
  plaques, 86
Pleuritis, 111
Plummer's disease, 209
Pneumoconioses, 83–87
Pneumomediastinum, 85
  asthma and, 83
Pneumonia
  aspiration, 91–93
  atypical infectious, 99–100
  bacterial, 69
  chlamydial, 100

Pneumonia—*Continued*
  eosinophilic, 93
  interstitial, 96
  Klebsiella, 69
  Mycoplasma, 99–100
  Pneumocystic carinii, 100, 101
  Pseudomonas, 69
  round, 77, 78
  staphylococcal, 69
  viral, 99–100
Pneumonitis
  chemical, 92
  hypersensitivity, 86–87
Pneumoperitoneum, 2–5, 6
  double wall sign, 5
Pneumothorax, 84
  asthma and, 83
  atelectasis and, 70
Podagra, gouty arthritis and, 162, 164
Polyarteritis, 93
Polyarticular juvenile chronic arthritis, 155
Polycystic kidney disease
  adult, 127–128, 129
  infantile, 127–128
Polyostotic fibrous dysplasia, 183
Polyp, 16–17, 24
  pseudo, 27, 28
Polyposis syndromes, 20
Portal hypertension, 30
  polycystic disease and, 127, 128
Postpartum infection, 252
Potter's syndrome, multicystic kidney and, 128
Precocious puberty, fibrous dysplasia and, 183
Pregnancy
  biliary complications in, 250
  cardiac complications in, 251
  ectopic, 213
  liver complications in, 250
  neoplasms in, 252
  neurologic complications in, 252
  pancreatic complications in, 250
  postpartum infection, 252
  renal complications of, 249
  respiratory complications in, 251
  thromboembolism in, 251
Progressive massive fibrosis, in coal worker's pneumoconiosis, 85
Prostate
  adenocarcinoma of, causing osteoblastic metastasis, 206
  cancer of, 147–150
    adenocarcinoma, 147
    incidence of, 147
    prognosis of, 147–148
    staging of, 147–150
Prosthetic valves, 58, 59
Proteinosis, alveolar, 102
Protrusio acetabuli deformity, 158
Pseudarthrosis, 159
Pseudofracture, of Paget's disease, 174
Pseudogout, CPPD and, 162
Pseudohypoparathyroidism, 177
Pseudomembranous colitis, 22, 24
Pseudomyxoma peritonei, 40
Pseudopolyps, 27
Pseudopseudohypoparathyroidism, 177
Pseudotumor, hemophiliac, 182
Pseudotumor cerebri, 229
  in pregnancy, 252
Psoas, abscess of, 192
Psoriatic arthritis, 159–160
  vs. rheumatoid arthritis, 161

Pulmonary edema
  bat wing pattern in, 101–102
  butterfly pattern in, 101
  confluent bat wing pattern in, 68
  noncardiogenic, 101–102
Pulmonary embolism, 61–63, 102–104
  cold spot, 103
  with infarction, 103–104
  without infarction, 103
  lung scanning in, 103
  in pregnancy, 251
  Westermark's sign of, 103
Pulmonary eosinophilia, 93
Pulmonary hemorrhage, 98–99
Pulmonary hypertension, congestive
    heart failure and, 51
Pulmonary hypertensive heart disease,
    61–63
Pulmonary infarction, embolism and,
    103–104
Pulmonary infiltrates with eosinophilia,
    93
Pulmonary venous congestion, 54
Pulmonary venous hypertension, 57
Pulmonary-renal syndrome, 98, 99
Pyelonephritis, 117–119
Pyelonephrosis
  acute, 117–118
  chronic, 118, 119
  xanthogranulomatous, 119
Pyogenic diskitis, 191
Pyogenic hematogenous osteomyelitis,
    187–189
Pyogenic infectious spondylitis, 190–
    192
Pyogenic septic arthritis, 189–190
Pyrophosphate arthropathy, 162–163

Quadriplegia, 241, 244

Rachitic rosary, 175
Radiation injuries
  esophagitis, 10
  genitourinary obstruction and, 122
  of respiratory system, 95
  risk-benefit ratio, 143
  small bowel ischemia and, 21
  teratogenicity, 252
Radiographic contrast material,
    aspiration of, 92–93
Radiolabelled red blood cells
  in cardiovascular disease, 51
  in liver tumors, 31
Radionuclide scintigraphy
  in biliary disorders, 34
  in breast cancer, 144
  in cardiovascular disease, 51, 53
  in cerebral ischemia, 217
  in cirrhosis, 30
  in fibrous dysplasia, 184
  in gallbladder disease, 34
  in hypertrophic osteoarthropathy,
    184–185
  in Meckel's diverticulum, 20, 21
  in neoplasms, 195
  in osteonecrosis, 186
  in Paget's disease, 178–179
  in prostate carcinoma, 149
  in pulmonary embolism, 103, 104
  in pyogenic hematogenous
    osteomyelitis, 187
  in sarcoidosis, 94
  in spinal cord pathologies, 239
  in substernal thyroid, 105

Radius
  hypertrophic osteoarthropathy of, 184
  rickets and, 175
Rectum
  sessile adenomatous polyp of, 24
  ulcerative colitis of, 28
  villous adenomas of, 25
Reflex sympathetic dystrophy
    syndrome, osteoarthritis and, 173,
    174
Reflux esophagitis, 8–10
  scleroderma and, 11
Reflux uropathy, 117
Regional enteritis. See Crohn's disease
Reiter's syndrome, 160–162
  vs. rheumatoid arthritis, 161
  syndesmophytes and, 158
Renal artery, aneurysm of, 136–137
Renal cell carcinoma, 134–136
Renal colic, 124–125
Renal cysts, 125–130
  "bouquet of flowers," 130, 131
  medullary sponge kidney, 130–131
  multicystic, 130
  polycystic, 127–128
  simple, 125–127
    computed tomography in, 126, 127
    needle aspiration in, 126–127
    radiographic features of, 125–126
    ultrasonography in, 126
Renal failure, 136
  acute, in pregnancy, 249, 250
  chest x-ray in, 53
  chronic, in pregnancy, 249
Renal function, decreased, 136
Renal osteodystrophy,
    hyperparathyroidism and, 177
Renal tubular necrosis
  in pregnancy, 249
  renal transplantation and, 138
Renal vein thrombosis, 249, 250
Reproductive disease, 213–215
Respiratory tract disease, 67–111
  AIDS, 100–101
  aspiration pneumonia, 91–93
  atypical infectious pneumonias, 99–
    100
  bacterial pneumonia patterns, 69
  basic principles, 67–72
  bronchiectasis, 90–91
  chronic obstructive pulmonary
    disease, 81–83
  consolidation, 67–69
  drug-induced, 94–95
  fungal, 87–90
  interstitial, 69–70, 96–98
  lung neoplasms, 72–76
  mediastinal masses, 104–109
  noncardiogenic pulmonary edema,
    101–102
  oxygen toxicity, 95
  pleural, 109–111
  pneumoconioses, 83–87
  in pregnancy, 251
  pulmonary embolism, 102–104
  pulmonary eosinophilia, 93
  pulmonary hemorrhage, 98–99
  radiation injuries, 95
  sarcoidosis, 93–94
  silhouette sign in, 67–69
  silo filler's disease, 96
  solitary pulmonary nodule, 76–79
  tuberculosis, 87–89
  upper airway, 79–81
Reticulum cell sarcoma, 204
Retinitis pigmentosa, 235

Retroperitoneal fibrosis, 40
  genitourinary obstruction and, 122,
    123
Retroperitoneal lymphadenopathy, 146
Rheumatic heart disease, 55, 56–57
Rheumatoid arthritis, 151–154
  coal worker's pneumoconiosis and, 85
  collagen vascular disease and, 96
Rib
  fibrous dysplasia of, 183–184
  hyperparathyroidism and, 177
  prostatic carcinoma metastases to, 149
Rickets, 175–177
Rokitansky-Aschoff sinuses, 36
Rubella infection, of bone, 195

Saber sheath trachea, 81
Sacroiliac joint
  ankylosing spondylitis of, 157, 159
  Reiter's syndrome of, 161
Sacroiliitis, 157
  psoriatic arthritis and, 159
Salmonellosis, 22, 24
Sarcoidosis, 93–94, 185
  adenopathy of, 93
  hydroxyapatite crystals in, 165
  lung parenchymal involvement in, 94
Sarcoma, Paget's disease and, 179
"Sausage digit," 160
Schmorl's nodes, osteoporosis and, 173
Schwannoma, 243
Scleroderma, 97
  esophagus in, 11
  hydroxyapatite crystals in, 165
Sclerosing cholangitis, 35
Seizures, in pregnancy, 252
Septic arthritis
  pyogenic, 189–190
  sickle cell disease and, 180
  tuberculous, 192
Sequestrum, in pyogenic hematogenous
    osteomyelitis, 187, 189
Seronegative spondyloarthropathies,
    157–162
  ankylosing spondylitis, 157–159
  inflammatory bowel disease and, 159
  psoriatic arthritis, 159–160
  Reiter's syndrome, 160–162
  spondyloarthritis, 159
Sexually transmitted disease, Reiter's
    syndrome and, 160–161
Shigellosis, 22, 24
Shock lung, in pregnancy, 251
Short bowel syndrome, 21
Shoulder
  ankylosing spondylitis of, 158
  CPPD of, 163
  HADD of, 165, 166
  musculotendinous rotator cuff, 165
Sickle cell disease, 179–181
  papillary necrosis in, 124
Sickle cell trait, 180
Sickle cell-hemoglobin C disease, 180–
    181
Sigmoid colon, volvulus, 2, 4
Silhouette sign, in respiratory disease,
    67–69
Silicosis, 83–85
Silo filler's disease, 96
Skeletal tuberculosis, 192
Skeleton. See also Spine
  leprosy of, 193
  metastatic carcinoma of, 206
  syphilis of, 193
  tuberculosis of, 192

Skull
  depressed fracture of, 232–233
  eosinophilic granuloma of, 199
  fibrous dysplasia of, 183, 184
  hemolytic anemia and, 182
  nondepressed fracture of, 232
  osteoporosis circumscripta of, 178
  Paget's disease of, 180
  sickle cell disease and, 179–180
  thalassemia major and, 181
Small bowel
  adhesions, 3
  diseases of, 19–23
  diverticulosis, 20
  examination methods, 19
  infection of, 19–20
  ischemia, 21, 23
  malabsorption syndrome, 21, 22
  Meckel's diverticulum, 20–21, 22
  neoplasms of, 20, 21
  obstruction of, 2, 3–4
Soft tissue
  calcification of, 177
  hypertrophic osteoarthropathy and,
    184
Solitary bone cyst, 198, 199
Solitary pulmonary nodule, 76–79
Solitary thyroid nodule, 209, 210
Spherocytosis, hereditary, 182
Spine
  ankylosing hyperostosis of, 171
  ankylosing spondylitis of, 158
  apophyseal joint osteoarthritis of, 171,
    172
  arteriovenous malformation, 241
  "bamboo," 158
  bony outgrowth of, differential
    diagnosis of, 163
  cervical. See Cervical spine
  compression fracture of, 173
  cysts, 240
  degenerative joint disease of, 168–171
  diastematomyelia, 239, 240
  diffuse idiopathic skeletal
    hyperostosis of, 171
  diplomyelia, 240
  epidural pathology of, 244–245
  hematogenous infections of, 190–191
  intervertebral osteochondrosis of, 171
  intradural extramedullary pathology,
    243–244
  intramedullary pathology of, 239–
    242
  lumbar. See Lumbar spine
  lumbosacral. See Lumbosacral spine
  neoplasms, 240–241
  osseous epidural pathology of, 244–
    245
  osteophytosis, 168–171
  osteoporotic fracture of, 173
  pathology of, 239–246
  prostatic carcinoma metastases, 149–
    150
  psoriatic arthritis of, 159–160
  sickle cell disease of, 180
  spondylosis deformans of, 168–171
  synovial apophyseal joints of, 171
  tethered cord, 240
  thoracic. See Thoracic spine
  transverse myelitis, 241
  trauma to, 245–246
Spinopontinecerebellar degeneration,
  235, 236
Spleen, lymphoma of, 146
Spondylitis, pyogenic infectious, 190–
  192

Spondyloarthritis
  with inflammatory bowel disease, 159
  juvenile-onset, 155
  psoriatic, syndesmophytes and, 158
  seronegative, 157–162
Spondylosis, 246–247
Spondylosis deformans, 168–171
St. Jude's valve prosthesis, 58, 59
Staghorn calculus, 124
Stanford dissecting aortic aneurysm, 63
Starr-Edwards prosthetic valve, 58, 59
Still's disease, 155
Stomach
  adenocarcinoma of, 12
  carcinoma of, 17
  diseases of, 14–19
  fungating carcinoma of, 17
  Hodgkin's lymphoma and, 144, 145
  infiltrating carcinoma of, 17
  inflammation of, 14–16
  leiomyoma of, 17
  lymphoma of, 17
  malignant ulcer of, 15
  polyps of, 16–17
  volvulus, 18–19
Strawberry gallbladder, 36
Struvite stones, 124
Subarachnoid cyst, 229
Subarachnoid hemorrhage, 220
Subarachnoid space, 239
Subchondral cyst
  osteoarthritis and, 168
  rheumatoid arthritis and, 151
Subchondral sclerosis, osteoarthritis
  and, 167–168
Subclavian artery, 219
Subclavin steal syndrome, 220
Subdiaphragmatic air, 1
Subdural empyema, 237
Subdural hematoma, 233–234
Subdural hygroma, 237
Superior sulcus tumor, 73–74
Suprarenal adenoma, 212
Swan neck deformity in, rheumatoid
  arthritis, 154
Syndesmophytes, ankylosing
  spondylitis and, 158
Syphilis
  acquired, 194, 195
  congenital, 193–195
  fusiform aortic aneurysm in, 63
Syrinx, 240

Tabes dorsalis, syphilis and, 193
Technetium imaging, in pulmonary
  embolism, 103
Teratoma, 105, 228
Testes, disorders of, 213
Thalassemia, 181–182
Thallium-201 imaging, in cardiovascular
  disease, 51
Thermography, in breast cancer, 143–
  144
Thoracic radiographs, in cardiovascular
  disease, 45, 46–47
Thoracic spine, 239
  disk herniation, 246
  meningioma of, 243
  ochronosis of, 166, 167
  tuberculosis of, 192
Thoracolumbar spine, tuberculosis of,
  192
Thorax, emphysema and, 82
Thorotrast, 40
Thromboembolism, in pregnancy, 251
Thrombophlebitis, in pregnancy, 251

Thumb, sarcoidosis of, 185
Thymoma, 104–105
Thyroid
  cancer of, 211
    lung cancer and, 75
  cold nodules, 209
  disorders of, 209–211
  solitary nodule, 209, 210
  substernal, 105
Thyroiditis, 209, 210
Tibia
  fibrous dysplasia of, 183
  hyperparathyroidism and, 177
  hypertrophic osteoarthropathy of, 184
  Paget's disease of, 179
  sickle cell disease and, 181
  staphylococcal osteomyelitis of, 188,
    189
Tibiotalar slant
  hemophilia and, 182
  sickle cell disease and, 180
Toxemia of pregnancy, 250
  neurologic disorders of, 252
Toxic megacolon, 2
Toxoplasmosis, 238
Trachea
  saber sheath, 81
  stenosis of, 80
Tracheobronchomegaly, 80–81
Tracheoesophageal fistula, chronic
  aspiration and, 92
Transillumination, in breast cancer, 143
Transitional cell carcinoma, 136
Transplantation, renal, 138
Trauma
  osteoarthritis and, 167, 168
  osteoporosis and, 173, 174
Trichobezoar, 18
Trophoblastic disease, 252
Tuberculosis
  atypical, 89
  chronic pyelonephritis and, 119
  of colon, 24
  genitourinary, 120
  miliary, 89
  osteoarticular, 192
  primary infection, 87–88
  reactivation, 88–89
Tumoral calcinosis, secondary, 177

Ulcer collar, 14
Ulcerative colitis, 28–29, 157
  toxic megacolon and, 2
Ulna
  hypertrophic osteoarthropathy of, 184
  rickets and, 175
Ultrasound
  in acute pancreatitis, 250
  in angiomyolipoma, 131
  in breast cancer, 143
  in cervical carcinoma, 215
  in empyema, 111
  in gallstones, 250
  in genitourinary obstruction, 121
  in hepatic abscess, 30
  in hypernephroma, 135–136
  in jaundice, 34
  in medullary sponge kidney, 130
  in multicystic kidney disease, 129–
    130
  in pelvic inflammatory disease, 213
  in polycystic kidney disease, 127–128
  in prostate carcinoma, 148
  in pyelonephritis, 118
  in renal transplantation, 138
  in simple renal cysts, 126

Ultrasound—*Continued*
  in thyroid follicular carcinoma, 211
  in thyroid nodules, 209, 211
  in thyroid papillary carcinoma, 211
  in trophoblastic disease, 252
  in ureteroceles, 115
  in xanthogranulomatous
     pyelonephritis, 119, 120
Upper airway disease, 79–81
Ureter
  calculus, 125
  cicatrization of, 119, 120
  columnization, 124, 125
  congenital stenosis of, 121–122
  fibrous polyps, 120
  obstruction of, 115, 120–122
  posterior valves, 123
  transitional cell carcinoma of, 136
Ureterocele, 115, 116
Ureteropelvic junction, obstruction,
    120–122
Ureterovesicular junction, obstruction of
  renal transplantation and, 138
Urethritis, Reiter's syndrome and, 160
Uric acid stones, 124
Urinary tract disease. *See* Genitourinary
    disease
Urine, intrarenal reflux, 117
Uroepithelial carcinoma, 136
Urography
  in obstructive disease, 120–122
  in pyelonephritis, 118

Urography—*Continued*
  in renal adenoma, 131
  in renal infarction, 138
  in tuberculosis, 120
Uropathy, reflex, 117
Uterus, disorders of, 215

Valvular heart disease, calcification in,
    58
Vasa recta, necrosis, 123
Vasculitis, cerebral, 220, 221
Vena cava, superior
  obstruction of, 107, 108
  thrombosis, 64
Venous thrombosis, 64, 65
  cerebral, 200, 222
  cesarean section and, 251
Ventilation-perfusion study, in
    pulmonary hypertensive heart
    disease, 61
Ventricular septal defect, 51, 52
Ventriculitis, 237
Vertebra
  of fish, 181
  infection of, mediastinal mass and,
    108
  osteomyelits of, 191
  plana, 200
Vertebral end plate, sickle cell disease
    and, 180
Vesicoureteral reflux, 117

Viral infection
  of bone and joint, 195
  of esophagus, 11, 12
  in pregnancy, 250
Voiding cystourethrography, 130
von Hippel-Lindau disease, renal cysts
    in, 127
von Recklinghausen's
    neurofibromatosis, 96–98
  mediastinal mass in, 107, 109
  multiple nerve tumors in, 243

Warfarin toxicity, 99
Water-bath breast scanner, 143
Webs, esophageal, 14
Wegener's granulomatosis, 93, 96
Whipple's disease, 157
Wilms' tumor, 131–133
Wilson's disease, 165–167, 236
Wimberger's sign, in syphilis, 194
Wrist
  CPPD of, 163, 164
  juvenile chronic arthritis of, 156
  rheumatoid arthritis of, 153

Xanthogranulomatous pyelonephrosis,
    119
Xeromammography, 140

Zenker's diverticulum, 14
Zollinger-Ellison syndrome, 19